2025

Changes | An Insider's View

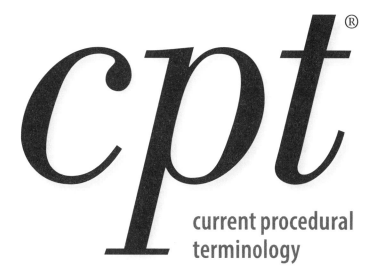

cpt®

current procedural
terminology

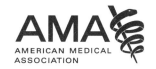

AMA

AMERICAN MEDICAL
ASSOCIATION

Contents

Contents

Contents

Foreword

The American Medical Association (AMA) is pleased to offer *CPT® Changes 2025: An Insider's View (CPT Changes)*. Since this book was first published in 2000, it has served as the definitive text on additions, revisions, and deletions to the CPT code set.

In developing this book, our intention was to provide CPT users with a glimpse of the logic, rationale, and proposed function of the changes in the CPT code set that resulted from the decisions of the CPT Editorial Panel and the yearly update process. The AMA staff members have the unique perspective of being both participants in the CPT editorial process and users of the CPT code set.

CPT Changes is intended to bridge understanding between clinical decisions made by the CPT Editorial Panel regarding appropriate service or procedure descriptions with functional interpretations of coding guidelines, code intent, and code combinations, which are necessary for users of the CPT code set. A new edition of this book, like the codebook, is published annually.

To assist CPT users in applying the new and revised CPT codes, this book includes clinical examples that describe the typical patient who might undergo the procedure and detailed descriptions of the procedure. Both of these are required as a part of the CPT code–change proposal process, which are used by the CPT Editorial Panel in crafting language, guidelines, and parenthetical notes associated with the new or revised codes. In addition, many of the clinical examples and descriptions of the procedures are used in the AMA/Specialty Society Relative Value Scale (RVS) Update (RUC) process to conduct surveys on physician work and to develop work relative value recommendations to the Centers for Medicare & Medicaid Services (CMS) as part of the Medicare physician fee schedule (MPFS).

We are confident that the information provided in *CPT Changes* will prove to be a valuable resource to CPT users, not only as they apply changes for the year of publication, but also as a resource for frequent reference as they continue their education in CPT coding. The AMA makes every effort to be a voice of clarity and consistency in an otherwise confusing system of health care claims and payment, and *CPT Changes 2025: An Insider's View* demonstrates our continued commitment to assist users of the CPT code set.

Using This Book

This book is designed to serve as a reference guide to understanding the changes contained in the Current Procedural Terminology (CPT®) 2025 code set and is not intended to replace the CPT codebook. Every effort is made to ensure accuracy; however, if differences exist, you should always defer to the information in the *CPT® 2025* codebook.

The Symbols

This book uses the same coding conventions as those used in the CPT nomenclature.

● Indicates a new procedure number was added to the CPT nomenclature

▲ Indicates a code revision has resulted in a substantially altered procedure descriptor

+ Indicates a CPT add-on code

⊘ Indicates a code that is exempt from the use of modifier 51 but is not designated as a CPT add-on procedure or service

►◄ Indicates revised guidelines, cross-references, and/or explanatory text

✗ Indicates a code for a vaccine that is pending FDA approval

\# Indicates a resequenced code. Note that rather than deleting and renumbering, resequencing allows existing codes to be relocated to an appropriate location for the code concept, regardless of the numeric sequence. Numerically placed references (ie, Code is out of numerical sequence. See...) are used as navigational alerts in the CPT codebook to direct the user to the location of an out-of-sequence code. Therefore, remember to refer to the CPT codebook for these references.

★ Indicates a telemedicine code

⚤ Indicates a duplicate PLA test

↑↓ Indicates a Category I PLA

◀ Indicates Audio-only Telemedicine Services

Whenever possible, complete segments of text from the CPT codebook are provided; however, in some instances, only pertinent text is included.

The Rationale

After listing each change or series of changes from the CPT codebook, a rationale is provided. The rationale is intended to provide a brief clarification and explanation of the changes. Nevertheless, it is important to note that they may not address every question that may arise as a result of the changes.

Reading the Clinical Examples

The clinical examples and their procedural descriptions, which reflect typical clinical situations found in the healthcare setting, are included in this text with many of the codes to provide practical situations for which the new and/or revised codes in the CPT 2025 code set would be appropriately reported. It is important to note that these examples do not suggest limiting the use of a code; instead, they are meant to represent the typical patient and service or procedure, as previously stated. In addition, they do not describe the universe of patients for whom the service or procedure would be appropriate. It is important also to note that third-party payer reporting policies may differ.

Summary of Additions, Deletions, and Revisions and Indexes

A **summary of additions, deletions, and revisions** for the section is presented in a tabular format at the beginning of each section. This table provides readers with the ability to quickly search and have an overview of all of the new, revised, and deleted codes for 2025. In addition to the tabular review of changes, the coding index individually lists all of the new, revised, and deleted codes with each code's status (new, revised, deleted) in parentheses. For more information about these indexes, please read the **Instructions for the Use of the Changes Indexes** on page 271.

CPT Codebook Conventions and Styles

Similar to the CPT codebook, the guidelines and revised and new CPT code descriptors and parenthetical notes in *CPT Changes 2025* are set in green type. Any revised text, guidelines, and/or headings are indicated with the ▶◀ symbols. To match the style used in the codebook, the revised or new text symbol is placed at the beginning and end of a paragraph or section that contains revisions, and the use of green text visually indicates new and/or revised content. Similarly, each section's and subsections' (Surgery) complete code range is listed in the tabs, regardless of whether these codes are discussed in this book. In addition, all of the different level of headings in the codebook are also picked up, as appropriate, and set in the same style and color. Besides matching the convention and style used in the CPT codebook, the Rationales are placed within a shaded box to distinguish them from the rest of the content for quick and easy reference.

Introduction

Current Procedural Terminology (CPT®), Fourth Edition, is a set of codes, descriptions, and guidelines intended to describe procedures and services performed by physicians and other qualified health care professionals, or entities. Each procedure or service is identified with a five-digit code. The use of CPT codes simplifies the reporting of procedures and services. In the CPT code set, the term "procedure" is used to describe services, including diagnostic tests.

Inclusion of a descriptor and its associated five-digit code number in the CPT Category I code set is based on whether the procedure or service is consistent with contemporary medical practice and is performed by many practitioners in clinical practice in multiple locations. Inclusion in the CPT code set of a procedure or service, or proprietary name, does not represent endorsement by the American Medical Association (AMA) of any particular diagnostic or therapeutic procedure or service or proprietary test or manufacturer. Inclusion or exclusion of a procedure or service, or proprietary name, does not imply any health insurance coverage or reimbursement policy.

▶The main body of the Category I section is listed in six sections. Each section is divided into subsections with anatomic, procedural, condition, or descriptor subheadings. The procedures and services with their identifying codes are presented in numeric order with the exception of the resequenced codes and the entire **Evaluation and Management** section (98000-98016, 99202-99499), which appears at the beginning of the listed procedures. The evaluation and management codes are used by most physicians in reporting a significant portion of their services.◀

Rationale

In accordance with the establishment of codes 98000-98016, the Introduction has been revised to reflect these changes.

Refer to the codebook and the Rationale for codes 98000-98016 for a full discussion of these changes.

Release of CPT Codes

The CPT code set is published annually in late summer or early fall as both electronic data files and books. The release of CPT data files occurs annually between August 31 and early September. The release of the CPT Professional publication comes several weeks later. However, to meet the needs of a rapidly changing health care environment, the CPT code set is periodically updated throughout the year on a set schedule. Each update has both a release date and an effective date. The interval between the release of the update and the effective date is considered an implementation period and is intended to allow physicians and other providers, payers, and vendors to incorporate CPT changes into their systems. Changes to the CPT code set are meant to be applied prospectively from the effective date. The following table outlines the complete CPT code set update calendar.

New CPT codes have been created to streamline services related to the novel coronavirus. It is imperative to check the AMA CPT public website at https://www.ama-assn.org/practice-management/cpt/covid-19-coding-and-guidance throughout the year to obtain the necessary frequent updates to the CPT code set.

CPT Code Set Update Calendar

CPT Category/Section	Release Timeline	Effective Timeline
Category I Category II	August 31	January 1
Category III	January 1	July 1
	July 1	January 1
▶Immune Globulins, Serum, or Recombinant Products Vaccines, Toxoids	April 1	July 1
	July 1	October 1
	October 1*	January 1◀
Molecular Pathology Tier 2 Administrative MAAA	April 1	July 1
	July 1	October 1
	October 1*	January 1
PLA	January 1	April 1
	April 1	July 1
	July 1	October 1
	October 1	January 1

*Note that the release date may be delayed by several days due to the timing of the CPT Panel fall meeting.

Rationale

The CPT Code Set Update Calendar in the **Introduction** section of the CPT code set has been revised to accommodate more frequent releases and updated content for immune globulin and vaccine codes.

The revision involves updating the release and effective dates of immune globulins, serums, or recombinant products, vaccines, and toxoids. Previously, these codes were released at six-month intervals (ie, January 1st/July 1st or July 1st/January 1st). However, in acknowledgment of the advances in medicine, technology, and immunization needs, these dates have been revised to allow for more frequent releases of these codes.

Instructions for Use of the CPT Codebook

▶Select the CPT code of the procedure or service that accurately identifies the procedure or service performed. Do not select a CPT code that merely approximates the procedure or service provided. If no such specific code exists, then report the procedure or service using the appropriate unlisted procedure or service code. When using an unlisted code, any modifying or extenuating circumstances should be adequately and accurately documented in the medical record. Furthermore, all the language within a code descriptor should be assessed when selecting the appropriate procedure or service. This includes information directly in the descriptor that may be enclosed in parentheses.◀

It is equally important to recognize that as techniques in medicine and surgery have evolved, new types of services, including minimally invasive surgery, as well as endovascular, percutaneous, and endoscopic interventions have challenged the traditional distinction of Surgery vs Medicine. Thus, the listing of a service or procedure in a specific section of this book should not be interpreted as strictly classifying the service or procedure as "surgery" or "not surgery" for insurance or other purposes. The placement of a given service in a specific section of the book may reflect historical or other considerations (eg, placement of the percutaneous peripheral vascular endovascular interventions in the Surgery/Cardiovascular System section, while the percutaneous coronary interventions appear in the Medicine/Cardiovascular section).

Rationale

The Instructions for Use of the CPT Codebook subsection in the **Introduction** section has been revised. Instructions have been added to state that all language in a code descriptor, including information in parentheses, is essential to the descriptor and should not be considered optional when determining appropriate code selection.

Before the CPT 2025 code set, there was no definitive language that stressed the importance of all language included within a descriptor or the parentheses directly in a descriptor. The new notation should help clarify and make clear the importance of assessing all provided language to minimize the possibility of misinterpreting the descriptor.

★ = Telemedicine   ◀ = Audio-only   ✛ = Add-on code   ⊬ = FDA approval pending   # = Resequenced code   ⊘ = Modifier 51 exempt

Evaluation and Management

Summary of Additions, Deletions, and Revisions

The summary of changes shows the actual changes that have been made to the code descriptors.

New codes appear with a bullet (●) and are indicated as "Code added." Revised codes are preceded with a triangle (▲). Within revised codes, or if a code symbol has been deleted, the deleted language and code symbol appear with a ~~strikethrough~~, while new text appears <u>underlined</u>.

The ⁄ symbol is used to identify codes for vaccines that are pending FDA approval. The # symbol is used to identify codes that have been resequenced. CPT add-on codes are annotated by the ✚ symbol. The ⊘ symbol is used to identify codes that are exempt from the use of modifier 51. The ★ symbol is used to identify codes that may be used for reporting telemedicine services. The ✖ symbol is used to identify a proprietary laboratory analyses (PLA) test that has an identical descriptor as another PLA test. A PLA code that satisfies Category I code criteria and has been accepted by the CPT Editorial Panel is annotated with the ↑↓ symbol. The ◀ symbol is used to identify codes that may be used to report audio-only telemedicine services when appended by modifier 93 (**see Appendix T**).

Code	Description
#●98000	Code added
#●98001	Code added
#●98002	Code added
#●98003	Code added
#●98004	Code added
#●98005	Code added
#●98006	Code added
#●98007	Code added
#●98008	Code added
#●98009	Code added
#●98010	Code added
#●98011	Code added
#●98012	Code added
#●98013	Code added
#●98014	Code added
#●98015	Code added
#●98016	Code added

Code	Description
99441	~~Telephone evaluation and management service by a physician or other qualified health care professional who may report evaluation and management services provided to an established patient, parent, or guardian not originating from a related E/M service provided within the previous 7 days nor leading to an E/M service or procedure within the next 24 hours or soonest available appointment; 5-10 minutes of medical discussion~~
99442	~~11-20 minutes of medical discussion~~
99443	~~21-30 minutes of medical discussion~~

★=Telemedicine　◀=Audio-only　✚=Add-on code　✔=FDA approval pending　#=Resequenced code　⊘=Modifier 51 exempt

Evaluation and Management (E/M) Services Guidelines

E/M Guidelines Overview

The E/M guidelines have sections that are common to all E/M categories and sections that are category specific. Most of the categories and many of the subcategories of service have special guidelines or instructions unique to that category or subcategory. Where these are indicated, eg, "Hospital Inpatient and Observation Care," special instructions are presented before the listing of the specific E/M services codes. It is important to review the instructions for each category or subcategory. These guidelines are to be used by the reporting physician or other qualified health care professional to select the appropriate level of service. These guidelines do not establish documentation requirements or standards of care. The main purpose of documentation is to support care of the patient by current and future health care team(s). These guidelines are for services that require a face-to-face encounter with the patient and/or family/caregiver. (For 99211 and 99281, the face-to-face services may be performed by clinical staff.)

▶In the **Evaluation and Management** section (98000-98016, 99202-99499), there are many code categories. Each category may have specific guidelines, or the codes may include specific details. These E/M guidelines are written for the following categories:

- Office or Other Outpatient Services
- Telemedicine Services
- Hospital Inpatient and Observation Care Services
- Consultations
- Emergency Department Services
- Nursing Facility Services
- Home or Residence Services
- Prolonged Service With or Without Direct Patient Contact on the Date of an Evaluation and Management Service◀

Rationale

In accordance with the establishment of codes 98000-98016, the E/M Guidelines Overview subsection has been revised to reflect these changes.

Refer to the codebook and the Rationale for codes 98000-98016 for a full discussion of these changes.

Evaluation and Management

Office or Other Outpatient Services

New Patient

99202 **Office or other outpatient visit** for the evaluation and management of a new patient, which requires a medically appropriate history and/or examination and straightforward medical decision making.

When using total time on the date of the encounter for code selection, 15 minutes must be met or exceeded.

99203 **Office or other outpatient visit** for the evaluation and management of a new patient, which requires a medically appropriate history and/or examination and low level of medical decision making.

When using total time on the date of the encounter for code selection, 30 minutes must be met or exceeded.

99204 **Office or other outpatient visit** for the evaluation and management of a new patient, which requires a medically appropriate history and/or examination and moderate level of medical decision making.

When using total time on the date of the encounter for code selection, 45 minutes must be met or exceeded.

99205 **Office or other outpatient visit** for the evaluation and management of a new patient, which requires a medically appropriate history and/or examination and high level of medical decision making.

When using total time on the date of the encounter for code selection, 60 minutes must be met or exceeded.

(For services 75 minutes or longer, use prolonged services code 99417)

Established Patient

99212 **Office or other outpatient visit** for the evaluation and management of an established patient, which requires a medically appropriate history and/or examination and straightforward medical decision making.

When using total time on the date of the encounter for code selection, 10 minutes must be met or exceeded.

99213 **Office or other outpatient visit** for the evaluation and management of an established patient, which requires a medically appropriate history and/or examination and low level of medical decision making.

When using total time on the date of the encounter for code selection, 20 minutes must be met or exceeded.

99214 **Office or other outpatient visit** for the evaluation and management of an established patient, which requires a medically appropriate history and/or examination and moderate level of medical decision making.

When using total time on the date of the encounter for code selection, 30 minutes must be met or exceeded.

99215 **Office or other outpatient visit** for the evaluation and management of an established patient, which requires a medically appropriate history and/or examination and high level of medical decision making.

When using total time on the date of the encounter for code selection, 40 minutes must be met or exceeded.

(For services 55 minutes or longer, use prolonged services code 99417)

Rationale

In accordance with the establishment of codes 98000-98016 for reporting telemedicine office visits, the telemedicine symbol (★) has been removed from codes 99202-99205 and 99212-99215 because they will no longer be reported for telemedicine office visits.

Refer to the codebook and the Rationale for codes 98000-98016 for a full discussion of these changes.

►Telemedicine Services◄

►Telemedicine services are synchronous, real-time, interactive encounters between a physician or other qualified health care professional (QHP) and a patient utilizing either combined audio-video or audio-only telecommunication. Unless specifically stated in the code descriptor, level selection for telemedicine services is based on either the level of medical decision making (MDM) or the total time for E/M services performed on the date of the encounter, as defined for each service. Telemedicine services are used in lieu of an in-person service when medically appropriate to address the care of the patient and when the patient and/or family/caregiver agree to this format of care. Telemedicine services are not used to report routine telecommunications related to a previous encounter (eg, to communicate laboratory results). They may be used for follow-up of a previous encounter, when a follow-up E/M service is required, in the same manner as in-person E/M services are used. For example, telemedicine services may be used for a patient requiring re-assessment for response or complications related to the treatment plan of a previous visit. Except for 98016, these services do not require a specific time interval from the last in-person or telemedicine visit and may be initiated by a physician or other QHP as well as

★ = Telemedicine ◄ = Audio-only ✚ = Add-on code ✔ = FDA approval pending # = Resequenced code ⊘ = Modifier 51 exempt

by a patient and/or family/caregiver. However, the telemedicine services must be performed on a separate calendar date from another E/M service. When performed on the same date as another E/M service, the elements and time of these services are summed and reported in aggregate, ensuring that any overlapping time is only counted once. If the minimum time for reporting a telemedicine service has not been achieved, time spent with the patient may still count toward the total time on the date of the encounter of an in-person E/M service.

For audio-only telemedicine services for established patients with 5 to 10 minutes of medical discussion, report brief communication technology service (eg, virtual check-in) code 98016. Code 98016 is reported for established patients only. The service is patient-initiated and intended to evaluate whether a more extensive visit type is required (eg, an office or other outpatient E/M service [99212, 99213, 99214, 99215]). Video

technology is not required for audio-only visits. When the patient-initiated check-in leads to an E/M service on the same calendar date, and when time is used to select the level of that E/M service, the time from 98016 may be added to the time of the E/M service for the total time on the date of the encounter.

For services that are asynchronous (ie, not live in real-time), see **Online Digital Evaluation and Management Services** (99421, 99422, 99423). Do not report telemedicine services for oversight of clinical staff (eg, chronic care management [CCM]). Do not count the time performing telemedicine services toward time performing CCM (99437, 99491) or principal care management services (99424, 99425). See Table 2, Telemedicine and Non-Face-to-Face Services.

For 98000-98015, the level of service is selected based on MDM or total time on the date of the encounter. For

►**Table 2: Telemedicine and Non-Face-to-Face Services**

Service	New/Established	Synchronous	Level/Unit Reported	Service Reported	Other E/M Notations
Synchronous audio-video (98000-98007)	Both	Yes	MDM or total time on the date of the service. No minimum required time, unless level selected by time.	Per single calendar date	Do not report with same-day in-person E/M
Synchronous audio-only (98008-98015)	Both	Yes	MDM or total time on the date of the service. Must be more than 10 minutes of medical discussion.	Per single calendar date	Do not report with same-day in-person E/M
Brief synchronous communication technology service (98016)	Established	Yes	A single 5- to 10-minute medical discussion	Per single calendar date	Not related to E/M in prior 7 days or leading to E/M in next 24 hours
Online digital E/M (99421-99423)	Established	No	Minutes during 7-day period	Per 7 days	Not related to E/M in prior 7 days or leading to E/M in next 24 hours
Interprofessional telephone/Internet/EHR consultations (99446-99451)	Both	Not required	Minutes during 7-day period	Per 7 days	No in-person encounter within 14 days
Interprofessional telephone/Internet/EHR consultations (99452)	Both	Not required	Minutes during a single day	Per 14 days	No in-person encounter within 14 days
Care management and remote treatment management (99424, 99425, 99437, 99484, 99491)	Established	Not required	Minutes	Per calendar month	Physician or QHP time excluded on date of other E/M
All services (98000-98016, 99421-99425, 99437, 99446-99452, 99484, 99491)			Same time is not counted twice◄		

Evaluation / Management 99202-99499

audio-only codes 98008, 98009, 98010, 98011, 98012, 98013, 98014, 98015, the service must exceed 10 minutes of medical discussion. Code 98016 describes services for established patients with 5 to 10 minutes of medical discussion and is based only on the time of medical discussion and not MDM. Do not count time for establishing the connection or arranging the appointment, even when performed by the physician or other QHP. Services of less than five minutes are not reported.

For audio-only codes 98008, 98009, 98010, 98011, 98012, 98013, 98014, 98015, medical discussion is synchronous (real-time) interactive verbal communication and does not include online digital communication (except when via a telecommunication technology device for the deaf). The meaning of MDM has the meaning used in the E/M Guidelines and is a cognitive process by the physician or other QHP.

If during the encounter, audio-video connections are lost and only audio is restored, report the service that accounted for the majority of the time of the interactive portion of the service. Ten minutes of medical discussion or patient observation must be exceeded in order to report the audio-only service.◀

▶Synchronous Audio-Video Evaluation and Management Services◀

▶Codes 98000, 98001, 98002, 98003, 98004, 98005, 98006, 98007 may be reported for new or established patients. Synchronous audio and video telecommunication is required. These services may be reported based on total time on the date of the encounter or MDM.◀

▶New Patient◀

#● **98000**   **Synchronous audio-video visit** for the evaluation and management of a new patient, which requires a medically appropriate history and/or examination and straightforward medical decision making.

When using total time on the date of the encounter for code selection, 15 minutes must be met or exceeded.

#● **98001**   **Synchronous audio-video visit** for the evaluation and management of a new patient, which requires a medically appropriate history and/or examination and low medical decision making.

When using total time on the date of the encounter for code selection, 30 minutes must be met or exceeded.

#● **98002**   **Synchronous audio-video visit** for the evaluation and management of a new patient, which requires a medically appropriate history and/or examination and moderate medical decision making.

When using total time on the date of the encounter for code selection, 45 minutes must be met or exceeded.

#● **98003**   **Synchronous audio-video visit** for the evaluation and management of a new patient, which requires a medically appropriate history and/or examination and high medical decision making.

When using total time on the date of the encounter for code selection, 60 minutes must be met or exceeded.

▶(For services 75 minutes or longer, use prolonged services code 99417)◀

Clinical Example (98000)

Synchronous audio-video visit for a new patient with a self-limited problem.

Description of Procedure (98000)

Prior to Visit: Review any medical records and data. Communicate with other members of the health care team regarding the visit.

Day of Visit: Confirm the patient's identity. Review the medical history forms completed by the patient. Obtain a medically appropriate history, including pertinent components of history of present illness, review of systems, social history, family history, and allergies, and reconcile the patient's medications. Perform a medically appropriate visual examination. Synthesize the relevant history and visual examination to formulate a differential diagnosis and treatment plan (requiring straightforward medical decision making). Discuss the treatment plan with the patient and the patient's family. Provide patient education, and respond to questions from the patient and/or the patient's family. Document the encounter in the medical record. Perform electronic data capture and reporting to comply with the quality payment program and other electronic mandates.

After Visit: Answer follow-up questions from the patient and/or the patient's family, and respond to treatment failures that may occur after the visit. Coordinate follow-up or orders with office staff.

Clinical Example (98001)

Synchronous audio-video visit for a new patient with a stable chronic illness or acute uncomplicated injury.

Description of Procedure (98001)

Prior to Visit: Review any medical records and data. Query the prescription monitoring program, health information exchange, and other registries, as required. Communicate with other members of the health care team regarding the visit.

Day of Visit: Confirm the patient's identity. Review the medical history forms completed by the patient. Obtain a medically appropriate history, including pertinent components of history of present illness, review of systems, social history, family history, and allergies, and reconcile the patient's medications. Perform a medically appropriate visual examination. Synthesize the relevant history, visual examination, and data elements to formulate a differential diagnosis, diagnostic strategy, and treatment plan (requiring low level of medical decision making). Discuss the treatment options with the patient and the patient's family, incorporating their values in the creation of the plan. Provide patient education and respond to questions from the patient and/or the patient's family. Electronically prescribe all chronic and new medications after verifying the preferred pharmacy, making changes as needed based on the payer formulary. Arrange for diagnostic testing and referral if necessary. Document the encounter in the medical record. In concert with the clinical staff, complete prior authorizations for medications and other orders, when performed. Perform electronic data capture and reporting to comply with quality payment programs and other electronic mandates.

After Visit: Answer follow-up questions from the patient and/or the patient's family, and respond to treatment failures or complications or adverse reactions to medications that may occur after the visit. Review and analyze interval testing results. Communicate results to and plan modifications with the patient and/or the patient's family. Respond to queries from the pharmacy regarding changes in medications due to formulary or other issues.

Clinical Example (98002)

Synchronous audio-video visit for a new patient with a progressing illness or acute injury that requires medical management or potential surgical treatment.

Description of Procedure (98002)

Prior to Visit: Review any medical records and data. Query the prescription monitoring program, health information exchange, and other registries, as required. Communicate with other members of the health care team regarding the visit.

Day of Visit: Confirm the patient's identity. Review the medical history forms completed by the patient. Obtain a medically appropriate history, including pertinent components of history of present illness, review of systems, social history, family history, and allergies, and reconcile the patient's medications. Perform a medically appropriate visual examination. Synthesize the relevant history, visual examination, and data elements to formulate a differential diagnosis, diagnostic strategy, and treatment plan (requiring moderate level of medical

decision making). Discuss the treatment options with the patient and that patient's family, incorporating their values in the creation of the plan. Provide patient education, and respond to questions from the patient and/or the patient's family. Electronically prescribe all chronic and new medications after verifying the preferred pharmacy, making changes as needed based on the payer formulary. Arrange for diagnostic testing and referral if necessary. Document the encounter in the medical record. In concert with the clinical staff, complete prior authorizations for medications and other orders, when performed. Perform electronic data capture and reporting to comply with quality payment programs and other electronic mandates.

After Visit: Answer follow-up questions from the patient and/or the patient's family, and respond to treatment failures or complications or adverse reactions to medications that may occur after the visit. Review and analyze interval testing results. Communicate results to and plan modifications with the patient and/or the patient's family. Respond to queries from the pharmacy regarding changes in medications due to formulary or other issues.

Clinical Example (98003)

Synchronous audio-video visit for a new patient with a chronic illness with severe exacerbation, or an acute illness/injury, that poses an acute threat to life or bodily function.

Description of Procedure (98003)

Prior to Visit: Review any medical records and data. Query the prescription monitoring program, health information exchange, and other registries, as required. Communicate with other members of the health care team regarding the visit.

Day of Visit: Confirm the patient's identity. Review the medical history forms completed by the patient. Obtain a medically appropriate history, including pertinent components of history of present illness, review of systems, social history, family history, and allergies, and reconcile the patient's medications. Perform a medically appropriate visual examination. Synthesize the relevant history, visual examination, and data elements to formulate a differential diagnosis, diagnostic strategy, and treatment plan (requiring high level of medical decision making). Discuss the treatment options with the patient and the patient's family, incorporating their values in creation of the plan. Provide patient education, and respond to questions from the patient and/or the patient's family. Electronically prescribe all chronic and new medications after verifying preferred pharmacy, making changes as needed based on payer formulary. Arrange for diagnostic testing and referral if necessary. Document the encounter in the medical record. In concert with the clinical staff, complete prior authorizations for medications and other orders, when performed. Perform electronic data capture and reporting to comply with quality payment program and other electronic mandates.

After Visit: Answer follow-up questions from the patient and/or the patient's family, and respond to treatment failures or complications or adverse reactions to medications that may occur after the visit. Review and analyze interval testing results. Communicate results to and plan modifications with the patient and/or the patient's family. Respond to queries from the pharmacy regarding changes in medications due to formulary or other issues.

▶Established Patient◀

#● 98004 **Synchronous audio-video visit** for the evaluation and management of an established patient, which requires a medically appropriate history and/or examination and straightforward medical decision making.

When using total time on the date of the encounter for code selection, 10 minutes must be met or exceeded.

#● 98005 **Synchronous audio-video visit** for the evaluation and management of an established patient, which requires a medically appropriate history and/or examination and low medical decision making.

When using total time on the date of the encounter for code selection, 20 minutes must be met or exceeded.

#● 98006 **Synchronous audio-video visit** for the evaluation and management of an established patient, which requires a medically appropriate history and/or examination and moderate medical decision making.

When using total time on the date of the encounter for code selection, 30 minutes must be met or exceeded.

#● 98007 **Synchronous audio-video visit** for the evaluation and management of an established patient, which requires a medically appropriate history and/or examination and high medical decision making.

When using total time on the date of the encounter for code selection, 40 minutes must be met or exceeded.

▶(For services 55 minutes or longer, use prolonged services code 99417)◀

Clinical Example (98004)

Synchronous audio-video visit for an established patient with a self-limited problem.

Description of Procedure (98004)

Prior to Visit: If necessary, review interval correspondence, referral notes, and medical records generated since the last visit. Communicate with other members of the health care team regarding the visit.

Day of Visit: Confirm the patient's identity. Review the medical history form completed by the patient and prior clinical note. Obtain a medically appropriate history. Update pertinent components of history of present illness, review of systems, social history, family history, and allergies, and reconcile the patient's medications. Perform a medically appropriate visual examination. Synthesize the relevant history and visual examination to formulate a differential diagnosis and treatment plan (requiring straightforward medical decision making). Discuss the treatment plan with the patient and the patient's family. Provide patient education, and respond to questions from the patient and/or the patient's family. Document the encounter in the medical record. Perform electronic data capture and reporting to comply with quality payment programs and other electronic mandates.

After Visit: Answer follow-up questions from the patient and/or the patient's family, and respond to treatment failures that may occur after the visit. Coordinate follow-up or orders with office staff.

Clinical Example (98005)

Synchronous audio-video visit for an established patient with a stable chronic illness or acute uncomplicated illness or injury.

Description of Procedure (98005)

Prior to Visit: Review interval correspondence, referral notes, medical records, and diagnostic data generated since the last visit. Query the prescription monitoring program, health information exchange, and other registries, as required. Communicate with other members of the health care team regarding the visit.

Day of Visit: Confirm the patient's identity. Review the medical history form completed by the patient and prior clinical note. Obtain a medically appropriate history, including the response to any treatment initiated or continued at the last visit. Update pertinent components of the social history, family history, review of systems, and allergies that have changed since the last visit. Reconcile the medication list. Perform a medically appropriate visual examination. Synthesize the relevant history, visual examination, and data elements to update differential diagnosis, diagnostic strategy, and treatment plan (requiring low level of medical decision making). Discuss treatment options with the patient and the patient's family, incorporating their values in creation of the plan. Provide patient education, and respond to questions from the patient and/or the patient's family.

★ = Telemedicine   ◀ = Audio-only   ✚ = Add-on code   ⟋ = FDA approval pending   # = Resequenced code   ⦰ = Modifier 51 exempt

Electronically prescribe medications, making changes as needed based on payer formulary. Arrange diagnostic testing and referral if necessary. Document the encounter in the medical record. In concert with the clinical staff, complete prior authorizations for medications and other orders, when performed. Perform electronic data capture and reporting to comply with quality payment programs and other electronic mandates.

After Visit: Answer follow-up questions from the patient and/or the patient's family, and respond to treatment failures or complications or adverse reactions to medications that may occur after the visit. Review and analyze interval testing results. Communicate results to and plan modifications with the patient and/or the patient's family. Respond to queries from the pharmacy regarding changes in medications due to formulary or other issues.

Clinical Example (98006)

Synchronous audio-video visit for an established patient with a progressing illness or acute injury that requires medical management or potential surgical treatment.

Description of Procedure (98006)

Prior to Visit: Review interval correspondence, referral notes, medical records, and diagnostic data generated since the last visit. Query the prescription monitoring program, health information exchange, and other registries, as required. Communicate with other members of the health care team regarding the visit.

Day of Visit: Confirm the patient's identity. Review the medical history form completed by the patient and the prior clinical note. Obtain a medically appropriate history, including the response to any treatment initiated or continued at the last visit. Update pertinent components of the social history, family history, review of systems, and allergies that have changed since the last visit. Reconcile the medication list. Perform a medically appropriate visual examination. Synthesize the relevant history, visual examination, and data elements to update differential diagnosis, diagnostic strategy, and treatment plan (requiring moderate level of medical decision making). Discuss treatment options with the patient and the patient's family, incorporating their values in creation of the plan. Provide patient education, and respond to questions from the patient and/or the patient's family. Electronically prescribe medications, making changes as needed based on the payer formulary. Arrange diagnostic testing and referral if necessary. Document the encounter in the medical record. In concert with the clinical staff, complete prior authorizations for medications and other orders, when performed. Perform electronic data capture and reporting to comply with quality payment programs and other electronic mandates.

After Visit: Answer follow-up questions from the patient and/or the family, and respond to treatment failures or complications or adverse reactions to medications that may occur after the visit. Review and analyze interval testing results. Communicate results to and plan modifications with the patient and/or the patient's family. Respond to queries from the pharmacy regarding changes in medications due to formulary or other issues.

Clinical Example (98007)

Synchronous audio-video visit for an established patient with a chronic illness with severe exacerbation, or an acute illness/injury, that poses an acute threat to life or bodily function.

Description of Procedure (98007)

Prior to Visit: Review interval correspondence, referral notes, medical records, and diagnostic data generated since the last visit. Query the prescription monitoring program, health information exchange, and other registries, as required. Communicate with other members of the health care team regarding the visit.

Day of Visit: Confirm the patient's identity. Review the medical history form completed by the patient and prior clinical note. Obtain a medically appropriate history, including the response to any treatment initiated or continued at the last visit. Update pertinent components of the social history, family history, review of systems, and allergies that have changed since the last visit. Reconcile the medication list. Perform a medically appropriate visual examination. Synthesize the relevant history, visual examination, and data elements to update differential diagnosis, diagnostic strategy, and treatment plan (requiring high level of medical decision making). Discuss treatment options with the patient and the patient's family, incorporating their values in the creation of the plan. Provide patient education, and respond to questions from the patient and/or the patient's family. Electronically prescribe medications, making changes as needed based on the payer formulary. Arrange diagnostic testing and referral if necessary. Document the encounter in the medical record. In concert with the clinical staff, complete prior authorizations for medications and other orders, when performed. Perform electronic data capture and reporting to comply with quality payment programs and other electronic mandates.

After Visit: Answer follow-up questions from the patient and/or the patient's family, and respond to treatment failures or complications or adverse reactions to medications that may occur after the visit. Review and analyze interval testing results. Communicate results to and plan modifications with the patient and/or the patient's family. Respond to queries from the pharmacy regarding changes in medications due to formulary or other issues.

▶Synchronous Audio-Only Evaluation and Management Services◀

▶Codes 98008, 98009, 98010, 98011, 98012, 98013, 98014, 98015 may be reported for new or established patients. They require more than 10 minutes of medical discussion. For services of 5 to 10 minutes of medical discussion, report 98016, if appropriate. If 10 minutes of medical discussion is exceeded, total time on the date of the encounter or MDM may be used for code level selection.◀

▶New Patient◀

 # ● 98008   **Synchronous audio-only visit** for the evaluation and management of a new patient, which requires a medically appropriate history and/or examination, straightforward medical decision making, and more than 10 minutes of medical discussion.

When using total time on the date of the encounter for code selection, 15 minutes must be met or exceeded.

 # ● 98009   **Synchronous audio-only visit** for the evaluation and management of a new patient, which requires a medically appropriate history and/or examination, low medical decision making, and more than 10 minutes of medical discussion.

When using total time on the date of the encounter for code selection, 30 minutes must be met or exceeded.

 # ● 98010   **Synchronous audio-only visit** for the evaluation and management of a new patient, which requires a medically appropriate history and/or examination, moderate medical decision making, and more than 10 minutes of medical discussion.

When using total time on the date of the encounter for code selection, 45 minutes must be met or exceeded.

 # ● 98011   **Synchronous audio-only visit** for the evaluation and management of a new patient, which requires a medically appropriate history and/or examination, high medical decision making, and more than 10 minutes of medical discussion.

When using total time on the date of the encounter for code selection, 60 minutes must be met or exceeded.

▶(For services 75 minutes or longer, use prolonged services code 99417)◀

Clinical Example (98008)

Synchronous audio-only visit for a new patient with a self-limited problem.

Description of Procedure (98008)

Prior to Visit: Review any medical records and data. Communicate with other members of the health care team regarding the visit.

Day of Visit: Confirm the patient's identity. Review the medical history forms completed by the patient. Obtain a medically appropriate history, including pertinent components of history of present illness, review of systems, social history, family history, and allergies, and reconcile the patient's medications. Assess the patient's condition with available information to formulate a differential diagnosis and treatment plan (requiring straightforward medical decision making). Discuss the treatment plan with the patient and the patient's family. Provide patient education, and respond to questions from the patient and/or the patient's family. Document the encounter in the medical record. Perform electronic data capture and reporting to comply with quality payment programs and other electronic mandates.

After Visit: Answer follow-up questions from the patient and/or the patient's family, and respond to treatment failures that may occur after the visit. Coordinate follow-up or orders with office staff.

Clinical Example (98009)

Synchronous audio-only visit for a new patient with a stable chronic illness or acute uncomplicated illness or injury.

Description of Procedure (98009)

Prior to Visit: Review any medical records and data. Query the prescription monitoring program, health information exchange, and other registries, as required. Communicate with other members of the health care team regarding the visit.

Day of Visit: Confirm the patient's identity. Review the medical history forms completed by the patient. Obtain a medically appropriate history, including pertinent components of history of present illness, review of systems, social history, family history, and allergies, and reconcile the patient's medications. Assess the patient's condition with available information to formulate a differential diagnosis and treatment plan (requiring low level of medical decision making). Discuss the treatment options with the patient and the patient's family, incorporating their values in the creation of the plan. Provide patient education, and respond to questions from the patient and/or the patient's family. Electronically prescribe all chronic and new medications after verifying the preferred pharmacy, making changes as needed based on the payer formulary. Arrange for diagnostic testing and referral if necessary. Document the encounter in the medical record. In concert with the clinical staff, complete prior authorizations for medications and other orders, when performed. Perform electronic data capture and reporting to comply with quality payment programs and other electronic mandates.

After Visit: Answer follow-up questions from the patient and/or the patient's family, and respond to treatment failures or complications or adverse reactions to medications that may occur after the visit. Review and analyze interval testing results. Communicate results to and plan modifications with the patient and/or the patient's family. Respond to queries from the pharmacy regarding changes in medications due to formulary or other issues.

Clinical Example (98010)

Synchronous audio-only visit for a new patient with a progressing illness or acute injury that requires medical management or potential surgical treatment.

Description of Procedure (98010)

Prior to Visit: Review any medical records and data. Query the prescription monitoring program, health information exchange, and other registries, as required. Communicate with other members of the health care team regarding the visit.

Day of Visit: Confirm the patient's identity. Review the medical history forms completed by the patient. Obtain a medically appropriate history, including pertinent components of history of present illness, review of systems, social history, family history, and allergies, and reconcile the patient's medications. Assess the patient's condition with available information to formulate a differential diagnosis and treatment plan (requiring moderate level of medical decision making). Discuss the treatment options with the patient and the patient's family, incorporating their values in the creation of the plan. Provide patient education, and respond to questions from the patient and/or the patient's family. Electronically prescribe all chronic and new medications after verifying the preferred pharmacy, making changes as needed based on the payer formulary. Arrange for diagnostic testing and referral if necessary. Document the encounter in the medical record. In concert with the clinical staff, complete prior authorizations for medications and other orders, when performed. Perform electronic data capture and reporting to comply with quality payment programs and other electronic mandates.

After Visit: Answer follow-up questions from the patient and/or the patient's family, and respond to treatment failures or complications or adverse reactions to medications that may occur after the visit. Review and analyze interval testing results. Communicate results to and plan modifications with the patient and/or the patient's family. Respond to queries from the pharmacy

regarding changes in medications due to formulary or other issues.

Clinical Example (98011)

Synchronous audio-only visit for a new patient with a chronic illness with severe exacerbation, or an acute illness/injury, that poses an acute threat to life or bodily function.

Description of Procedure (98011)

Prior to Visit: Review any medical records and data. Query the prescription monitoring program, health information exchange, and other registries, as required. Communicate with other members of the health care team regarding the visit.

Day of Visit: Confirm the patient's identity. Review the medical history forms completed by the patient. Obtain a medically appropriate history, including pertinent components of history of present illness, review of systems, social history, family history, and allergies, and reconcile the patient's medications. Assess the patient's condition with available information to formulate a differential diagnosis and treatment plan (requiring high level of medical decision making). Discuss the treatment options with the patient and the patient's family, incorporating their values in creation of the plan. Provide patient education, and respond to questions from the patient and/or the patient's family. Electronically prescribe all chronic and new medications after verifying preferred pharmacy, making changes as needed based on payer formulary. Arrange for diagnostic testing and referral if necessary. Document the encounter in the medical record. In concert with the clinical staff, complete prior authorizations for medications and other orders, when performed. Perform electronic data capture and reporting to comply with quality payment programs and other electronic mandates.

After Visit: Answer follow-up questions from the patient and/or the patient's family, and respond to treatment failures or complications, or adverse reactions to medications that may occur after the visit. Review and analyze interval testing results. Communicate results to and plan modifications with the patient and/or the patient's family. Respond to queries from the pharmacy regarding changes in medications due to formulary or other issues.

►Established Patient◄

\#● **98012**   **Synchronous audio-only visit** for the evaluation and management of an established patient, which requires a medically appropriate history and/or examination, straightforward medical decision making, and more than 10 minutes of medical discussion.

When using total time on the date of the encounter for code selection, 10 minutes must be exceeded.

▶(Do not report 98012 for home and outpatient INR monitoring when reporting 93792, 93793)◀

▶(Do not report 98012 when using 99374, 99375, 99377, 99378, 99379, 99380 for the same call[s])◀

▶(Do not report 98012 during the same month with 99487, 99489)◀

▶(Do not report 98012 when performed during the service time of 99495, 99496)◀

#● **98013**　**Synchronous audio-only visit** for the evaluation and management of an established patient, which requires a medically appropriate history and/or examination, low medical decision making, and more than 10 minutes of medical discussion.

When using total time on the date of the encounter for code selection, 20 minutes must be met or exceeded.

▶(Do not report 98013 for home and outpatient INR monitoring when reporting 93792, 93793)◀

▶(Do not report 98013 when using 99374, 99375, 99377, 99378, 99379, 99380 for the same call[s])◀

▶(Do not report 98013 during the same month with 99487, 99489)◀

▶(Do not report 98013 when performed during the service time of 99495, 99496)◀

#● **98014**　**Synchronous audio-only visit** for the evaluation and management of an established patient, which requires a medically appropriate history and/or examination, moderate medical decision making, and more than 10 minutes of medical discussion.

When using total time on the date of the encounter for code selection, 30 minutes must be met or exceeded.

▶(Do not report 98014 for home and outpatient INR monitoring when reporting 93792, 93793)◀

▶(Do not report 98014 when using 99374, 99375, 99377, 99378, 99379, 99380 for the same call[s])◀

▶(Do not report 98014 during the same month with 99487, 99489)◀

▶(Do not report 98014 when performed during the service time of 99495, 99496)◀

#● **98015**　**Synchronous audio-only visit** for the evaluation and management of an established patient, which requires a medically appropriate history and/or examination, high medical decision making, and more than 10 minutes of medical discussion.

When using total time on the date of the encounter for code selection, 40 minutes must be met or exceeded.

▶(Do not report 98015 for home and outpatient INR monitoring when reporting 93792, 93793)◀

▶(Do not report 98015 when using 99374, 99375, 99377, 99378, 99379, 99380 for the same call[s])◀

▶(Do not report 98015 during the same month with 99487, 99489)◀

▶(Do not report 98015 when performed during the service time of 99495, 99496)◀

▶(For services 55 minutes or longer, use prolonged services code 99417)◀

Clinical Example (98012)

Synchronous audio-only visit for an established patient with a self-limited problem.

Description of Procedure (98012)

Prior to Visit: If necessary, review interval correspondence, referral notes, and medical records generated since the last visit. Communicate with other members of the health care team regarding the visit.

Day of Visit: Confirm the patient's identity. Review the medical history form completed by the patient and prior clinical note. Obtain a medically appropriate history. Update pertinent components of history of present illness, review of systems, social history, family history, and allergies, and reconcile the patient's medications. Assess the patient's condition with available information to formulate a differential diagnosis and treatment plan (requiring straightforward medical decision making). Discuss the treatment plan with the patient and the patient's family. Provide patient education, and respond to questions from the patient and/or the patient's family. Document the encounter in the medical record. Perform electronic data capture and reporting to comply with quality payment programs and other electronic mandates.

After Visit: Answer follow-up questions from the patient and/or the patient's family, and respond to treatment failures that may occur after the visit. Coordinate follow-up or orders with office staff.

Clinical Example (98013)

Synchronous audio-only visit for an established patient with a stable chronic illness or acute uncomplicated illness or injury.

Description of Procedure (98013)

Prior to Visit: Review interval correspondence, referral notes, medical records, and diagnostic data generated since the last visit. Query the prescription monitoring program, health information exchange, and other registries, as required. Communicate with other members of the health care team regarding the visit.

Day of Visit: Confirm the patient's identity. Review the medical history form completed by the patient and prior clinical note. Obtain a medically appropriate history, including the response to any treatment initiated or continued at the last visit. Update pertinent components of the social history, family history, review of systems, and allergies that have changed since the last visit. Reconcile the medication list. Assess the patient's condition with available information to formulate a differential diagnosis and treatment plan (requiring low level of medical decision making). Discuss treatment options with the patient and the patient's family, incorporating their values in the creation of the plan. Provide patient education, and respond to questions from the patient and/or the patient's family. Electronically prescribe medications, making changes as needed based on the payer formulary. Arrange diagnostic testing and referral if necessary. Document the encounter in the medical record. In concert with the clinical staff, complete prior authorizations for medications and other orders, when performed. Perform electronic data capture and reporting to comply with quality payment programs and other electronic mandates.

After Visit: Answer follow-up questions from the patient and/or the patient's family, and respond to treatment failures or complications or adverse reactions to medications that may occur after the visit. Review and analyze interval testing results. Communicate results to and plan modifications with the patient and/or the patient's family. Respond to queries from the pharmacy regarding changes in medications due to formulary or other issues.

Clinical Example (98014)

Synchronous audio-only visit for an established patient with a progressing illness or acute injury that requires medical management or potential surgical treatment.

Description of Procedure (98014)

Prior to Visit: Review interval correspondence, referral notes, medical records, and diagnostic data generated since the last visit. Query the prescription monitoring program, health information exchange, and other registries, as required. Communicate with other members of the health care team regarding the visit.

Day of Visit: Confirm the patient's identity. Review the medical history form completed by the patient and prior clinical note. Obtain a medically appropriate history, including the response to any treatment initiated or continued at the last visit. Update pertinent components of the social history, family history, review of systems, and allergies that have changed since the last visit. Reconcile the medication list. Assess the patient's condition with available information to formulate a differential diagnosis and treatment plan (requiring moderate level of medical decision making). Discuss treatment options with the patient and the patient's

family, incorporating their values in creation of the plan. Provide patient education, and respond to questions from the patient and/or the patient's family. Electronically prescribe medications, making changes as needed based on payer formulary. Arrange diagnostic testing and referral if necessary. Document the encounter in the medical record. In concert with the clinical staff, complete prior authorizations for medications and other orders, when performed. Perform electronic data capture and reporting to comply with quality payment programs and other electronic mandates.

After Visit: Answer follow-up questions from the patient and/or the patient's family, and respond to treatment failures or complications or adverse reactions to medications that may occur after the visit. Review and analyze interval testing results. Communicate results to and plan modifications with the patient and/or the patient's family. Respond to queries from the pharmacy regarding changes in medications due to formulary or other issues.

Clinical Example (98015)

Synchronous audio-only visit for an established patient with a chronic illness with severe exacerbation, or an acute illness/injury, that poses an acute threat to life or bodily function.

Description of Procedure (98015)

Prior to Visit: Review interval correspondence, referral notes, medical records, and diagnostic data generated since the last visit. Query the prescription monitoring program, health information exchange, and other registries, as required. Communicate with other members of the health care team regarding the visit.

Day of Visit: Confirm the patient's identity. Review the medical history form completed by the patient and prior clinical note. Obtain a medically appropriate history, including the response to any treatment initiated or continued at the last visit. Update pertinent components of the social history, family history, review of systems, and allergies that have changed since the last visit. Reconcile the medication list. Assess the patient's condition with available information to formulate a differential diagnosis and treatment plan (requiring high level of medical decision making). Discuss treatment options with the patient and the patient's family, incorporating their values in the creation of the plan. Provide patient education, and respond to questions from the patient and/or the patient's family. Electronically prescribe medications, making changes as needed based on the payer formulary. Arrange diagnostic testing and referral if necessary. Document the encounter in the medical record. In concert with the clinical staff, complete prior authorizations for medications and other orders, when performed. Perform electronic data capture and reporting to comply with quality payment programs and other electronic mandates.

After Visit: Answer follow-up questions from the patient and/or the patient's family, and respond to treatment failures or complications or adverse reactions to medications that may occur after the visit. Review and analyze interval testing results. Communicate results to and plan modifications with the patient and/or the patient's family. Respond to queries from the pharmacy regarding changes in medications due to formulary or other issues.

▶Brief Synchronous Communication Technology Service (eg, Virtual Check-In)◀

▶Code 98016 is reported for established patients only. The service is patient-initiated and intended to evaluate whether a more extensive visit type is required (eg, an office or other outpatient E/M service [99212, 99213, 99214, 99215]). Video technology is not required. Code 98016 describes a service of shorter duration than the audio-only services and has other restrictions that are related to the intended use as a "virtual check-in" or triage to determine if another E/M service is necessary. When the patient-initiated check-in leads to an E/M service on the same calendar date, and when time is used to select the level of that E/M service, the time from 98016 may be added to the time of the E/M service for total time on the date of the encounter.◀

#● **98016**   **Brief communication technology-based service** (eg, virtual check-in) by a physician or other qualified health care professional who can report evaluation and management services, provided to an established patient, not originating from a related evaluation and management service provided within the previous 7 days nor leading to an evaluation and management service or procedure within the next 24 hours or soonest available appointment, 5-10 minutes of medical discussion

▶(Do not report 98016 in conjunction with 98000-98015)◀

▶(Do not report services of less than 5 minutes of medical discussion)◀

Rationale

A new subsection, "Telemedicine Services," has been added to the Evaluation and Management section with new guidelines and 17 new codes for reporting synchronous (ie, real-time) evaluation and management (E/M) services.

Prior to 2025, audio-video telemedicine office or other outpatient E/M services were reported using codes 99202-99205 (new patient) and 99211-99215 (established patient) with modifier 95, *Synchronous Telemedicine Service Rendered via a Real-Time Interactive Audio and Video Telecommunications System,* appended. The new codes better reflect the resources needed to provide these services.

The Relative Value Scale Update Committee (RUC)/Current Procedural Terminology (CPT) (RUC/CPT) E/M Workgroup (Workgroup) performed an assessment of available data for audio-video and audio-only office visits and surveyed medical specialty societies. The Workgroup's findings indicated that PE for clinical staff time is applicable to both audio-video and audio-only office visits; therefore, a coding solution was needed to accurately reflect the clinical staff time associated with these services. For 2025, codes 98000-98007 have been established for synchronous **(real-time) audio-video** E/M office services. Codes 98008-98015 have been established for synchronous **(real-time) audio-only** E/M services. With the establishment of these codes, codes 99441-99443 for telephone services have been deleted and a cross-reference parenthetical note added directing users to new codes 98008-98016. These telemedicine service codes describe real-time, interactive encounters between the physician or other qualified health care professional and the patient. Both the audio-video and the audio-only codes have the same categories (new and established patients) and structure as the office or other outpatient codes 99202-99205 and 99211-99215.

Code 98016 has been established for a brief synchronous communication technology service (eg, a virtual check-in). Note that this service is reported for an established patient and is initiated by the patient to determine if a more extensive E/M service is necessary. Code 98016 is similar to Healthcare Common Procedure Coding System (HCPCS) Level II code G2252.

New guidelines have been added to define the services described in these new codes and explain the appropriate reporting of these services. It is important to note that when a telemedicine office visit is performed on the same date as another E/M service, the elements and time of these services are summed together to avoid duplicate reporting. The new guidelines include a Telemedicine and Non-Face-to-Face Services table, which provides additional guidance for reporting codes 98000-98016 and other online and non-face-to-face E/M services codes. Parenthetical notes have been added throughout the new subsection to provide instructions on the appropriate reporting of these new codes, too.

Clinical Example (98016)

An established patient contacts the office to request an evaluation regarding the necessity of being seen for symptoms of concern to the patient.

Description of Procedure (98016)

Prior to Visit: Review any medical records and data. Communicate with other members of the health care team regarding the visit.

Day of Visit: Confirm the patient's identity. Review the medical history forms completed by the patient. Obtain a medically appropriate history, including pertinent components of history of present illness, review of systems, social history, family history, and allergies, and reconcile the patient's medications. Assess the patient's condition with available information to formulate a differential diagnosis and treatment plan (requiring straightforward medical decision making). Discuss the treatment plan with the patient and the patient's family. Provide patient education, and respond to questions from the patient and/or the patient's family. Document the encounter in the medical record. Perform electronic data capture and reporting to comply with quality payment programs and other electronic mandates.

After visit: Answer follow-up questions from the patient and/or the patient's family, and respond to treatment failures that may occur after the visit. Coordinate follow-up or orders with office staff.

Hospital Observation Services

Observation Care Discharge Services

(99217 has been deleted. To report observation care discharge services, see 99238, 99239)

Prolonged Services

Prolonged Service With or Without Direct Patient Contact on the Date of an Evaluation and Management Service

#★✚ 99417   **Prolonged outpatient evaluation and management service(s)** time with or without direct patient contact beyond the required time of the primary service when the primary service level has been selected using total time, each 15 minutes of total time (List separately in addition to the code of the outpatient **Evaluation and Management** service)

▶(Use 99417 in conjunction with 98003, 98007, 98011, 98015, 99205, 99215, 99245, 99345, 99350, 99483)◀

(Use 99417 in conjunction with 99483, when the total time on the date of the encounter exceeds the typical time of 99483 by 15 minutes or more)

(Do not report 99417 on the same date of service as 90833, 90836, 90838, 99358, 99359, 99415, 99416)

(Do not report 99417 for any time unit less than 15 minutes)

Rationale

In accordance with the establishment of telemedicine codes 98003, 98007, 98011, and 98015, the inclusionary parenthetical note for add-on code 99417 has been revised with the addition of these codes.

Refer to the codebook and the Rationale for codes 98000-98016 for a full discussion of these changes.

Case Management Services

Medical Team Conferences

Medical team conferences include face-to-face participation by a minimum of three qualified health care professionals from different specialties or disciplines (each of whom provide direct care to the patient), with or without the presence of the patient, family member(s), community agencies, surrogate decision maker(s) (eg, legal guardian), and/or caregiver(s). The participants are actively involved in the development, revision, coordination, and implementation of health care services needed by the patient. Reporting participants shall have performed face-to-face evaluations or treatments of the patient, independent of any team conference, within the previous 60 days.

Physicians or other qualified health care professionals who may report evaluation and management services should report their time spent in a team conference with the patient and/or family/caregiver present using evaluation and management (E/M) codes. These introductory guidelines do not apply to services reported using E/M codes (see E/M Services Guidelines). However, the individual must be directly involved with the patient, providing face-to-face services outside of the conference visit with other physicians, and qualified health care professionals, or agencies.

Reporting participants shall document their participation in the team conference as well as their contributed information and subsequent treatment recommendations.

No more than one individual from the same specialty may report 99366-99368 at the same encounter.

Individuals should not report 99366-99368 when their participation in the medical team conference is part of a facility or organizational service contractually provided by the organization or facility.

▶The team conference starts at the beginning of the review of an individual patient and ends at the conclusion of the review. Time related to record keeping and report generation is not reported. The reporting participant shall be present for all time reported. The time reported is not limited to the time that the participant is communicating to the other team members or patient and/or family/caregiver. Time reported for medical team conferences may not be used in the determination of time for other services such as care plan oversight (99374-99380), prolonged services (99358, 99359), psychotherapy, or any E/M service. For team conferences where the patient is present for any part of the duration of the conference, nonphysician qualified health care professionals report the team conference face-to-face code 99366.◀

Rationale

The terms "physician" and "other qualified health care professional (QHP)" appear in many places in the CPT code set. In 2012, the CPT code set was updated to provide a definition of "physician or other QHP" in the introductory guidelines. The CPT 2013 code set was extensively revised to standardize the terminology and ensure neutral reporting across the code set. A small section of codes focuses on services provided by QHPs who are considered "nonphysicians" within the coding nomenclature. In some cases, the reference to "nonphysician QHP" is stated inconsistently across the code set. Revisions have been made to the CPT 2025 code set to standardize the use of "nonphysician qualified health care professional" in those areas that were misaligned.

It is important to note that the CPT code set will continue to adhere to the definition provided in the **Instructions for Use of the CPT Codebook** subsection, which defines *physician or other qualified health care professional* as follows:

A "physician or other qualified health care professional" is an individual who is qualified by education, training, licensure/regulation (when applicable), and facility privileging (when applicable) who performs a professional service within his/her scope of practice and independently reports that professional service. These professionals are distinct from "clinical staff." A clinical staff member is a person who works under the supervision of a physician or other QHP and who is allowed by law, regulation, and facility policy to perform or assist in the performance of a specified professional service but who does not individually report that professional service. Other policies may also affect who may report specific services.

Throughout the CPT code set, the use of terms such as "physician," "qualified health care professional," or "individual" is not intended to indicate that other entities may not report the service. In selected instances, specific instructions may define a service as limited to professionals or limited to other entities (eg, hospital or home health agency).

To address misaligned and inconsistent use of terminology, numerous revisions and deletions have been made throughout the CPT code set to incorporate the consistent use of "nonphysician qualified health care professional," wherever applicable:

- Revisions to guidelines in various sections, including E/M, Radiology, and Medicine, to support standardization and consistency throughout the guidelines.

- Revisions to codes 98960-98962, 98966-98968, and 98970-98972.

- Revisions to section headers in the Medicine subsection. In conjunction with these revisions, other updates to various parenthetical notes to support standardization and consistency were made as well.

In conjunction with these changes, editorial changes have been made throughout guidelines in the Medicine subsection and the guidelines for non-face-to-face nonphysician services by replacing "E/M" with "assessment and management."

Care Plan Oversight Services

Care plan oversight services are reported separately from codes for office/outpatient, hospital, home or residence (including assisted living facility, group home, custodial care facility, residential substance abuse treatment facility, rest home), nursing facility, or non-face-to-face services. The complexity and approximate time of the care plan oversight services provided within a 30-day period determine code selection. Only one individual may report services for a given period of time to reflect the sole or predominant supervisory role with a particular patient. These codes should not be reported for supervision of patients in nursing facilities or under the care of home health agencies, unless they require recurrent supervision of therapy.

The work involved in providing very low intensity or infrequent supervision services is included in the pre- and post-encounter work for home, office/outpatient and nursing facility or domiciliary visit codes.

> (For care plan oversight services provided in rest home [eg, assisted living facility] or home, see care management services codes 99437, 99491, or principal care management codes 99424, 99425, and for hospice agency, see 99377, 99378)

> ▶(Do not report 99374-99380 for time reported with 98012, 98013, 98014, 98015, 98016, 98966, 98967, 98968, 99421, 99422, 99423)◀

> (Do not report 99374-99378 during the same month with 99487, 99489)

99374 **Supervision** of a patient under care of home health agency (patient not present) in home, domiciliary or equivalent environment (eg, Alzheimer's facility) requiring complex and multidisciplinary care modalities involving regular development and/or revision of care plans by that individual, review of subsequent reports of patient status, review of related laboratory and other studies, communication (including telephone calls) for purposes of assessment or care decisions with health care professional(s), family member(s), surrogate decision maker(s) (eg, legal guardian) and/or key caregiver(s) involved in patient's care, integration of new information into the medical treatment plan and/or adjustment of medical therapy, within a calendar month; 15-29 minutes

99375   30 minutes or more

Rationale

In accordance with the deletion of codes 99441-99443 and the establishment of codes 98012-98016, the exclusionary parenthetical note preceding code 99374 has been revised to reflect these changes.

Refer to the codebook and the Rationale for codes 98012-98016 for a full discussion of these changes.

Preventive Medicine Services

The following codes are used to report the preventive medicine evaluation and management of infants, children, adolescents, and adults.

The extent and focus of the services will largely depend on the age of the patient.

If an abnormality is encountered or a preexisting problem is addressed in the process of performing this preventive medicine evaluation and management service, and if the problem or abnormality is significant enough to require additional work to perform the key components of a problem-oriented evaluation and management service, then the appropriate office/outpatient code 99202, 99203, 99204, 99205, 99211, 99212, 99213, 99214, 99215 should also be reported. Modifier 25 should be added to the office/outpatient code to indicate that a significant, separately identifiable evaluation and management service was provided on the same day as the preventive medicine service. The appropriate preventive medicine service is additionally reported.

An insignificant or trivial problem/abnormality that is encountered in the process of performing the preventive medicine evaluation and management service and which does not require additional work and the performance of the key components of a problem-oriented E/M service should not be reported.

The "comprehensive" nature of the preventive medicine services codes 99381-99397 reflects an age- and gender-appropriate history/exam and is **not** synonymous with the "comprehensive" examination required in evaluation and management codes 99202-99350.

Codes 99381-99397 include counseling/anticipatory guidance/risk factor reduction interventions which are provided at the time of the initial or periodic comprehensive preventive medicine examination. (Refer to 99401, 99402, 99403, 99404, 99411, and 99412 for reporting those counseling/anticipatory guidance/risk factor reduction interventions that are provided at an encounter separate from the preventive medicine examination.)

(For behavior change intervention, see 99406, 99407, 99408, 99409)

▶Immunization/vaccine/toxoid products, immunization administrations, ancillary studies involving laboratory, radiology, other procedures, or screening tests (eg, vision, hearing, developmental) identified with a specific CPT code are reported separately. For immunization administration and immunization risk/benefit counseling, see 90460, 90461, 90471-90474, 90480, 96380, 96381. For immunization/vaccine/toxoid products, see 90380, 90381, 90476-90759, 91304, 91318, 91319, 91320, 91321, 91322.◀

Rationale

The guidelines within the Preventive Medicine Services subsection have been revised to: (1) include the addition of existing codes for immune globulin products for respiratory syncytial virus (RSV) (90380, 90381); (2) accommodate the addition of new codes for reporting immune globulin administration for RSV (96380, 96381); (3) reflect the removal of previously deleted COVID-19 product codes (91300-91317) and administration codes (0001A-0174A); (4) add a reference to a new code for COVID-19 vaccine administration (90480); (5) add new codes for reporting COVID-19 vaccine products (91318-91322); and (6) retain the use of code 91304 for Novavax vaccine product.

In addition, the term "immunization" has been included within these guidelines to be congruent with the new terminology added to the code set that clarifies the use of immune globulins in addition to vaccines/toxoids for immunizations.

Refer to the codebook and the Rationale for codes 90380, 90381, 90480, 96380, and 96381 for a full discussion of these changes.

Counseling Risk Factor Reduction and Behavior Change Intervention

Other Preventive Medicine Services

99421   Code is out of numerical sequence. See 99412-99447

99422   Code is out of numerical sequence. See 99412-99447

99423   Code is out of numerical sequence. See 99412-99447

Non-Face-to-Face Services

Telephone Services

►(99441, 99442, 99443 have been deleted. To report, see 98008, 98009, 98010, 98011, 98012, 98013, 98014, 98015, 98016)◄

Rationale

In accordance with the establishment of codes 98008-98016, telephone service codes 99441-99443 and their associated guidelines and parenthetical notes have been deleted. A deletion parenthetical note has been added that directs users to the new codes.

Refer to the codebook and the Rationale for codes 98008-98016 for a full discussion of these changes.

Online Digital Evaluation and Management Services

Online digital evaluation and management (E/M) services (99421, 99422, 99423) are patient-initiated services with physicians or other qualified health care professionals (QHPs). Online digital E/M services require physician or other QHP's evaluation, assessment, and management of the patient. These services are not for the nonevaluative electronic communication of test results, scheduling of appointments, or other communication that does not include E/M. While the patient's problem may be new to the physician or other QHP, the patient is an established patient. Patients initiate these services through Health Insurance Portability and Accountability Act (HIPAA)-compliant secure platforms, such as electronic health record (EHR) portals, secure email, or other digital applications, which allow digital communication with the physician or other QHP.

Online digital E/M services are reported once for the physician's or other QHP's cumulative time devoted to the service during a seven-day period. The seven-day period begins with the physician's or other QHP's initial, personal review of the patient-generated inquiry. Physician's or other QHP's cumulative service time includes review of the initial inquiry, review of patient records or data pertinent to assessment of the patient's problem, personal physician or other QHP interaction with clinical staff focused on the patient's problem, development of management plans, including physician- or other QHP generation of prescriptions or ordering of tests, and subsequent communication with the patient through online, telephone, email, or other digitally supported communication, which does not otherwise represent a separately reported E/M service. All professional decision making, assessment, and subsequent management by physicians or other QHPs in the same group practice contribute to the cumulative service time of the patient's online digital E/M service. Online digital E/M services require permanent documentation storage (electronic or hard copy) of the encounter.

►If within seven days of the initiation of an online digital E/M service, a separately reported E/M visit occurs, then the physician or other QHP work devoted to the online digital E/M service is incorporated into the separately reported E/M visit. This includes E/M services that are provided through synchronous telemedicine visits using interactive audio and video telecommunication equipment. To report synchronous audio-video E/M services, see 98000, 98001, 98002, 98003, 98004, 98005, 98006, 98007. To report synchronous audio-only E/M services, see 98008, 98009, 98010, 98011, 98012, 98013, 98014, 98015, 98016.◄

If the patient initiates an online digital inquiry for the same or a related problem within seven days of a previous E/M service, then the online digital visit is not reported. If the online digital inquiry is related to a surgical procedure and occurs during the postoperative period of a previously completed procedure, then the online digital E/M service is not reported separately.

If the patient generates the initial online digital inquiry for a new problem within seven days of a previous E/M visit that addressed a different problem, then the online digital E/M service may be reported separately.

If the patient presents a new, unrelated problem during the seven-day period of an online digital E/M service, then the physician's or other QHP's time spent on evaluation, assessment, and management of the additional problem is added to the cumulative service time of the online digital E/M service for that seven-day period.

▶(For online digital assessment and management services provided by a nonphysician qualified health care professional who may not report E/M services, see 98970, 98971, 98972)◀

 # 99421   **Online digital evaluation and management service,** for an established patient, for up to 7 days, cumulative time during the 7 days; 5-10 minutes

Rationale

In support of the establishment of codes 98000-98016, the Online Digital Evaluation and Management Services subsection guidelines have been revised to reflect these changes. Refer to the codebook and the Rationale for codes 98000-98016 for a full discussion of these changes.

In addition, in accordance with efforts to standardize the phrase "nonphysician qualified health care professional" throughout the CPT 2025 code set, the guidelines preceding code 99421 have been revised. Refer to the codebook and the Rationale for the Medical Team Conferences subsection guidelines in the E/M section for a full discussion of these changes.

Interprofessional Telephone/ Internet/Electronic Health Record Consultations

The consultant should use codes 99446, 99447, 99448, 99449, 99451 to report interprofessional telephone/ Internet/electronic health record consultations. An interprofessional telephone/Internet/electronic health record consultation is an assessment and management service in which a patient's treating (eg, attending or primary) physician or other qualified health care professional requests the opinion and/or treatment advice of a physician or other qualified health care professional with specific specialty expertise (the consultant) to assist the treating physician or other qualified health care professional in the diagnosis and/or management of the patient's problem without patient face-to-face contact with the consultant.

The patient for whom the interprofessional telephone/ Internet/electronic health record consultation is requested may be either a new patient to the consultant or an established patient with a new problem or an exacerbation of an existing problem. However, the consultant should not have seen the patient in a face-to-face encounter within the last 14 days. When the telephone/Internet/ electronic health record consultation leads to a transfer of care or other face-to-face service (eg, a surgery, a hospital visit, or a scheduled office evaluation of the patient) within the next 14 days or next available appointment date of the consultant, these codes are not reported.

Review of pertinent medical records, laboratory studies, imaging studies, medication profile, pathology specimens, etc is included in the telephone/Internet/electronic health record consultation service and should not be reported separately when reporting 99446, 99447, 99448, 99449, 99451. The majority of the service time reported (greater than 50%) must be devoted to the medical consultative verbal or Internet discussion. If greater than 50% of the time for the service is devoted to data review and/or analysis, 99446, 99447, 99448, 99449 should not be reported. However, the service time for 99451 is based on total review and interprofessional-communication time.

If more than one telephone/Internet/electronic health record contact(s) is required to complete the consultation request (eg, discussion of test results), the entirety of the service and the cumulative discussion and information review time should be reported with a single code. Codes 99446, 99447, 99448, 99449, 99451 should not be reported more than once within a seven-day interval.

The written or verbal request for telephone/Internet/ electronic health record advice by the treating/requesting physician or other qualified health care professional should be documented in the patient's medical record, including the reason for the request. Codes 99446, 99447, 99448, 99449 conclude with a verbal opinion report and written report from the consultant to the treating/requesting physician or other qualified health care professional. Code 99451 concludes with only a written report.

▶Telephone/Internet/electronic health record consultations of less than five minutes should not be reported. Consultant communications with the patient and/or family may be reported using 98012, 98013, 98014, 98015, 98016, 98966, 98967, 98968, 99421, 99422, 99423, and the time related to these services is not used in reporting 99446, 99447, 99448, 99449. Do not report 99358, 99359 for any time within the service period, if reporting 99446, 99447, 99448, 99449, 99451.◀

When the sole purpose of the telephone/Internet/electronic health record communication is to arrange a transfer of care or other face-to-face service, these codes are not reported.

The treating/requesting physician or other qualified health care professional may report 99452, if spending 16-30 minutes in a service day preparing for the referral and/or communicating with the consultant. Do not report 99452 more than once in a 14-day period. If the telephone/Internet/electronic health record referral service(s) and an E/M service are performed on the same day by the treating/requesting physician or other qualified health care professional and total time is used to select the level of E/M service, the time spent providing the referral service is added to the time spent on the day of the encounter performing the E/M service. If MDM is used to select the level of E/M service, the work of performing the referral service is considered part of the MDM. Do not report 99452 separately on the same date an E/M service is reported.

▶(For telephone services provided by a physician or other qualified health care professional to a patient, see 98008, 98009, 98010, 98011, 98012, 98013, 98014, 98015, 98016)◀

▶(For telephone services provided by a nonphysician qualified health care professional who may not report evaluation and management services, see 98966, 98967, 98968)◀

(For online digital E/M services provided by a physician or other qualified health care professional to a patient, see 99421, 99422, 99423)

Rationale

In accordance with the deletion of codes 99441-99443 and the establishment of codes 98008-98016, the Interprofessional Telephone/Internet/Electronic Health Record Consultations subsection guidelines and the cross-reference parenthetical note for telephone services provided by a physician or other QHP to a patient have been revised to reflect these changes.

In addition, in accordance with efforts to standardize the term "nonphysician qualified health care professional" throughout the CPT 2025 code set, a parenthetical note within the Interprofessional Telephone/Internet/Electronic Health Record Consultations subsection has also been revised.

Refer to the codebook and the Rationale for the Medical Team Conferences subsection guidelines in the E/M section and the Rationale for codes 98008-98016 for a full discussion of these changes.

Care Management Services

Chronic Care Management Services

 # 99490 **Chronic care management services** with the following required elements:

- multiple (two or more) chronic conditions expected to last at least 12 months, or until the death of the patient,
- chronic conditions that place the patient at significant risk of death, acute exacerbation/decompensation, or functional decline,
- comprehensive care plan established, implemented, revised, or monitored;

first 20 minutes of clinical staff time directed by a physician or other qualified health care professional, per calendar month.

#+ 99439 each additional 20 minutes of clinical staff time directed by a physician or other qualified health care professional, per calendar month (List separately in addition to code for primary procedure)

(Use 99439 in conjunction with 99490)

(Chronic care management services of less than 20 minutes duration in a calendar month are not reported separately)

(Chronic care management services of 60 minutes or more and requiring moderate or high complexity medical decision making may be reported using 99487, 99489)

(Do not report 99439 more than twice per calendar month)

(Do not report 99439, 99490 in the same calendar month with 90951-90970, 99374, 99375, 99377, 99378, 99379, 99380, 99424, 99425, 99426, 99427, 99437, 99487, 99489, 99491, 99605, 99606, 99607)

▶(Do not report 99439, 99490 for service time reported with 93792, 93793, 98012, 98013, 98014, 98015, 98016, 98960, 98961, 98962, 98966, 98967, 98968, 98970, 98971, 98972, 99071, 99078, 99080, 99091, 99358, 99359, 99366, 99367, 99368, 99421, 99422, 99423, 99605, 99606, 99607)◀

 # 99491 **Chronic care management services** with the following required elements:

- multiple (two or more) chronic conditions expected to last at least 12 months, or until the death of the patient,
- chronic conditions that place the patient at significant risk of death, acute exacerbation/decompensation, or functional decline,
- comprehensive care plan established, implemented, revised, or monitored;

first 30 minutes provided personally by a physician or other qualified health care professional, per calendar month.

★=Telemedicine   ◀=Audio-only   +=Add-on code   ✗=FDA approval pending   #=Resequenced code   ⊘=Modifier 51 exempt

#+ 99437   each additional 30 minutes by a physician or other qualified health care professional, per calendar month (List separately in addition to code for primary procedure)

(Use 99437 in conjunction with 99491)

(Do not report 99437 for less than 30 minutes)

(Do not report 99437, 99491 in the same calendar month with 90951-90970, 99374, 99375, 99377, 99378, 99379, 99380, 99424, 99425, 99426, 99427, 99439, 99487, 99489, 99490, 99605, 99606, 99607)

►(Do not report 99437, 99491 for service time reported with 93792, 93793, 98012, 98013, 98014, 98015, 98016, 98960, 98961, 98962, 98966, 98967, 98968, 98970, 98971, 98972, 99071, 99078, 99080, 99091, 99358, 99359, 99366, 99367, 99368, 99421, 99422, 99423, 99495, 99496, 99605, 99606, 99607)◄

Rationale

In accordance with the deletion of codes 99441-99443 and the establishment of codes 98012-98016, the exclusionary parenthetical notes following codes 99437 and 99439 have been revised to reflect these changes.

Refer to the codebook and the Rationale for codes 98012-98016 for a full discussion of these changes.

Complex Chronic Care Management Services

99487   **Complex chronic care management services** with the following required elements:

- multiple (two or more) chronic conditions expected to last at least 12 months, or until the death of the patient,
- chronic conditions that place the patient at significant risk of death, acute exacerbation/decompensation, or functional decline,
- comprehensive care plan established, implemented, revised, or monitored,
- moderate or high complexity medical decision making;

first 60 minutes of clinical staff time directed by a physician or other qualified health care professional, per calendar month.

(Complex chronic care management services of less than 60 minutes duration in a calendar month are not reported separately)

+ 99489   each additional 30 minutes of clinical staff time directed by a physician or other qualified health care professional, per calendar month (List separately in addition to code for primary procedure)

(Report 99489 in conjunction with 99487)

(Do not report 99489 for care management service of less than 30 minutes)

(Do not report 99487, 99489 during the same calendar month with 90951-90970, 99374, 99375, 99377, 99378, 99379, 99380, 99424, 99425, 99426, 99427, 99437, 99439, 99490, 99491)

►(Do not report 99487, 99489 for service time reported with 93792, 93793, 98012, 98013, 98014, 98015, 98016, 98960, 98961, 98962, 98966, 98967, 98968, 98970, 98971, 98972, 99071, 99078, 99080, 99091, 99358, 99359, 99366, 99367, 99368, 99421, 99422, 99423, 99605, 99606, 99607)◄

Rationale

In accordance with the deletion of codes 99441-99443 and the establishment of codes 98012-98016, the exclusionary parenthetical note following code 99489 has been revised to reflect these changes.

Refer to the codebook and the Rationale for codes 98012-98016 for a full discussion of these changes.

Principal Care Management Services

99424   **Principal care management services,** for a single high-risk disease, with the following required elements:

- one complex chronic condition expected to last at least 3 months, and that places the patient at significant risk of hospitalization, acute exacerbation/decompensation, functional decline, or death,
- the condition requires development, monitoring, or revision of disease-specific care plan,
- the condition requires frequent adjustments in the medication regimen and/or the management of the condition is unusually complex due to comorbidities,
- ongoing communication and care coordination between relevant practitioners furnishing care;

first 30 minutes provided personally by a physician or other qualified health care professional, per calendar month.

#+ 99425   each additional 30 minutes provided personally by a physician or other qualified health care professional, per calendar month (List separately in addition to code for primary procedure)

(Use 99425 in conjunction with 99424)

(Principal care management services of less than 30 minutes duration in a calendar month are not reported separately)

(Do not report 99424, 99425 in the same calendar month with 90951-90970, 99374, 99375, 99377, 99378, 99379, 99380, 99426, 99427, 99437, 99439, 99473, 99474, 99487, 99489, 99490, 99491)

▶(Do not report 99424, 99425 for service time reported with 93792, 93793, 98012, 98013, 98014, 98015, 98016, 98960, 98961, 98962, 98966, 98967, 98968, 98970, 98971, 98972, 99071, 99078, 99080, 99091, 99358, 99359, 99366, 99367, 99368, 99421, 99422, 99423, 99605, 99606, 99607)◄

99426   **Principal care management services,** for a single high-risk disease, with the following required elements:

- one complex chronic condition expected to last at least 3 months, and that places the patient at significant risk of hospitalization, acute exacerbation/ decompensation, functional decline, or death,

- the condition requires development, monitoring, or revision of disease-specific care plan,

- the condition requires frequent adjustments in the medication regimen and/or the management of the condition is unusually complex due to comorbidities,

- ongoing communication and care coordination between relevant practitioners furnishing care;

first 30 minutes of clinical staff time directed by physician or other qualified health care professional, per calendar month.

#+ **99427**   each additional 30 minutes of clinical staff time directed by a physician or other qualified health care professional, per calendar month (List separately in addition to code for primary procedure)

(Use 99427 in conjunction with 99426)

(Do not report 99427 more than twice per calendar month)

(Do not report 99426, 99427 in the same calendar month with 90951-90970, 99374, 99375, 99377, 99378, 99379, 99380, 99424, 99425, 99437, 99439, 99473, 99474, 99487, 99489, 99490, 99491)

▶(Do not report 99426, 99427 for service time reported with 93792, 93793, 98012, 98013, 98014, 98015, 98016, 98960, 98961, 98962, 98966, 98967, 98968, 98970, 98971, 98972, 99071, 99078, 99080, 99091, 99358, 99359, 99366, 99367, 99368, 99421, 99422, 99423, 99605, 99606, 99607)◄

Rationale

In accordance with the deletion of codes 99441-99443 and the establishment of codes 98012-98016, the exclusionary parenthetical notes following codes 99425 and 99427 have been revised to reflect these changes.

Refer to the codebook and the Rationale for codes 98012-98016 for a full discussion of these changes.

★=Telemedicine   ◀=Audio-only   ✚=Add-on code   ✗=FDA approval pending   #=Resequenced code   ⊘=Modifier 51 exempt

Anesthesia Guidelines

Anesthesia Services

▶Services rendered in the office, home, or hospital; consultation; and other medical services are listed in the **Evaluation and Management Services** section (98000-98016, 99202-99499 series) on page 15. "Special Services, Procedures and Reports" (99000-99082 series) are listed in the **Medicine** section.◀

Rationale

In accordance with the establishment of codes 98000-98016, the Anesthesia Services subsection guidelines have been revised to reflect these changes.

Refer to the codebook and the Rationale for codes 98000-98016 for a full discussion of these changes.

Notes

Surgery

Summary of Additions, Deletions, and Revisions

The summary of changes shows the actual changes that have been made to the code descriptors.

New codes appear with a bullet (●) and are indicated as "Code added." Revised codes are preceded with a triangle (▲). Within revised codes, or if a code symbol has been deleted, the deleted language and code symbol appear with a ~~strikethrough~~, while new text appears <u>underlined</u>.

The ✔ symbol is used to identify codes for vaccines that are pending FDA approval. The # symbol is used to identify codes that have been resequenced. CPT add-on codes are annotated by the ✚ symbol. The ⊘ symbol is used to identify codes that are exempt from the use of modifier 51. The ★ symbol is used to identify codes that may be used for reporting telemedicine services. The ✖ symbol is used to identify a proprietary laboratory analyses (PLA) test that has an identical descriptor as another PLA test. A PLA code that satisfies Category I code criteria and has been accepted by the CPT Editorial Panel is annotated with the ↑↓ symbol. The ◀ symbol is used to identify codes that may be used to report audio-only telemedicine services when appended by modifier 93 (**see Appendix T**).

Code	Description
●**15011**	Code added
✚●**15012**	Code added
●**15013**	Code added
✚●**15014**	Code added
●**15015**	Code added
✚●**15016**	Code added
●**15017**	Code added
✚●**15018**	Code added
~~**15819**~~	~~Cervicoplasty;~~
▲**21630**	Radical resection of sternum~~;~~
~~**21632**~~	~~Radical resection of sternum; with mediastinal lymphadenectomy~~
▲**25447**	Arthroplasty, ~~interposition,~~ intercarpal or carpometacarpal joints; <u>interposition (eg, tendon)</u>
●**25448**	Code added
~~**33471**~~	~~Valvotomy, pulmonary valve, closed heart; via pulmonary artery~~
~~**33737**~~	~~open heart, with inflow occlusion~~
~~**33813**~~	~~Obliteration of aortopulmonary septal defect; without cardiopulmonary bypass~~
▲**33814**	Obliteration of aortopulmonary septal defect<u>, with cardiopulmonary bypass</u>~~; with cardiopulmonary bypass~~
#●**38225**	Code added
#●**38226**	Code added
#●**38227**	Code added

Code	Description
#●38228	Code added
~~47802~~	~~U-tube hepaticoenterostomy~~
●49186	Code added
●49187	Code added
●49188	Code added
●49189	Code added
●49190	Code added
~~49203~~	~~Excision or destruction, open, intra-abdominal tumors, cysts or endometriomas, 1 or more peritoneal, mesenteric, or retroperitoneal primary or secondary tumors; largest tumor 5 cm diameter or less~~
~~49204~~	~~largest tumor 5.1-10.0 cm diameter~~
~~49205~~	~~largest tumor greater than 10.0 cm diameter~~
~~50135~~	~~complicated (eg, secondary operation, congenital kidney abnormality)~~
▲51020	Cystotomy or cystostomy, with fulguration and/or insertion of radioactive material~~; with fulguration and/or insertion of radioactive material~~
~~51030~~	~~Cystotomy or cystostomy; with cryosurgical destruction of intravesical lesion~~
●51721	Code added
●53865	Code added
●53866	Code added
~~54438~~	~~Replantation, penis, complete amputation including urethral repair~~
●55881	Code added
●55882	Code added
~~58957~~	~~Resection (tumor debulking) of recurrent ovarian, tubal, primary peritoneal, uterine malignancy (intra-abdominal, retroperitoneal tumors), with omentectomy, if performed~~
▲58958	Resection (tumor debulking) of recurrent ovarian, tubal, primary peritoneal, uterine malignancy (intra-abdominal, retroperitoneal tumors), with omentectomy, if performed, with pelvic lymphadenectomy and limited para-aortic lymphadenectomy~~; with pelvic lymphadenectomy and limited para-aortic lymphadenectomy~~
●60660	Code added
➕●60661	Code added
●61715	Code added
#●64466	Code added
#●64467	Code added
#●64468	Code added
#●64469	Code added
#●64473	Code added
#●64474	Code added
●66683	Code added

★ = Telemedicine   ◀ = Audio-only   ➕ = Add-on code   𝑵 = FDA approval pending   # = Resequenced code   ⊘ = Modifier 51 exempt

Surgery Guidelines

Services

▶Services rendered in the office, home, or hospital, consultations, and other medical services are listed in the **Evaluation and Management Services** section (98000-98016, 99202-99499) beginning on page 15. "Special Services, Procedures and Reports" (99000-99082) are listed in the **Medicine** section.◀

Rationale

In accordance with the establishment of codes 98000-98016, the Services subsection in the Surgery Guidelines has been revised to reflect these changes.

Refer to the codebook and the Rationale for codes 98000-98016 for a full discussion of these changes.

Surgery

Integumentary System

Repair (Closure)

Skin Replacement Surgery

▶Skin replacement surgery consists of ***surgical preparation*** and topical placement of an ***autograft*** (including tissue cultured autograft and skin cell suspension autograft [SCSA]) or ***skin substitute graft*** (ie, homograft, allograft, xenograft). The graft is anchored using the individual's choice of fixation. When services are performed in the office, routine dressing supplies are not reported separately.◀

The following definition should be applied to those codes that reference "100 sq cm or 1% of body area of infants and children" when determining the involvement of body size: The measurement of 100 sq cm is applicable to adults and children 10 years of age and older; and percentages of body surface area apply to infants and children younger than 10 years of age. The measurements apply to the size of the recipient area.

Procedures involving wrist and/or ankle are reported with codes that include arm or leg in the descriptor.

When a primary procedure requires a skin substitute or skin autograft for definitive skin closure (eg, orbitectomy, radical mastectomy, deep tumor removal), use 15100-15278 in conjunction with primary procedure.

For biological implant for soft tissue reinforcement, use 15777 in conjunction with primary procedure.

The supply of skin substitute graft(s) should be reported separately in conjunction with 15271-15278.

Definitions

Surgical preparation codes 15002-15005 for skin replacement surgery describe the initial services related to preparing a clean and viable wound surface for placement of an autograft, flap, skin substitute graft or for negative pressure wound therapy. In some cases, closure may be possible using adjacent tissue transfer (14000-14061) or complex repair (13100-13153). In all cases, appreciable nonviable tissue is removed to treat a burn, traumatic wound or a necrotizing infection. The clean wound bed may also be created by incisional release of a scar contracture resulting in a surface defect from separation of tissues. The intent is to heal the wound by primary intention, or by the use of negative pressure wound therapy. Patient conditions may require the closure or application of graft, flap, or skin substitute to be delayed, but in all cases the intent is to include these treatments or

negative pressure wound therapy to heal the wound. Do not report 15002-15005 for removal of nonviable tissue/debris in a chronic wound (eg, venous or diabetic) when the wound is left to heal by secondary intention. See active wound management codes (97597, 97598) and debridement codes (11042-11047) for this service. For necrotizing soft tissue infections in specific anatomic locations, see 11004-11008.

Select the appropriate code from 15002-15005 based upon location and size of the resultant defect. For multiple wounds, sum the surface area of all wounds from all anatomic sites that are grouped together into the same code descriptor. For example, sum the surface area of all wounds on the trunk and arms. Do not sum wounds from different groupings of anatomic sites (eg, face and arms). Use 15002 or 15004, as appropriate, for excisions and incisional releases resulting in wounds up to and including 100 sq cm of surface area. Use 15003 or 15005 for each additional 100 sq cm or part thereof. For example: Surgical preparation of a 20 sq cm wound on the right hand and a 15 sq cm wound on the left hand would be reported with a single code, 15004. Surgical preparation of a 75 sq cm wound on the right thigh and a 75 sq cm wound on the left thigh would be reported with 15002 for the first 100 sq cm and 15003 for the second 50 sq cm. If all four wounds required surgical preparation on the same day, use modifier 59 with 15002, and 15004.

▶***Skin Cell Suspension Autograft (SCSA)*** involves harvesting of skin and preparing a suspension of autologous skin cells for direct spray-on application for treatment of conditions such as thermal burn wounds, traumatic avulsion (eg, degloving), surgical excision (eg, necrotizing tissue infection), or resection (eg, skin cancer).

Codes 15011, 15012 are used to report the harvest of epidermal and dermal skin (eg, 0.006-0.008 inch depth). The harvested skin may be divided into smaller portions for processing. The expansion ratio of harvested skin to prepare a SCSA is typically 1:80. For example, 25 sq cm of harvested skin will produce a quantity of skin cells sufficient to cover a defect measuring up to 2000 sq cm.

Codes 15013, 15014 are used to report the preparation of the SCSA, which requires enzymatic processing, manual mechanical disaggregation of skin cells, and filtration of the final suspension.

Codes 15013, 15014 are not reported if the harvested skin is nonmanually processed (ie, using automation).

Codes 15015, 15016, 15017, 15018 are used to report the spray-on application of the SCSA to the wound and the donor site when performed. Application of a primary dressing with choice of fixation (eg, surgical glue, sutures, staples) is included in 15015, 15016, 15017, 15018.

For surgical preparation of the recipient site prior to application of the SCSA, see 15002, 15003, 15004, 15005.

Placement of a separate additional autograft (eg, split-thickness, full-thickness autograft) prior to application of SCSA is separately reportable with 15040-15261, as appropriate.

Repair of donor site requiring skin graft or local flaps is considered a separate procedure.

Autografts/tissue cultured autografts (other than SCSA) include the harvest and/or application of an autologous skin graft. Repair of donor sites requiring skin graft or local flaps is reported separately. Removal of current graft and/or simple cleansing of the wound is included, when performed. Do not report 97602. Debridement is considered a separate procedure only when gross contamination requires prolonged cleansing, when appreciable amounts of devitalized or contaminated tissue are removed, or when debridement is carried out separately without immediate primary closure. ◄

Select the appropriate code from 15040-15261 based upon type of autograft and location and size of the defect. The measurements apply to the size of the recipient area. For multiple wounds, sum the surface area of all wounds from all anatomic sites that are grouped together into the same code descriptor. For example, sum the surface area of all wounds on the trunk and arms. Do not sum wounds from different groupings of anatomic sites (eg, face and arms).

Skin substitute grafts include non-autologous human skin (dermal or epidermal, cellular and acellular) grafts (eg, homograft, allograft), non-human skin substitute grafts (ie, xenograft), and biological products that form a sheet scaffolding for skin growth. These codes are not to be reported for application of non-graft wound dressings (eg, gel, powder, ointment, foam, liquid) or injected skin substitutes. Application of non-graft wound dressings is not separately reportable. Removal of current graft and/or simple cleansing of the wound is included, when performed. Do not report 97602. Debridement is considered a separate procedure only when gross contamination requires prolonged cleansing, when appreciable amounts of devitalized or contaminated tissue are removed, or when debridement is carried out separately without immediate primary closure.

Select the appropriate code from 15271-15278 based upon location and size of the defect. For multiple wounds, sum the surface area of all wounds from all anatomic sites that are grouped together into the same code descriptor. For example, sum the surface area of all wounds on the trunk and arms. Do not sum wounds from different groupings of anatomic sites (eg, face and arms). The supply of skin substitute graft(s) should be

reported separately in conjunction with 15271, 15272, 15273, 15274, 15275, 15276, 15277, 15278. For biologic implant for soft tissue reinforcement, use 15777 in conjunction with code for primary procedure.

Surgical Preparation

15002   Surgical preparation or creation of recipient site by excision of open wounds, burn eschar, or scar (including subcutaneous tissues), or incisional release of scar contracture, trunk, arms, legs; first 100 sq cm or 1% of body area of infants and children

(For linear scar revision, see 13100-13153)

+ 15003   each additional 100 sq cm, or part thereof, or each additional 1% of body area of infants and children (List separately in addition to code for primary procedure)

(Use 15003 in conjunction with 15002)

15004   Surgical preparation or creation of recipient site by excision of open wounds, burn eschar, or scar (including subcutaneous tissues), or incisional release of scar contracture, face, scalp, eyelids, mouth, neck, ears, orbits, genitalia, hands, feet and/or multiple digits; first 100 sq cm or 1% of body area of infants and children

+ 15005   each additional 100 sq cm, or part thereof, or each additional 1% of body area of infants and children (List separately in addition to code for primary procedure)

► *Skin Cell Suspension Autograft* ◄

● **15011**   Harvest of skin for skin cell suspension autograft; first 25 sq cm or less

+● **15012**   each additional 25 sq cm or part thereof (List separately in addition to code for primary procedure)

►(Use 15012 in conjunction with 15011)◄

● **15013**   Preparation of skin cell suspension autograft, requiring enzymatic processing, manual mechanical disaggregation of skin cells, and filtration; first 25 sq cm or less of harvested skin

+● **15014**   each additional 25 sq cm of harvested skin or part thereof (List separately in addition to code for primary procedure)

►(Use 15014 in conjunction with 15013)◄

● **15015**   Application of skin cell suspension autograft to wound and donor sites, including application of primary dressing, trunk, arms, legs; first 480 sq cm or less

+● **15016**   each additional 480 sq cm or part thereof (List separately in addition to code for primary procedure)

►(Use 15016 in conjunction with 15015)◄

● **15017** Application of skin cell suspension autograft to wound and donor sites, including application of primary dressing, face, scalp, eyelids, mouth, neck, ears, orbits, genitalia, hands, feet, and/or multiple digits; first 480 sq cm or less

✚● **15018** each additional 480 sq cm or part thereof (List separately in addition to code for primary procedure)

▶(Use 15018 in conjunction with 15017)◀

Rationale

A new subsection of codes (15011-15018) has been added to the Skin Replacement Surgery subsection to report skin cell suspension autograft (SCSA) procedures. The Skin Replacement Surgery guidelines have been revised by adding a definition for SCSA and instructions for the appropriate reporting of codes 15011-15018.

Before 2025, the Skin Replacement Surgery subsection included codes for autografts and tissue cultured autografts (15040-15261) that describe the harvest and/or application of an autologous skin graft and codes for skin substitute grafts (15271-15278) that describe non-autologous human skin grafts, nonhuman skin substitute grafts, and biological products, which form a sheet of scaffolding for skin growth. The work involved in SCSA procedures was not accurately described in the existing codes for autografts, tissue cultured autografts, or skin substitute grafts. SCSA is an autograft of autologous skin cells that is applied as a direct spray-on application. New codes have been established to report the skin harvesting, autograft preparation, and application of SCSA.

Codes 15011 and 15012 describe the harvesting of epidermal and dermal skin for use in an autograft. Code 15011 is reported for the first 25 sq cm or less of skin, and add-on code 15012 is reported with code 15011 for each additional 25 sq cm of skin or part thereof. Codes 15013 and 15014 describe the preparation of SCSA. It is important to note that SCSA preparation requires enzymatic processing, manual mechanical disaggregation of skin cells, and filtration. If harvested skin is processed using automation rather than a manual process as described here, then it would not be appropriate to report codes 15013 and 15014 for the autograft preparation. Code 15013 is reported for the first 25 sq cm or less of harvested skin, and add-on code 15014 is reported with 15013 for each additional 25 sq cm or part thereof of harvested skin.

Codes 15015-15018 describe the spray-on application of the SCSA to the wound and donor sites. Application of the primary dressing with fixation (eg, surgical glue, sutures, staples) is included in codes 15015-15018 and not reported separately. Codes 15015 and 15016 are reported

for the treatment of the trunk, arms, or legs. Code 15015 is reported for the first 480 sq cm or less of wound and donor sites, and add-on code 15016 is reported with 15015 for each additional 480 sq cm of wound and donor sites or part thereof. Codes 15017 and 15018 are reported for the treatment of the face, scalp, eyelids, mouth, neck, ears, orbits, genitalia, hands, feet, and/or multiple digits. Code 15017 is reported for the first 480 sq cm or less of wound and donor sites, and add-on code 15018 is reported with code 15015 for each additional 480 sq cm of wound and donor sites or part thereof.

The Skin Replacement Surgery subsection guidelines have been revised with definitions and instructions regarding SCSA procedures. The new instructions state that surgical preparation of the recipient site prior to the application of the SCSA, placement of a separate additional autograft prior to the application of the SCSA, and repair of a donor site requiring a skin graft or local flaps are separately reported.

Clinical Example (15011)

A 35-year-old male sustained partial-thickness thermal burns measuring 1800 sq cm on his trunk and arms. A very thin (0.006 to 0.008 in thick) 24 sq cm epidermal/dermal skin graft is harvested.

Description of Procedure (15011)

Measure and sum the components of the wound. The surgeon computes the required donor-site size needed to prepare a meshed, split-thickness autograft (reported separately). Using a complex series of calculations, the surgeon computes the required donor-site size and total volume of the skin cell suspension autograft (SCSA) and selects the donor site. Prepare and tumesce the donor site with serial infiltration of crystalloid solution to ensure even harvest of the thin and delicate donor skin graft. Position the patient to ensure that the donor area is taut. The physician uses a dermatome to harvest a split-thickness graft (0.010 to 0.015 in deep) from a healthy portion of skin (reported separately). For the SCSA procedures, the physician uses a dermatome to harvest a separate, very thin skin graft (0.006 to 0.008 in deep) from the donor site, taking the epidermis along with a thin dermal layer.

Clinical Example (15012)

At the time of the skin cell suspension autograft (SCSA) procedure, a 35-year-old male sustained partial-thickness thermal burns measuring 3600 sq cm on his trunk and arms. An additional, very thin (0.006 to 0.008 in thick) 24 sq cm epidermal/dermal skin graft is harvested. [**Note:** This is an add-on code. Only consider the additional work related to the harvesting of skin for SCSA.]

Description of Procedure (15012)

The physician uses a dermatome to harvest a split-thickness graft (0.010 to 0.015 in thick) from a healthy portion of skin (reported separately). For the SCSA procedures, the physician uses a dermatome to harvest a very thin skin graft (0.006 to 0.008 in deep) from the donor site, taking the epidermis along with a thin dermal layer.

Clinical Example (15013)

A 35-year-old male sustained partial-thickness thermal burns measuring 1800 sq cm on his trunk and arms. Four 2 x 3-cm strips of very thin (0.006 to 0.008 in thick) epidermal/dermal skin graft undergo enzymatic processing, manual mechanical disaggregation of skin cells, and filtration to produce a skin cell suspension.

Description of Procedure (15013)

Separate the skin cell suspension autograft (SCSA)-harvested skin into sections measuring 2 x 3 cm. The number of sections needed depends on the size of the area to be treated. Place one or two sections of the SCSA-harvested skin in the SCSA device, where the sections are enzymatically incubated for 15 to 20 minutes each. Following incubation, the physician removes the treated skin and mechanically disaggregates a small portion of the skin on the scraping tray to confirm that the enzyme has broken down the skin and the cells can be easily separated. If the skin cells do not separate easily, return the skin to the enzyme for 10 minutes, and then reassess the tissue. After confirming that the cells separate easily, rinse the tissue with a buffer solution. Then place the tissue dermal side down on the mechanical scraping tray. The physician then vigorously scrapes the epidermal cells while altering the orientation of the skin to ensure complete disaggregation. Carefully rinse the scraping tray with buffer to capture all fully disaggregated skin cells into one area for collection. Then the surgeon carefully draws up the SCSA from the tray into a separate syringe. Dispense and filter the SCSA through the cell strainer.

Clinical Example (15014)

At the time of the skin cell suspension autograft (SCSA) procedure, a 35-year-old male sustained partial-thickness thermal burns measuring 3600 sq cm on his trunk and arms. Four 2 x 3-cm strips of very thin (0.006 to 0.008 in thick) epidermal/dermal skin graft undergo enzymatic processing, manual mechanical disaggregation of skin cells, and filtration to produce a skin cell suspension. [**Note:** This is an add-on code. Only consider the additional work related to the preparation of SCSA.]

Description of Procedure (15014)

The SCSA-harvested skin is separated into sections measuring 2 x 3 cm. The number of sections needed depends on the size of the area to be treated. Place one or two sections of the SCSA-harvested skin in the SCSA device, where the sections are enzymatically incubated for 15 to 20 minutes each. Following incubation, the physician removes the treated skin and mechanically disaggregates a small portion of the skin on the scraping tray to confirm that the enzyme has broken down the skin and the cells can be easily separated. If the skin cells do not separate easily, return the skin to the enzyme for 10 minutes, and then reassess the tissue. After confirming that the cells separate easily, rinse the tissue with a buffer solution. Then place the tissue dermal side down on the mechanical scraping tray. The physician then vigorously scrapes the epidermal cells while altering the orientation of the skin to ensure complete disaggregation. Carefully rinse the scraping tray with buffer to capture all fully disaggregated skin cells into one area for collection. The surgeon then carefully draws up the SCSA from the tray into a separate syringe. Dispense and filter the SCSA through the cell strainer. Draw the filtered SCSA into a new syringe that is prepared for application.

Clinical Example (15015)

A 35-year-old male sustained partial-thickness thermal burns measuring 3600 sq cm on his trunk and arms. A skin cell suspension autograft (SCSA) is applied to 480 sq cm of the wound bed.

Description of Procedure (15015)

The physician applies the meshed split-thickness skin graft (STSG) [separately coded] to the first 480 sq cm of the wound bed and secures it using the surgeon's fixation of choice (eg, surgical glue, sutures, or staples). Contour the primary dressing and partially affix at the lower aspect of the wound bed without covering the wound using the surgeon's fixation of choice (eg, surgical glue, sutures, or staples). The physician then applies the SCSA, which is layered by aerosolization, over the top of the first 480 sq cm of the STSG and donor sites. Then completely secure the primary dressing over the wound bed using the surgeon's fixation of choice. Apply secondary dressings in layers over the primary dressing and cover with thick absorbent gauze and elastic bandage.

Clinical Example (15016)

At the time of the skin cell suspension autograft (SCSA) procedure, a 35-year-old male sustained partial-thickness thermal burns measuring 3600 sq cm on his trunk and arms. A SCSA is applied to an additional 480 sq cm of the wound bed. [**Note:** This is an add-on code. Only consider the additional work related to the application of SCSA to wound and donor sites.]

Description of Procedure (15016)

Following the initial layered split-thickness skin graft (STSG) [separately coded] and SCSA procedure of 480 sq cm [separately reported with base code 15015], the physician applies the meshed split-thickness skin graft to the additional 480 sq cm of the wound bed and secures it using the surgeon's fixation of choice (eg, surgical glue, sutures, or staples). Contour the primary dressing and partially affix at the lower aspect of the wound bed without covering the wound using the surgeon's fixation of choice (eg, surgical glue, sutures, or staples). The physician applies the SCSA, which is layered by aerosolization, over the top of the meshed STSG and donor sites. Then completely secure the primary dressing over the wound bed using the surgeon's fixation of choice. Apply secondary dressings in layers over the primary dressing and cover with thick absorbent gauze and elastic bandage.

Clinical Example (15017)

A 78-year-old female sustained an acute, partial-thickness thermal burn measuring 1800 sq cm on her head. A skin cell suspension autograft (SCSA) is applied to 480 sq cm of the wound bed.

Description of Procedure (15017)

The physician applies the meshed split-thickness skin graft (STSG) [separately coded] to the first 480 sq cm of the wound bed and secures it using the surgeon's fixation of choice (eg, surgical glue, sutures, or staples). Contour the primary dressing and partially affix at the lower aspect of the wound bed without covering the wound using the surgeon's fixation of choice (eg, surgical glue, sutures, or staples). The physician then applies the SCSA, which is layered by aerosolization, over the top of the first 480 sq cm of the STSG and donor sites. Then completely secure the primary dressing over the wound bed using the surgeon's fixation of choice. Apply the secondary dressings in layers over the primary dressing and cover with thick absorbent gauze and elastic bandage.

Clinical Example (15018)

A 78-year-old female sustained an acute, partial-thickness thermal burn measuring 1800 sq cm on her head at the time of the skin cell suspension autograft (SCSA) procedure. A SCSA is applied to an additional 480 sq cm of the wound bed. [**Note:** This is an add-on code. Only consider the additional work related to application of SCSA to wound and donor sites.]

Description of Procedure (15018)

Following the initial layered, split-thickness skin graft (STSG) [separately coded] and SCSA procedure of 480 sq cm [separately reported with base code 15017], the physician applies the meshed STSG to the additional 480 sq cm of the wound bed and secures it using the surgeon's fixation of choice (eg, surgical glue, sutures, or staples). Contour the primary dressing and partially affix at the lower aspect of the wound bed without covering the wound using the surgeon's fixation of choice (eg, surgical glue, sutures, or staples). The physician applies the SCSA, which is layered by aerosolization, over the top of the meshed STSG and donor sites. Then completely secure the primary dressing over the wound bed using the surgeon's fixation of choice. Apply the secondary dressings in layers over the primary dressing and cover with thick absorbent gauze and elastic bandage.

Autografts/Tissue Cultured Autograft

15040   Harvest of skin for tissue cultured skin autograft, 100 sq cm or less

Other Procedures

▶(15819 has been deleted)◄

Rationale

To ensure the CPT 2025 code set reflects current clinical practice, code 15819, *Cervicoplasty*, has been deleted due to low utilization. A parenthetical note has been added to indicate this deletion.

Breast

Mastectomy Procedures

19301   Mastectomy, partial (eg, lumpectomy, tylectomy, quadrantectomy, segmentectomy);

▶(For intraoperative assessment for abnormal [tumor] tissue, in-vivo, following partial mastectomy using computer-aided fluorescence imaging, use 19301 in conjunction with 0945T)◄

★ = Telemedicine   ◀ = Audio-only   ✚ = Add-on code   ✗ = FDA approval pending   # = Resequenced code   ⊘ = Modifier 51 exempt

Rationale

In accordance with the addition of Category III code 0945T, a parenthetical note has been added following code 19301.

Refer to the codebook and the Rationale for code 0945T for a full discussion of these changes.

19302   with axillary lymphadenectomy

(For placement of radiotherapy after loading balloon/brachytherapy catheters, see 19296-19298)

(Intraoperative placement of clip[s] is not separately reported)

(For the preparation of tumor cavity with placement of an intraoperative radiation therapy applicator concurrent with partial mastectomy, use 19294)

(For radiofrequency spectroscopy, real time, intraoperative margin assessment, at the time of partial mastectomy, with report, use 0546T)

(For 3-dimensional volumetric specimen imaging, use 0694T)

Musculoskeletal System

Neck (Soft Tissues) and Thorax

Excision

▲ **21630**   Radical resection of sternum

▶(21632 has been deleted)◀

Rationale

To ensure the CPT 2025 code set reflects current clinical practice, code 21632, *Radical resection of sternum; with mediastinal lymphadenectomy*, has been deleted due to low utilization. A parenthetical note has been added to indicate this deletion. In accordance with the deletion of code 21632, code 21630 has been revised with the removal of the semicolon because it is no longer a parent code.

Forearm and Wrist

Repair, Revision, and/or Reconstruction

25310   Tendon transplantation or transfer, flexor or extensor, forearm and/or wrist, single; each tendon

▶(Do not report 25310 in conjunction with 25447, 25448, when performed for intercarpal or carpometacarpal joint arthroplasty)◀

25312   with tendon graft(s) (includes obtaining graft), each tendon

▲ **25447**   Arthroplasty, intercarpal or carpometacarpal joints; interposition (eg, tendon)

▶(Do not report 25447 in conjunction with 25448)◀

▶(Do not report 25447 in conjunction with 25310, 26480, when performed for intercarpal or carpometacarpal joint arthroplasty)◀

(For wrist arthroplasty, use 25332)

● **25448**   suspension, including transfer or transplant of tendon, with interposition, when performed

▶(Do not report 25448 in conjunction with 25447)◀

▶(Do not report 25448 in conjunction with 25310, 26480, when performed for intercarpal or carpometacarpal joint arthroplasty)◀

Rationale

Code 25447 has been revised and code 25448 has been added to report joint arthroplasty (ie, intercarpal or carpometacarpal) procedures. In addition, several exclusionary parenthetical notes were added to instruct users on the appropriate reporting of these codes.

The American Medical Association (AMA)/Specialty Society Relative Value Scale (RVS) Update Committee (RUC) Relativity Assessment Workgroup (RAW) identified arthroplasty code 25447 as a service performed by the same physician on the same date of service as code 26480 more than 75% of the time. In response to this analysis, code 25447 has been revised and code 25448 has been established.

Code 25447 was originally created to report arthroplasty, interposition, intercarpal, or carpometacarpal joints. For the CPT 2025 code set, code 25447 has been revised by transposing the term "interposition" after the semicolon and adding the parenthetical phrase "(eg, tendon)."

Code 25448 has been established to report suspension arthroplasty, including the transfer or transplant of the tendon and the interposition of tendons when performed. As a result, interposition is not separately reported for this procedure when it is performed.

Exclusionary parenthetical notes have been added following codes 25310, 25447, 25448, and 26480 to restrict the reporting of duplicate services, such as transplantation as in code 25310 vs code 25448, or mutually exclusive services, such as the choice of arthroplasty, as in code 25447 vs arthroplasty and transfer or transplant of a tendon as in code 25448.

Clinical Example (25447)

A 72-year-old female, who has painful arthritis at the base of the thumb, undergoes excision of the trapezium with interposition of local tissue between the scaphoid and the base of the first metacarpal.

Description of Procedure (25447)

Make an incision over the base of the first metacarpal and trapezium. Perform a meticulous dissection, taking care to protect the branches of the superficial radial nerve and the crossing branch of the radial artery. Incise the capsule over the trapezium and the first carpometacarpal (CMC) joint and elevate the periosteum over the trapezium. Elevate the dissection proximally to identify and open the scaphotrapeziotrapezoid joint. Expose the trapezium via subperiosteal resection. Remove the trapezium in piecemeal fashion using osteotomes and a rongeur, taking care to protect the flexor carpi radialis (FCR). Clear the base of the first metacarpal of any osteophytes. Expose the FCR proximally through two transverse incisions in the distal forearm and split longitudinally. Transect the proximal radial slip of the FCR but leave it attached to its insertion on the second metacarpal. Pull the FCR radial slip into the distal wound, roll it up, and suture to itself. Secure the rolled FCR in the trapeziectomy void with a suture anchored in the depths of the trapeziectomy wound. Hold the first ray in an adducted position and pass a K-wire into the first metacarpal into the second metacarpal, if required. Thoroughly irrigate the wound. Repair the first CMC capsule, trapezial periosteum, and scaphotrapezial capsular flap in a vest-over-pants fashion. Close the wound in layers.

Clinical Example (25448)

A 68-year-old female, who has painful arthritis at the base of the thumb, undergoes arthroplasty with excision of the trapezium and suspension stabilization of the first metacarpal.

Description of Procedure (25448)

Make an incision over the base of the first metacarpal and trapezium. Perform a meticulous dissection, taking care to protect the branches of the superficial radial nerve and the crossing branch of the radial artery. Incise the capsule over the trapezium and the first carpometacarpal joint and elevate the periosteum over the trapezium. Extend the dissection proximally to identify and open the scaphotrapeziotrapezoid joint. Expose the trapezium via subperiosteal resection. Remove the trapezium in piecemeal fashion using osteotomes and a rongeur. Protect the flexor carpi radialis (FCR). Remove the first metacarpal base osteophytes. Create a bone tunnel in the base of the first metacarpal using

successively larger drills, followed by debridement for passage of the FCR tendon. Expose the FCR proximally through two transverse incisions in the distal forearm, and proximally transect either part or all of the tendon at the musculotendinous junction. Pull the proximally transected FCR into the distal wound. Then dissect or longitudinally split the tendon to its insertion at the base of the second metacarpal and tag the end(s) with a suture for passage. Pass a looped suture passer through the prepared drill hole in the base of the first metacarpal, and bring the FCR tendon through the hole. Align the first ray with the scaphoid and the trapezial and maintain the space height without distraction to position the tendon transfer. Tension and suture the two limbs of the FCR tendon to each other. Assess the transfer tension to ensure there is no collapse of the trapezial space and assess motion to ensure there is no impingement. Roll up and suture the remainder of the tendon to itself and then suture to the soft tissue in the depths of the wound. Close the capsule in a vest-over-pants fashion. Close the wound in layers.

Hand and Fingers

Repair, Revision, and/or Reconstruction

26480   Transfer or transplant of tendon, carpometacarpal area or dorsum of hand; without free graft, each tendon

▶(Do not report 26480 in conjunction with 25447, 25448, when performed for intercarpal or carpometacarpal joint arthroplasty)◀

26483   with free tendon graft (includes obtaining graft), each tendon

Rationale

In accordance with the revision of 25447 and establishment of code 25448, an exclusionary parenthetical note has been added following code 26480 to restrict the reporting of duplicated services.

Refer to the codebook and the Rationale for code 25448 for a full discussion of these changes.

Cardiovascular System

Heart and Pericardium

Pacemaker or Implantable Defibrillator

A pacemaker system with lead(s) includes a pulse generator containing electronics, a battery, and one or more leads. A lead consists of one or more electrodes, as well as conductor wires, insulation, and a fixation mechanism. Pulse generators are placed in a subcutaneous "pocket" created in either a subclavicular site or just above the abdominal muscles just below the ribcage. Leads may be inserted through a vein (transvenous) or they may be placed on the surface of the heart (epicardial). The epicardial location of leads requires a thoracotomy for insertion.

A single chamber pacemaker system with lead includes a pulse generator and one electrode inserted in either the atrium or ventricle. A dual chamber pacemaker system with two leads includes a pulse generator and one lead inserted in the right atrium and one lead inserted in the right ventricle. In certain circumstances, an additional lead may be required to achieve pacing of the left ventricle (bi-ventricular pacing). In this event, transvenous (cardiac vein) placement of the lead should be separately reported using code 33224 or 33225. For body surface–activation mapping to optimize electrical synchrony of a biventricular pacing or biventricular pacing-defibrillator system at the time of implant, also report 0695T with the appropriate code (ie, 33224, 33225, 33226). Epicardial placement of the lead should be separately reported using 33202, 33203.

A leadless cardiac pacemaker system includes a pulse generator with built-in battery and electrode for implantation in a cardiac chamber via a transvenous transcatheter approach. For implantation of a right ventricular leadless pacemaker system, use 33274. Insertion, replacement, or removal of a right ventricular leadless pacemaker system includes insertion of a catheter via transvenous access under fluoroscopic guidance into the right ventricle. For a complete dual-chamber leadless cardiac pacemaker system which is implanted in both the right ventricle and right atrium, or individual components of a dual-chamber leadless pacemaker system, see 0795T, 0796T, 0797T, 0798T, 0799T, 0800T, 0801T, 0802T, 0803T. Device evaluation at the time of leadless pacemaker insertion, replacement, or removal is included in 33274, 33275, 0795T, 0796T, 0797T, 0798T, 0799T, 0800T, 0801T, 0802T, 0803T, 0823T, 0824T, 0825T and is not separately reported. For subsequent leadless pacemaker device evaluation, see 93279, 93286, 93288, 93294, 93296, 0804T, 0826T.

For a single-chamber leadless cardiac pacemaker implanted in the right atrium that is not a component of a dual-chamber leadless pacemaker system, see 0823T, 0824T, 0825T.

Right heart catheterization (93451, 93453, 93456, 93457, 93460, 93461, 93593, 93594, 93596, 93597) may not be reported in conjunction with leadless pacemaker insertion and removal codes 33274, 33275, 0795T, 0796T, 0797T, 0798T, 0799T, 0800T, 0801T, 0802T, 0803T, 0823T, 0824T, 0825T, unless complete right heart catheterization is performed for an indication distinct from the leadless pacemaker procedure.

Like a pacemaker system, an implantable defibrillator system includes a pulse generator and electrodes. Three general categories of implantable defibrillators exist: transvenous implantable pacing cardioverter-defibrillator (ICD), subcutaneous implantable defibrillator (S-ICD), and substernal implantable cardioverter-defibrillator. Implantable pacing cardioverter-defibrillator devices use a combination of antitachycardia pacing, low-energy cardioversion or defibrillating shocks to treat ventricular tachycardia or ventricular fibrillation. The subcutaneous implantable defibrillator uses a single subcutaneous electrode to treat ventricular tachyarrhythmias. The substernal implantable cardioverter-defibrillator uses at least one substernal electrode to perform defibrillation, cardioversion, and antitachycardia pacing. Subcutaneous implantable defibrillators differ from transvenous implantable pacing cardioverter-defibrillators in that subcutaneous defibrillators do not provide antitachycardia pacing or chronic pacing. Substernal implantable defibrillators differ from both subcutaneous and transvenous implantable pacing cardioverter-defibrillators in that they provide antitachycardia pacing, but not chronic pacing.

Implantable defibrillator pulse generators may be implanted in a subcutaneous infraclavicular, axillary, or abdominal pocket. Removal of an implantable defibrillator pulse generator requires opening of the existing subcutaneous pocket and disconnection of the pulse generator from its electrode(s). A thoracotomy (or laparotomy in the case of abdominally placed pulse generators) is not required to remove the pulse generator.

The electrodes (leads) of an implantable defibrillator system may be positioned within the atrial and/or ventricular chambers of the heart via the venous system (transvenously), or placed on the surface of the heart (epicardial), or positioned under the skin overlying the heart (subcutaneous). Electrode positioning on the epicardial surface of the heart requires a thoracotomy or thoracoscopic placement of the leads. Epicardial placement of electrode(s) may be separately reported using 33202, 33203. The electrode (lead) of a subcutaneous implantable defibrillator system is tunneled under the skin to the left parasternal margin. Subcutaneous placement of electrode may be reported using 33270 or 33271. The electrode (lead) of a substernal implantable defibrillator system is tunneled subcutaneously and placed into the substernal anterior mediastinum without entering the pericardial cavity and may be reported using 0571T, 0572T. In certain circumstances, an additional electrode may be required to achieve pacing of the left ventricle (bi-ventricular pacing). In this event, transvenous (cardiac vein) placement of the electrode may be separately reported using 33224 or 33225.

Removal of a transvenous electrode(s) may first be attempted by transvenous extraction (33234, 33235, or 33244). However, if transvenous extraction is unsuccessful, a thoracotomy may be required to remove the electrodes (33238 or 33243). Use 33212, 33213, 33221, 33230, 33231, 33240 as appropriate, in addition to the thoracotomy or endoscopic epicardial lead placement codes (33202 or 33203) to report the insertion of the generator if done by the same physician during the same session. Removal of a subcutaneous implantable defibrillator electrode may be separately reported using 33272. For removal of a leadless pacemaker system without replacement, use 33275. For removal and replacement of a leadless pacemaker system during the same session, use 33274.

▶When the "battery" of a pacemaker system with lead(s) or implantable defibrillator is changed, it is actually the pulse generator that is changed. Removal of only the pacemaker or implantable defibrillator pulse generator is reported with 33233 or 33241. If only a pulse generator is inserted or replaced without any right atrial and/or right ventricular lead(s) inserted or replaced, report the appropriate code for only pulse generator insertion or replacement based on the number of final existing lead(s) (33227, 33228, 33229 and 33262, 33263, 33264). Do not report removal of a pulse generator (33233 or 33241) separately for this service. Insertion of a new pulse generator, when existing lead(s) are already in place and when no prior pulse generator is removed, is reported with 33212, 33213, 33221, 33230, 33231, 33240. When a pulse generator insertion involves the insertion or replacement of one or more right atrial and/or right ventricular lead(s) or subcutaneous lead(s), use system codes 33206, 33207, 33208 for pacemaker, 33249 for implantable pacing cardioverter-defibrillator, or 33270 for subcutaneous implantable defibrillator. When reporting the system insertion or replacement codes, removal of a pulse generator (33233 or 33241) may be reported separately, when performed. In addition, extraction of leads 33234, 33235 or 33244 for transvenous or 33272 for subcutaneous may be reported separately, when performed. An exception involves a pacemaker upgrade from single to dual system that includes removal of pulse generator, replacement of new

pulse generator, and insertion of new lead, reported with 33214. For insertion, removal, relocation, and repositioning of cardiac contractility modulation-defibrillation codes, see 0915T-0925T.◀

Revision of a skin pocket is included in 33206-33249, 33262, 33263, 33264, 33270, 33271, 33272, 33273. When revision of a skin pocket involves incision and drainage of a hematoma or complex wound infection, see 10140, 10180, 11042, 11043, 11044, 11045, 11046, 11047, as appropriate.

Relocation of a skin pocket for a pacemaker (33222) or implantable defibrillator (33223) is necessary for various clinical situations such as infection or erosion. Relocation of an existing pulse generator may be performed as a stand-alone procedure or at the time of a pulse generator or electrode insertion, replacement, or repositioning. When skin pocket relocation is performed as part of an explant of an existing generator followed by replacement with a new generator, the pocket relocation is reported separately. Skin pocket relocation includes all work associated with the initial pocket (eg, opening the pocket, incision and drainage of hematoma or abscess if performed, and any closure performed), in addition to the creation of a new pocket for the new generator to be placed.

Repositioning of a pacemaker electrode, implantable defibrillator electrode(s), or a left ventricular pacing electrode is reported using 33215, 33226, or 33273, as appropriate.

Device evaluation codes 93260, 93261, 93279-93298 for pacemaker system with lead(s) may not be reported in conjunction with pulse generator and lead insertion or revision codes 33206-33249, 33262, 33263, 33264, 33270, 33271, 33272, 33273. For leadless pacemaker systems, device evaluation codes 93279, 93286, 93288, 93294, 93296 may not be reported in conjunction with leadless pacemaker insertion and removal codes 33274, 33275. Defibrillator threshold testing (DFT) during transvenous implantable defibrillator insertion or replacement may be separately reported using 93640, 93641. DFT testing during subcutaneous implantable defibrillator system insertion is not separately reportable. DFT testing for transvenous or subcutaneous implantable defibrillator in follow-up or at the time of replacement may be separately reported using 93642 or 93644.

Radiological supervision and interpretation related to the pacemaker or implantable defibrillator procedure is included in 33206-33249, 33262, 33263, 33264, 33270, 33271, 33272, 33273, 33274, 33275. Fluoroscopy (76000, 77002), ultrasound guidance for vascular access (76937), right ventriculography (93566), and femoral venography (75820) are included in 33274, 33275, when performed). To report fluoroscopic guidance for diagnostic lead evaluation without lead insertion, replacement, or revision procedures, use 76000.

Surgery / Cardiovascular System 33016-39599

Rationale

The introductory guidelines in the Pacemaker or Implantable Defibrillator subsection of the Heart and Pericardium section have been revised to accommodate new Category III codes 0915T-0925T to report inserting, removing, relocating, and repositioning of a cardiac contractility modulation-defibrillation system.

Refer to the codebook and the Rationale for codes 0915T-0931T for a full discussion of these changes.

Electrophysiologic Operative Procedures

Incision

+ 33258   Operative tissue ablation and reconstruction of atria, performed at the time of other cardiac procedure(s), extensive (eg, maze procedure), without cardiopulmonary bypass (List separately in addition to code for primary procedure)

▶(Use 33258 in conjunction with 33130, 33250, 33300, 33310, 33320, 33321, 33330, 33365, 33420, 33501-33503, 33510-33516, 33533-33536, 33690, 33735, 33750, 33755, 33762, 33764, 33766, 33800-33803, 33820, 33822, 33824, 33840, 33845, 33851, 33852, 33875, 33877, 33915, 33925, 33981, 33982, when the procedure is performed without cardiopulmonary bypass)◀

Rationale

In accordance with the deletion of codes 33471, 33737, and 33813, the inclusionary parenthetical note following code 33258 has been revised to reflect these changes.

Refer to the codebook and the Rationale for codes 33471, 33737, and 33813 for a full discussion of these changes.

Implantable Hemodynamic Monitors

33289   Transcatheter implantation of wireless pulmonary artery pressure sensor for long-term hemodynamic monitoring, including deployment and calibration of the sensor, right heart catheterization, selective pulmonary catheterization, radiological supervision and interpretation, and pulmonary artery angiography, when performed

(Do not report 33289 in conjunction with 36013, 36014, 36015, 75741, 75743, 75746, 76000, 93451, 93453, 93456, 93457, 93460, 93461, 93568, 93569, 93573, 93593, 93594, 93596, 93597, 93598)

(For remote monitoring of an implantable wireless pulmonary artery pressure sensor, use 93264)

▶(For implantation of a wireless left atrial pressure sensor, use 0933T)◀

Rationale

To accommodate the addition of Category III code 0933T, a parenthetical note following code 33289 has been added.

Refer to the codebook and the Rationale for codes 0933T and 0934T for a full discussion of these changes.

Cardiac Valves

Pulmonary Valve

When cardiopulmonary bypass is performed in conjunction with TPVI, code 33477 may be reported with the appropriate add-on code for percutaneous peripheral bypass (33367), open peripheral bypass (33368), or central bypass (33369).

▶(33471 has been deleted)◀

Rationale

To ensure the CPT 2025 code set reflects current clinical practice, code 33471, *Valvotomy, pulmonary valve, closed heart, via pulmonary artery*, has been deleted due to low utilization. A parenthetical note has been added to indicate this deletion.

33474   Valvotomy, pulmonary valve, open heart, with cardiopulmonary bypass

Shunting Procedures

33735   Atrial septectomy or septostomy; closed heart (Blalock-Hanlon type operation)

33736   open heart with cardiopulmonary bypass

(Do not report modifier 63 in conjunction with 33735, 33736)

▶(33737 has been deleted)◀

Rationale

To ensure the CPT 2025 code set reflects current clinical practice, code 33737, *Atrial septectomy or septostomy; open heart, with inflow occlusion*, has been deleted due to low utilization. A parenthetical note has been added to indicate this deletion.

Aortic Anomalies

33802 Division of aberrant vessel (vascular ring);

33803   with reanastomosis

▶(33813 has been deleted)◀

▲ **33814** Obliteration of aortopulmonary septal defect, with cardiopulmonary bypass

---

Rationale

To ensure the CPT 2025 code set reflects current clinical practice, code 33813, *Obliteration of aortopulmonary septal defect; without cardiopulmonary bypass*, has been deleted due to low utilization. A parenthetical note has been added to indicate this deletion. In accordance with the deletion of code 33813, code 33814 has been revised because it is no longer a child code to code 33813.

Endovascular Repair of Congenital Heart and Vascular Defects

Codes 33894, 33895, 33897 describe transcatheter interventions for revascularization or repair for coarctation of the aorta. Code 33897 describes dilation of the coarctation using balloon angioplasty without stent placement. Codes 33894, 33895 describe stent placement to treat the coarctation. The procedure described in 33894 involves stent placement across one or more major side branches of the aorta. For reporting purposes, the major side branches of the thoracic aorta are the brachiocephalic, carotid, and subclavian arteries, and the major side branches of the abdominal aorta are the celiac, superior mesenteric, inferior mesenteric, and renal arteries.

Codes 33894, 33895, 33897 include all fluoroscopic guidance of the intervention, diagnostic congenital left heart catheterization, all catheter and wire introductions and manipulation, and angiography of the target lesion.

Codes 33894, 33895 include stent introduction, manipulation, positioning, and deployment, temporary pacemaker insertion for rapid pacing (33210) to facilitate stent positioning, when performed, as well as any additional stent delivery in tandem with the initial stent for extension purposes. Balloon angioplasty within the target-treatment zone, either before or after stent deployment, is not separately reportable. For balloon angioplasty of an additional coarctation of the aorta in a segment separate from the treatment zone for the coarctation stent, use 33897.

▶For balloon angioplasty or stenting of the aorta for lesions other than coarctation (eg, atherosclerosis) of the aorta in a segment separate from the coarctation treatment zone, see 37236, 37246.◀

For additional diagnostic right heart catheterization in the same setting as 33894, 33895, see 93593, 93594.

Other interventional procedures performed at the time of endovascular repair of coarctation of the aorta (33894, 33895) may be reported separately (eg, innominate, carotid, subclavian, visceral, iliac, or pulmonary artery balloon angioplasty or stenting, arterial or venous embolization), when performed before or after coarctation stent deployment.

33894 Endovascular stent repair of coarctation of the ascending, transverse, or descending thoracic or abdominal aorta, involving stent placement; across major side branches

33895   not crossing major side branches

(Do not report 33894, 33895 in conjunction with 33210, 34701, 34702, 34703, 34704, 34705, 34706, 36200, 75600, 75605, 75625, 93567, 93595, 93596, 93597)

▶(Do not report 33894, 33895 in conjunction with 33897, 37236, 37246, for balloon angioplasty or stenting of the aorta within the coarctation stent treatment zone)◀

▶(For balloon angioplasty or stenting of the aorta for lesions other than coarctation [eg, atherosclerosis] of the aorta in a segment separate from the coarctation treatment zone, see 37236, 37246)◀

(For additional atrial, ventricular, pulmonary, coronary, or bypass graft angiography in the same setting, see 93563, 93564, 93565, 93566, 93568)

(For additional congenital right heart catheterization at same setting as 33894, 33895, see 93593, 93594)

(For angiography of other vascular structures, use the appropriate code from the Radiology/Diagnostic Radiology section)

33897 Percutaneous transluminal angioplasty of native or recurrent coarctation of the aorta

▶(Do not report 33897 in conjunction with 33210, 34701, 34702, 34703, 34704, 34705, 34706, 36200, 75600, 75605, 75625, 93567, 93595, 93596, 93597)◀

(Do not report 33897 in conjunction with 33894, 33895 for balloon angioplasty of the aorta within the coarctation stent treatment zone)

▶(Do not report 33897 in conjunction with 37236, 37246 for stenting or additional balloon angioplasty of the aorta within the coarctation treatment zone)◀

▶(For balloon angioplasty or stenting of the aorta for lesions other than coarctation [eg, atherosclerosis] of the aorta in a segment separate from the coarctation treatment zone, see 37236, 37246)◀

(For additional congenital right heart diagnostic catheterization performed in same setting as 33897, see 93593, 93594)

(For angioplasty and other transcatheter revascularization interventions of additional upper or lower extremity vessels in same setting, use the appropriate code from the Surgery/Cardiovascular System section)

Rationale

The guidelines for the Endovascular Repair of Congenital Heart and Vascular Defects subsection and parenthetical notes following codes 33895 and 33897 have been revised and added to restrict reporting angioplasty for the purpose of clearing a blockage in the aorta vs opening the coarctation (narrowing) of the aorta within the same zone.

A guideline and several parenthetical notes have been revised and added to clarify when it is appropriate to separately report angioplasty and coarctation services. The intent is to restrict reporting both procedures (ie, angioplasty and coarctation) when a single service is used to address both problems. The changes that have been made demonstrate an intention to restrict the reporting of two services when one service is actually being provided. They also allow reporting when services are provided in different treatment "zones." The changes include the addition of the phrase "or stenting" within the guidelines and parenthetical notes where necessary and the addition of angioplasty procedure code 37236 to the guidelines for the Endovascular Repair of Congenital Heart and Vascular Defects subsection. An exclusionary parenthetical note has been added following code 33897, which only allows reporting both codes when services are performed in different treatment zones. A cross-reference parenthetical note has been added to direct users to report code 37236 or 37246 for balloon angioplasty or stenting of the aorta for lesions other than coarctation (eg, atherosclerosis) of the aorta in a segment separate from the coarctation treatment zone.

Finally, to coincide with the other changes, codes 37236 and 37246 have been removed from the exclusionary note following code 33897 to allow the reporting of angioplasty and stenting when those procedures are performed in zones separate from the coarctation treatment zone.

Pulmonary Artery

33922   Transection of pulmonary artery with cardiopulmonary bypass

(Do not report modifier 63 in conjunction with 33922)

+ 33924   Ligation and takedown of a systemic-to-pulmonary artery shunt, performed in conjunction with a congenital heart procedure (List separately in addition to code for primary procedure)

▶(Use 33924 in conjunction with 33474, 33475, 33476, 33477, 33478, 33600-33617, 33622, 33684-33688, 33692-33697, 33735-33767, 33770-33783, 33786, 33917, 33920, 33922, 33925, 33926, 33935, 33945)◀

Rationale

In accordance with the deletion of code 33471, the inclusionary parenthetical note following code 33924 has been revised to reflect this change.

Refer to the codebook and the Rationale for code 33471 for a full discussion of this change.

Arteries and Veins

Endovascular Revascularization (Open or Percutaneous, Transcatheter)

+ 37235   with transluminal stent placement(s) and atherectomy, includes angioplasty within the same vessel, when performed (List separately in addition to code for primary procedure)

(Use 37235 in conjunction with 37231)

▶Codes 37246, 37247, 37248, 37249 describe open or percutaneous transluminal balloon angioplasty (eg, conventional, low profile, cutting, drug-coated balloon). Codes 37246, 37247 describe transluminal balloon angioplasty in an artery, excluding the central nervous system (61630, 61635), coronary (92920-92944, 0913T), pulmonary (92997, 92998), and lower extremities for occlusive disease (37220-37235). Codes 37248 and 37249 describe transluminal balloon angioplasty in a vein excluding the dialysis circuit (36902, 36905, 36907) when approached through the ipsilateral dialysis access. Transluminal balloon angioplasty is inherent to stenting in the extracranial carotid and innominate arteries (37215, 37216, 37217, 37218), peripheral arteries (37220-37237), and in peripheral veins (37238, 37239) and, therefore, is not separately reportable. Multiple angioplasties performed in a single vessel, including treatment of separate and distinct lesions within a single vessel, are reported with a single code. If a lesion extends across the margins of one vessel into another, but can be treated with a single therapy, the intervention should be reported only once. When additional, separate and distinct ipsilateral or contralateral vessels are treated in the same session, 37247 and/or 37249 may be reported as appropriate.◀

Non-selective and/or selective catheterization (eg, 36005, 36010, 36011, 36012, 36200, 36215, 36216, 36217, 36218, 36245, 36246, 36247, 36248) is reported separately. Codes 37246, 37247, 37248, 37249 include radiological supervision and interpretation directly related to the intervention performed and imaging performed to document completion of the intervention. Extensive repair or replacement of an artery may be reported separately (eg, 35226, 35286). Intravascular ultrasound may be reported separately (ie, 37252, 37253). Mechanical thrombectomy and/or thrombolytic therapy, when performed, may be reported separately (eg, 37184, 37185, 37186, 37187, 37188, 37211, 37212, 37213, 37214).

Rationale

In accordance with the establishment of Category III codes 0913T and 0914T to report percutaneous transcatheter therapeutic drug delivery by intracoronary drug-delivery balloon, the guidelines for the Endovascular Revascularization (Open or Percutaneous, Transcatheter) subsection have been revised by adding code 0913T.

Refer to the codebook and the Rationale for codes 0913T and 0914T for a full discussion of these changes.

Hemic and Lymphatic Systems

Spleen

Laparoscopy

38129   Unlisted laparoscopy procedure, spleen

General

►Cellular and Gene Therapies◄

►Cellular and gene therapies involve the collection, processing and handling of cells or other tissues, genetic modification of those cells or tissues, and administration of the genetically modified cells or tissues with the intent to treat, modify, reverse, or cure a serious or life-threatening disease or condition.

Codes 38225, 38226, 38227, 38228 describe the various steps required to collect, prepare, transport, receive, and administer genetically modified T cells. The collection and handling code (38225) may be reported only once per day, regardless of the number of collections or quantity of cells collected. Similarly, the administration code (38228) may only be reported once per day, regardless of the number of units administered. The development of genetically modified cells is not reported with this family of codes.

Chimeric antigen receptor therapy (CAR-T) with genetically modified T cells begins with the collection of cells from the patient by peripheral blood leukocyte cell

harvesting. The cells are then cryopreserved and/or otherwise prepared for processing or shipping to a manufacturing or cell-processing facility, if applicable, where gene modification and expansion of the cells are performed. When gene modification and expansion of the cells by the manufacturer are complete, the genetically modified cells are returned to the physician or other qualified health care professional when additional preparation occurs, including thawing of the cryopreserved CAR-T cells, if necessary, before the cells are administered to the patient.

The procedure to administer CAR-T cells includes physician or other qualified health care professional monitoring of multiple physiologic parameters, verification of cell processing, evaluation of the patient during, as well as immediately before and after the administration of the CAR-T cells, direct supervision of clinical staff, and management of any adverse events during the administration. Care on the same date of service that is not directly related to the service of administration of the CAR-T cells (eg, care provided after the administration is complete, care for the patient's underlying condition or other medical problems) may be separately reported using the appropriate evaluation and management code with modifier 25. Management of uncomplicated adverse events (eg, nausea, urticaria) during the infusion is not reported separately.

The fluid used to administer the cells and other infusions for incidental hydration (eg, 96360, 96361) are not reported separately. Similarly, infusion(s) of any supportive medication(s) (eg, steroids) concurrently with the CAR-T cell administration are not reported separately. However, hydration or administration of medications (eg, antibiotics, opioids) unrelated to the CAR-T administration may be reported separately with modifier 59.◄

►(For administration of drugs, agents and biologic response modifiers, see Chemotherapy and Other Highly Complex Drug or Highly Complex Biologic Agent Administration)◄

►(For transplant services/procedures, see Bone Marrow or Stem Cell Services/Procedures)◄

#● **38225**   Chimeric antigen receptor T-cell (CAR-T) therapy; harvesting of blood-derived T lymphocytes for development of genetically modified autologous CAR-T cells, per day

#● **38226**   preparation of blood-derived T lymphocytes for transportation (eg, cryopreservation, storage)

#● **38227**   receipt and preparation of CAR-T cells for administration

#● **38228**   CAR-T cell administration, autologous

★ =Telemedicine   ◀ =Audio-only   ✚ =Add-on code   ✗ =FDA approval pending   # =Resequenced code   ⊘ =Modifier 51 exempt

Rationale

The Cellular and Gene Therapy subsection, guidelines, and parenthetical notes, as well as codes 0537T-0540T, which describe chimeric antigen receptor T cell (CAR-T) therapy services, have been deleted from the Category III section and converted to Category I codes. The complete section, instructions, and codes have been added to the Hemic and Lymphatic Systems and General subsections.

The guidelines in this new subsection include a definition of cellular and gene therapies and a summary of the intent of these services (ie, treat, modify, reverse, or cure a patient of a serious or life-threatening disease or condition using CAR-T therapy). The guidelines also provide a brief review of the different stages or efforts involved in the process. This includes the work of collecting T cells from a patient and the selection and separation of the appropriate cells for the procedure (38225); all processing of the cells, such as freezing, in preparation for transport to the modification facility (38226); and the receipt and preparation services when the modified T cells return from the modification facility (38227); administration of the genetically modified cells or tissue into the patient (38228); and any treatment or service necessary to monitor the patient during the administration session, to verify cell processing, to evaluate the patient before, during, and after the administration, and any other services provided to facilitate the administration of the cells to the patient, including supervision by clinical staff as they manage and monitor the patient for adverse events during the administration of the CAR-T cells.

The guidelines include specific instructions regarding services that may or may not be reported in conjunction with CAR-T therapy. This includes when to report treatment or services (including E/M services reported with modifier 25) for both non-CAR-T and CAR-T–related conditions (eg, after the treatment is complete). The management of uncomplicated adverse events during the infusion is not reported separately. Hydration necessary for the treatment or infusion of supportive medications during the instillation of the administered cells is not reported separately. However, hydration or medication administration unrelated to CAR-T administration may be separately reported with modifier 59. The guidelines also direct users to report the collection and handling of the cells (38225) and the administration of the modified cells or tissue (38228) only once per day.

Specific language in the guidelines clarifies that genetic modification of the cells or tissue to fight the disease or condition is not included as part of the services. This is because modification of the T cells by an outside facility or laboratory is accomplished separately from the collection, processing, handling, and administration of the

T cells. Similarly, the expansion of the cells (ie, growing more cells or tissue to be used for treatment outside of the body) is not included in these codes.

Parenthetical notes that have been added to the guidelines provide cross-references to the appropriate codes to report non-CAR-T services, such as chemotherapy administration and transplant services for bone marrow or stem cells. Parenthetical notes provided within the deleted Category III subsection note the conversion of CAR-T service codes to Category I codes and direct users to these new codes.

Clinical Example (38225)

A 67-year-old male, who has refractory diffuse large B-cell lymphoma, is referred for treatment with autologous chimeric antigen receptor T cell therapy.

Description of Procedure (38225)

The physician supervises the initial collection of blood-derived T lymphocytes and patient monitoring. The physician remains immediately available throughout the duration of the procedure. The physician evaluates the patient and manages any complications that occur.

Clinical Example (38226)

A 67-year-old male, who has refractory diffuse large B-cell lymphoma, is referred for treatment with autologous chimeric antigen receptor T cell (CAR-T) therapy.

Description of Procedure (38226)

Confirm proper labeling to identify the patient, date of collection, and assessment of the risk of infectious disease transmission. Receive batch record (BR) after product collection. Confirm that post-collection cell product was appropriately collected per facility-defined requirements. Review BR to confirm it includes product characteristics, infectious disease results, verified critical calculations, and performance of good documentation practices. Confirm that the patient information and donor identification number with BR are associated with the facility-defined CAR-T–specific treatment process checklist.

Clinical Example (38227)

A 67-year-old male, who has refractory diffuse large B-cell lymphoma, is referred for treatment with autologous chimeric antigen receptor T cell (CAR-T) therapy.

Description of Procedure (38227)

Confirm that documentation of all steps of the final review on the facility-defined CAR-T-specific treatment process checklist has been completed, including the following:

- Review and confirm the infusion order of cellular therapy products and confirm that the ordered product type matches the drug information as documented on the CAR-T–specific treatment process checklist.
- Review the commercial CAR-T certification of analysis to confirm that the batch record patient identifiers match with the product information.
- Confirm infusion cell dose is within acceptable limits, as described on the drug product label and package insert.
- Confirm patient infusion weight is within facility-defined change-range from the collection weight. If necessary, confirm that the drug-infusion dose is not out of specification, given the weight change.

The physician or other qualified health care professional oversees the thawing of cryopreserved, genetically modified cells for cellular therapy. These cells must be thawed in a controlled manner to ensure viability and stored in containers to minimize the risk of product cross-contamination.

Clinical Example (38228)

A 67-year-old male, who has refractory diffuse large B-cell lymphoma, is referred for treatment with autologous chimeric antigen receptor T cell therapy.

Description of Procedure (38228)

The physician supervises the initiation of the product infusion and is present for the first 15 to 30 minutes. The physician remains immediately available to manage toxicities and complications that occur during the infusion. The physician evaluates the patient at the end of the infusion.

Bone Marrow or Stem Cell Services/ Procedures

38204 Management of recipient hematopoietic progenitor cell donor search and cell acquisition

38205 Blood-derived hematopoietic progenitor cell harvesting for transplantation, per collection; allogeneic

38206 autologous

38222 biopsy(ies) and aspiration(s)

(Do not report 38222 in conjunction with 38220 and 38221)

(For bilateral procedure, report 38220, 38221, 38222 with modifier 50)

(For bone marrow biopsy interpretation, use 88305)

38225 Code is out of numerical sequence. See 38129-38205

38226 Code is out of numerical sequence. See 38129-38205

38227 Code is out of numerical sequence. See 38129-38205

38228 Code is out of numerical sequence. See 38129-38205

38230 Bone marrow harvesting for transplantation; allogeneic

Digestive System

Esophagus

Endoscopy

Esophagoscopy

43191 Esophagoscopy, rigid, transoral; diagnostic, including collection of specimen(s) by brushing or washing when performed (separate procedure)

▶(Do not report 43191 in conjunction with 43192, 43193, 43194, 43195, 43196, 43197, 43198, 43210, 43497, 0884T)◀

(For diagnostic transnasal esophagoscopy, see 43197, 43198)

(For diagnostic flexible transoral esophagoscopy, use 43200)

43195 with balloon dilation (less than 30 mm diameter)

▶(Do not report 43195 in conjunction with 43191, 43197, 43198, 0884T)◀

(If fluoroscopic guidance is performed, use 74360)

(For esophageal dilation with balloon 30 mm diameter or larger, see 43214, 43233)

(For dilation without endoscopic visualization, see 43450, 43453)

(For flexible transoral esophagoscopy with balloon dilation [less than 30 mm diameter], use 43220)

43196 with insertion of guide wire followed by dilation over guide wire

▶(Do not report 43196 in conjunction with 43191, 43197, 43198, 0884T)◀

(If fluoroscopic guidance is performed, use 74360)

(For flexible transoral esophagoscopy with insertion of guide wire followed by dilation over guide wire, use 43226)

43200 Esophagoscopy, flexible, transoral; diagnostic, including collection of specimen(s) by brushing or washing, when performed (separate procedure)

▶(Do not report 43200 in conjunction with 43197, 43198, 43201-43232, 43497, 0884T)◀

(For diagnostic rigid transoral esophagoscopy, use 43191)

(For diagnostic flexible transnasal esophagoscopy, use 43197)

(For diagnostic flexible esophagogastroduodenoscopy, use 43235)

43220   with transendoscopic balloon dilation (less than 30 mm diameter)

▶(Do not report 43220 in conjunction with 43197, 43198, 43200, 43212, 43226, 43229, 0884T)◀

(If fluoroscopic guidance is performed, use 74360)

(For rigid transoral esophagoscopy with balloon dilation [less than 30 mm diameter], use 43195)

(For esophageal dilation with balloon 30 mm diameter or larger, use 43214)

(For dilation without endoscopic visualization, see 43450, 43453)

▶(For esophagoscopy with predilation followed by therapeutic drug delivery by drug-coated balloon catheter, use 0884T)◀

 # 43213   with dilation of esophagus, by balloon or dilator, retrograde (includes fluoroscopic guidance, when performed)

▶(Do not report 43213 in conjunction with 43197, 43198, 43200, 74360, 76000, 0884T)◀

(For transendoscopic balloon dilation of multiple strictures during the same session, report 43213 with modifier 59 for each additional stricture dilated)

 # 43214   with dilation of esophagus with balloon (30 mm diameter or larger) (includes fluoroscopic guidance, when performed)

▶(Do not report 43214 in conjunction with 43197, 43198, 43200, 74360, 76000, 0884T)◀

43226   with insertion of guide wire followed by passage of dilator(s) over guide wire

(Do not report 43226 in conjunction with 43229 for the same lesion)

▶(Do not report 43226 in conjunction with 43197, 43198, 43200, 43212, 43220, 0884T)◀

(If fluoroscopic guidance is performed, use 74360)

(For rigid transoral esophagoscopy with insertion of guide wire followed by dilation over guide wire, use 43196)

▶(For esophagoscopy with predilation followed by therapeutic drug delivery by drug-coated balloon catheter, use 0884T)◀

Rationale

In accordance with the establishment of Category III codes 0884T-0886T, several parenthetical notes following codes 43191, 43195, 43196, 43200, 43220, 43213, 43214, and 43226 (digestive system esophagoscopy) have been added or revised with code 0884T, which describes transoral flexible esophagoscopy with mechanical dilation followed by therapeutic drug delivery by a drug-coated balloon catheter.

Refer to the codebook and the Rationale for Category III codes 0884T-0886T for a full discussion of these changes.

Colon and Rectum

Endoscopy

45300   Proctosigmoidoscopy, rigid; diagnostic, with or without collection of specimen(s) by brushing or washing (separate procedure)

45303   with dilation (eg, balloon, guide wire, bougie)

▶(Do not report 45300, 45303 in conjunction with 0886T)◀

(For radiological supervision and interpretation, use 74360)

45330   Sigmoidoscopy, flexible; diagnostic, including collection of specimen(s) by brushing or washing, when performed (separate procedure)

▶(Do not report 45330 in conjunction with 45331-45342, 45346, 45347, 45349, 45350, 0886T)◀

45340   with transendoscopic balloon dilation

▶(Do not report 45340 in conjunction with 45330, 45346, 45347, 0886T)◀

(If fluoroscopic guidance is performed, use 74360)

▶(For sigmoidoscopy with predilation followed by therapeutic drug delivery by drug-coated balloon catheter, use 0886T)◀

(For transendoscopic balloon dilation of multiple strictures during the same session, use 45340 with modifier 59 for each additional stricture dilated)

45378   Colonoscopy, flexible; diagnostic, including collection of specimen(s) by brushing or washing, when performed (separate procedure)

▶(Do not report 45378 in conjunction with 45379-45393, 45398, 0885T)◀

(For colonoscopy with decompression [pathologic distention], use 45393)

Surgery / Digestive System **40490-49999**

45386   with transendoscopic balloon dilation

▶(Do not report 45386 in conjunction with 45378, 45388, 45389, 0885T)◀

(If fluoroscopic guidance is performed, use 74360)

▶(For colonoscopy with predilation followed by therapeutic drug delivery by drug-coated balloon catheter, use 0885T)◀

(For transendoscopic balloon dilation of multiple strictures during the same session, report 45386 with modifier 59 for each additional stricture dilated)

Rationale

To accommodate the establishment of Category III codes 0884T-0886T, several parenthetical notes following codes 45303, 45330, 45340, 45378, and 45386 (colon and rectum endoscopy) have been revised and added to reflect the new codes.

Refer to the codebook and the Rationale for Category III codes 0884T-0886T for a full discussion of these changes.

Biliary Tract

Repair

47801   Placement of choledochal stent

▶(47802 has been deleted)◀

Rationale

To ensure the CPT 2025 code set reflects current clinical practice, code 47802, *U-tube hepaticoenterostomy*, has been deleted due to low utilization. A parenthetical note has been added to indicate this deletion.

47900   Suture of extrahepatic biliary duct for pre-existing injury (separate procedure)

Abdomen, Peritoneum, and Omentum

Excision, Destruction

Code 49185 describes sclerotherapy of a fluid collection (eg, lymphocele, cyst, or seroma) through a percutaneous access. It includes contrast injection(s), sclerosant injection(s), sclerosant dwell time, diagnostic study, imaging guidance (eg, ultrasound, fluoroscopy), and radiological supervision and interpretation, when performed. Code 49185 may be reported once per day for each lesion treated through a separate catheter. Do not report 49185 more than once if treating multiple lesions through the same catheter. Codes for access to and drainage of the collection may be separately reportable according to location (eg, 10030, 10160, 49405, 49406, 49407, 50390).

▶Codes 49186, 49187, 49188, 49189, 49190 describe excision or destruction of intra-abdominal primary or secondary tumor(s) or cyst(s) via an open approach. Excision or destruction of intra-abdominal primary or secondary tumor(s) or cyst(s) via an open approach includes cytoreduction, debulking, or other methods of removal of the tumor(s) or cyst(s). Codes 49186, 49187, 49188, 49189, 49190 are reported based on the sum of the maximum length of each tumor or cyst excised or destroyed (eg, ultrasound desiccation). Only the tumor(s) and cyst(s) are measured, not the tissue (eg, mesentery) in which the tumor(s) and cyst(s) may be implanted. If only a portion of a tumor or cyst is excised or destroyed, then only the excised or destroyed portion is measured. The tumor(s) and cyst(s) should be measured in situ before excision or destruction and documented in the operative report. Measurement includes only the tumor(s) and cyst(s) and not the margins. Codes 49186, 49187, 49188, 49189, 49190 are reported when the resected or destroyed intra-abdominal tumor(s) and cyst(s) do not directly arise from a resected organ (eg, small bowel mass, renal mass, liver mass) or soft tissue that may be separately reportable. When the tumors arise directly from an organ or soft tissue, only the organ or soft tissue resection or destruction procedure code from which the tumors arise is reported. For example, if a partial ascending colon resection, including small tumor implants, is performed and a separate excision of multiple small tumor implants in the mesentery of the descending colon is also performed, the appropriate colectomy code (eg, 44140) would be reported for the partial ascending colon resection and the excision of the tumor implants in the mesentery of the descending colon would be separately reported with an appropriate tumor excision code (49186, 49187, 49188, 49189, 49190). The implants that were part of the ascending colon resection would not be included in the measurement for reporting the tumor excision code (49186, 49187, 49188, 49189, 49190).

Open resection of recurrent ovarian, endometrial, tubal, or primary peritoneal gynecological malignancies without lymphadenectomy should be reported with 49186, 49187, 49188, 49189, 49190. All other open resection of initial or recurrent ovarian, endometrial, tubal, or primary peritoneal gynecologic malignancies should be reported with 58943, 58950, 58951, 58952, 58953, 58954, 58956, 58958, 58960.◀

(For lysis of intestinal adhesions, use 44005)

★ = Telemedicine   ◀ = Audio-only   + = Add-on code   ✐ = FDA approval pending   # = Resequenced code   ⊘ = Modifier 51 exempt

49180 Biopsy, abdominal or retroperitoneal mass, percutaneous needle

(If imaging guidance is performed, see 76942, 77002, 77012, 77021)

(For fine needle aspiration biopsy, see 10004, 10005, 10006, 10007, 10008, 10009, 10010, 10011, 10012, 10021)

(For evaluation of fine needle aspirate, see 88172, 88173)

49185 Sclerotherapy of a fluid collection (eg, lymphocele, cyst, or seroma), percutaneous, including contrast injection(s), sclerosant injection(s), diagnostic study, imaging guidance (eg, ultrasound, fluoroscopy) and radiological supervision and interpretation when performed

(Do not report 49185 in conjunction with 49424, 76080)

(For access/drainage with catheter, see 10030, 49405, 49406, 49407, 50390)

(For access/drainage with needle, see 10160, 50390)

(For pleurodesis, use 32560)

(For sclerosis of veins or endovenous ablation of incompetent extremity veins, see 36468, 36470, 36471, 36475, 36476, 36478, 36479)

(For sclerotherapy of a lymphatic/vascular malformation, use 37241)

(For treatment of multiple interconnected lesions treated through a single access, report 49185 once)

(For exchange of existing catheter, before or after injection of sclerosant, see 49423, 75984)

(For treatment of multiple lesions in a single day requiring separate access, use modifier 59 for each additional treated lesion)

● **49186** Excision or destruction, open, intra-abdominal (ie, peritoneal, mesenteric, retroperitoneal), primary or secondary tumor(s) or cyst(s), sum of the maximum length of tumor(s) or cyst(s); 5 cm or less

● **49187** 5.1 to 10 cm

● **49188** 10.1 to 20 cm

● **49189** 20.1 to 30 cm

● **49190** greater than 30 cm

▶(Do not report 49186, 49187, 49188, 49189, 49190 in conjunction with 49000, 49010, 49215, 58943, 58950, 58951, 58952, 58953, 58954, 58956, 58958, 58960)◀

▶(For excision of perinephric cyst, use 50290)◀

▶(49203, 49204, 49205 have been deleted. For open excision or destruction of intra-abdominal [ie, peritoneal, mesenteric, retroperitoneal] primary or secondary tumor[s] or cyst[s], see 49186, 49187, 49188, 49189, 49190)◀

▶(For excision or destruction of endometriomas, open method, use 58999)◀

49215 Excision of presacral or sacrococcygeal tumor

(Do not report modifier 63 in conjunction with 49215)

Rationale

Codes 49203-49205 and 58957 and their related parenthetical notes have been deleted, and Category I codes 49186-49190 have been established to report open excision or destruction of intra-abdominal (ie, peritoneal, mesenteric, retroperitoneal) primary or secondary tumors or cysts. In addition, guidelines and parenthetical notes have been added and revised to provide instruction regarding intended reporting and to accommodate the addition of the new codes. This procedure is for peritoneal surface malignancies (PSMs), which are terminal cancers with limited therapeutic options.

To accommodate the development of the new codes, codes 49203-49205, which are based on the excision or destruction of the single largest tumor, have been deleted.

The guidelines provide specific instructions on how codes 49186-49190 may be reported, which includes reporting based on the sum of the maximum length of each tumor or cyst excised or destroyed (eg, ultrasound desiccation) and not the tissue (eg, mesentery) in which the tumor(s) and cyst(s) may be implanted. In addition, if only a portion of a tumor or cyst is excised or destroyed, only the excised or destroyed portion is measured. The tumor(s) and cyst(s) should be measured in situ before the excision or destruction, and the measurements should not include the margins. Finally, if both an organ and tumor(s) are removed as part of the procedural resection, then any tumor removed as part of the organ removal is not separately reported. If a separate resection is performed that requires separate efforts to remove the tumor, that tumor resection may be separately reported using the new codes.

Cross-reference parenthetical notes have been added and revised throughout the CPT 2025 code set to accommodate the addition of the new codes by directing users to the appropriate codes for other procedures and clarifying when other codes may or may not be reported. Parenthetical notes have also been added to direct users to the appropriate codes to report for deleted codes that are now obsolete.

Clinical Example (49186)

A 45-year-old female presents with a 4-cm mesenteric mass involving the small bowel mesentery near the base. She undergoes a resection of the mass.

Description of Procedure (49186)

Make a skin incision using sharp dissection. Achieve hemostasis using electrocautery and small ligatures, as necessary. Identify and carefully divide the linea alba. Grasp, elevate, and carefully incise the peritoneum to avoid injury to the bowel. Enter the peritoneal cavity under direct vision. Clear adhesions using sharp dissection in order to expose all of the abdominal viscera. Perform a visual and manual complete exploration of the abdominal cavity and its contents. Place the nasogastric tube and confirm its position. Inspect the stomach and palpate for pathology. View the duodenum and palpate. Inspect the gallbladder and palpate for the presence of stones. Palpate the liver and the porta hepatis bimanually. Inspect the pancreas through the hepatogastric ligament and palpate for possible masses. Palpate the tail of the pancreas for possible lymphadenopathy. Inspect the small bowel and palpate from the ligament of Treitz to the ileocecal valve. Inspect the small bowel mesentery and palpate for the presence of lymphadenopathy.

A large mass is identified in the mesentery of the distal small bowel. Inspect and palpate the cecum and appendix, ascending, transverse, and descending colon. Inspect and palpate the cul-de-sac and pelvic contents. Carefully insert a self-retaining retractor, while avoiding injury or entrapment of abdominal contents. Confirm the location and extent of the primary lesion. Pack away the abdominal contents, with the exclusion of the right colon, using laparotomy pads, and place additional retractors for optimal exposure. Mobilize the right colon and distal small bowel lateral to medial by incising the line of Toldt. Identify the small bowel mesentery containing the mass and the corresponding loop of small bowel. Resect the 4-cm mass along with the corresponding mesentery, avoiding division of the blood supply to the corresponding small bowel loop and right colon. During this dissection, identify the right ureter and place a vessel loop for continual identification and protection of the ureter. Irrigate the abdominal cavity copiously with antibiotic solution. Obtain hemostasis. Inspect the abdomen for injury and the presence of any instruments or lap pads (ie, conduct a count). Remove and count all the retractor components to ensure all components are accounted for. Return the abdominal organs to normal anatomical position. Drape the omentum over the abdominal contents. Place drain(s) as required. Close the fascia with running suture. Conduct a second count of the instrument, needle, sponge, and lap pad. Irrigate and approximate the subcutaneous tissues and close the skin.

Clinical Example (49187)

A 62-year-old male has progressive colorectal carcinoma with limited peritoneal disease. Multiple implants, which measure 8 cm in total size, are removed from the peritoneal cavity.

Description of Procedure (49187)

Make a skin incision using sharp dissection. Achieve hemostasis using electrocautery and small ligatures, as necessary. Identify and carefully divide the linea alba. Grasp, elevate, and carefully incise the peritoneum to avoid injury to the bowel. Enter the peritoneal cavity under direct vision. Clear adhesions using sharp dissection in order to expose all of the abdominal viscera. Perform a visual and manual complete exploration of the abdominal cavity and its contents. Place the nasogastric tube and confirm its position. Inspect the stomach and palpate for pathology. View and palpate the duodenum. Inspect the gallbladder and palpate for the presence of stones. Palpate the liver and the porta hepatis bimanually. Inspect the pancreas through the hepatogastric ligament and palpate for possible masses. Palpate the tail of the pancreas for possible lymphadenopathy. Inspect the small bowel and palpate from the ligament of Treitz to the ileocecal valve. Inspect the small bowel mesentery and palpate for the presence of lymphadenopathy. Inspect and palpate the cecum and appendix, ascending, transverse, and descending colon. Inspect and palpate the cul-de-sac and pelvic contents. Examine the greater vessels of the abdomen and the urinary tract. Inspect all other intra-abdominal organs systematically. Following peritoneal and retroperitoneal exploration, perform excision and destruction of all macroscopic tumor deposits on parietal, omental, and peritoneal surfaces. Perform resection of the small lesions and multiple surface nodules of the omentum, visceral, and peritoneal surfaces. Desicate some lesions on the small intestine serosal surface with ultrasonic desiccation. The in situ measured total dimension of all excised tumors is documented as 8 cm. Copiously irrigate the abdominal cavity with antibiotic solution. Obtain hemostasis. Inspect the abdomen for injury and the presence of any instruments or lap pads (ie, conduct a count). Remove and count the retractor components to ensure all components are accounted for. Return the abdominal organs to normal anatomical position. Drape the omentum over the abdominal contents. As required, place drain(s). Close the fascia with running suture. Conduct a second count of the instrument, needle, sponge, and lap pad. Irrigate and approximate the subcutaneous tissues and close the skin.

★ = Telemedicine ◀ = Audio-only ✚ = Add-on code ⩫ = FDA approval pending # = Resequenced code ⊘ = Modifier 51 exempt

Clinical Example (49188)

A 70-year-old female, who was diagnosed with peritoneal mesothelioma with a 6-cm right lower quadrant mass and multiple intraperitoneal and retroperitoneal implants, undergoes a resection of the mass and excision and destruction of the implants.

Description of Procedure (49188)

Make a skin incision using sharp dissection. Achieve hemostasis using electrocautery and small ligatures, as necessary. Identify and carefully divide the linea alba. Grasp, elevate, and carefully incise the peritoneum to avoid injury to the bowel. Enter the peritoneal cavity under direct vision. Clear adhesions using sharp dissection in order to expose all of the abdominal viscera. Perform a visual and manual complete exploration of the abdominal cavity and its contents. Place the nasogastric tube and confirm its position. Inspect the stomach and palpate for pathology. View and palpate the duodenum. Inspect the gallbladder and palpate for the presence of stones. Palpate the liver and the porta hepatis bimanually. Inspect the pancreas through the hepatogastric ligament and palpate for possible masses. Palpate the tail of the pancreas for possible lymphadenopathy. Inspect the small bowel and palpate from the ligament of Treitz to the ileocecal valve. Inspect the small bowel mesentery and palpate for the presence of lymphadenopathy. Inspect and palpate the cecum and appendix, ascending, transverse, and descending colon. Inspect and palpate the cul-de-sac and pelvic contents. Examine the greater vessels of the abdomen and the urinary tract. Inspect all other intra-abdominal organs systematically. Following peritoneal and retroperitoneal exploration, perform resection of the large lower abdominal mass and multiple surface nodules of the omentum, visceral, and peritoneal surfaces. Perform resection of the small lesions and multiple surface nodules of the omentum, visceral, and peritoneal surfaces. The in situ measured total dimension of all excised tumors is documented as 19 cm. Irrigate the abdominal cavity copiously with an antibiotic solution. Obtain hemostasis. Inspect the abdomen for injury and the presence of any instruments or lap pads (ie, conduct a count). Remove the retractor components and ensure that all components are accounted for. Return the abdominal organs to normal anatomical position. Drape the omentum over the abdominal contents. Make a lateral incision and pull a closed suction drain through the abdominal wall and place in the resection bed. Suture the drain to the skin with monofilament suture. Place additional drains as required. Close the fascia with running suture. Conduct a second count of the instrument, needle, sponge, and lap pad. Irrigate and approximate the subcutaneous tissues and close the skin.

Clinical Example (49189)

A 55-year-old male, who has a 28-cm retroperitoneal sarcoma and no evidence of distant metastases, undergoes a resection of the sarcoma.

Description of Procedure (49189)

Make a skin incision using sharp dissection. Achieve hemostasis using electrocautery and small ligatures, as necessary. Identify and carefully divide the linea alba. Grasp, elevate, and carefully incise the peritoneum to avoid injury to the bowel. Enter the peritoneal cavity under direct vision. Clear adhesions using sharp dissection in order to expose all of the abdominal viscera. Perform a visual and manual complete exploration of the abdominal cavity and its contents. Place the nasogastric tube and confirm its position. Inspect the stomach and palpate for pathology. View and palpate the duodenum. Inspect the gallbladder and palpate for the presence of stones. Palpate the liver and the porta hepatis bimanually. Inspect the pancreas through the hepatogastric ligament and palpate for possible masses. Palpate the tail of the pancreas for possible lymphadenopathy. Inspect the small bowel and palpate from the ligament of Treitz to the ileocecal valve. Inspect the small bowel mesentery and palpate for the presence of lymphadenopathy. Inspect and palpate the cecum and appendix, ascending, transverse, and descending colon. Inspect and palpate the cul-de-sac and pelvic contents. Examine the greater vessels of the abdomen and the urinary tract. Inspect all other intra-abdominal organs systematically. Following peritoneal and retroperitoneal exploration, mobilize the ascending colon by dividing the peritoneal reflection and take down the hepatic flexure of the colon. Elevate the second portion of the duodenum and the head of the pancreas from the retroperitoneum to expose the vena cava and aorta. Mobilize the base of the small bowel mesentery to the third portion of the duodenum to further expose the vena cava and aorta. Identify the kidneys, vasculature, and ureters. Control the proximal aorta, iliac arteries, subrenal vena cava, and iliac veins superiorly and inferiorly to the retroperitoneal tumor. Resect the 28-cm tumor from the retroperitoneum with sequential ligation of inflow and outflow vasculature of the tumor. Irrigate the abdominal cavity copiously with an antibiotic solution. Obtain hemostasis. Inspect the abdomen for injury and the presence of any instruments or lap pads (ie, conduct a count). Remove the retractor components and ensure all the components are accounted for. Return the abdominal organs to the normal anatomical position. Drape the omentum over the abdominal contents. Make a lateral incision and pull a closed suction drain through the abdominal wall and place in the resection bed. Suture the drain to the skin with monofilament suture. Place additional drains as required. Close the fascia with running suture. Conduct a second count of the instrument, needle, sponge, and lap pad. Irrigate and approximate the subcutaneous tissues and close the skin.

Clinical Example (49190)

A 58-year-old female, who has a previous colon resection for appendiceal adenocarcinoma, develops extensive peritoneal carcinomatosis. She undergoes a tumor excision and destruction.

Description of Procedure (49190)

Makes a skin incision using sharp dissection. Achieve hemostasis using electrocautery and small ligatures, as necessary. Identify and carefully divide the linea alba. Grasp, elevate, and carefully incise the peritoneum to avoid injury to the bowel. Enter the peritoneal cavity under direct vision. Clear adhesions using sharp dissection in order to expose all of the abdominal viscera. Perform a visual and manual complete exploration of the abdominal cavity and its contents. Place the nasogastric tube and confirm its position. Inspect the stomach and palpate for pathology. View and palpate the duodenum. Inspect the gallbladder and palpate for the presence of stones. Palpate the liver and the porta hepatis bimanually. Inspect the pancreas through the hepatogastric ligament and palpate for possible masses. Palpate the tail of the pancreas for possible lymphadenopathy. Inspect and palpate the small bowel from the ligament of Treitz to the ileocecal valve. Inspect and palpate the small bowel mesentery for the presence of lymphadenopathy. Inspect and palpate the cecum and appendix, ascending, transverse, and descending colon. Inspect and palpate the cul-de-sac and pelvic contents. Examine the greater vessels of the abdomen and the urinary tract. Inspect all other intra-abdominal organs systematically. Following peritoneal and retroperitoneal exploration, perform cytoreduction of all macroscopic tumor deposits on parietal, omental, and peritoneal surfaces. Perform resection of multiple surface nodules of the omentum, visceral, and mesenteric surfaces. Mobilize the liver fully and resect the peritoneum from both diaphragms. Perform resection of the small lesions and multiple surface nodules of the omentum, visceral, and peritoneal surfaces. The in situ measured total dimension of all excised tumors is documented as 35 cm. Irrigate the abdominal cavity copiously with an antibiotic solution. Obtain hemostasis. Inspect the abdomen for injury and the presence of any instruments or lap pads (ie, conduct a count). Remove and ensure all retractor components are accounted for. Return the abdominal organs to normal anatomical position. Drape the omentum over the abdominal contents. Make a lateral incision and pull a closed suction drain through the abdominal wall and place in the resection bed. Suture the drain to the skin with monofilament suture. Place additional drains as required. Close the fascia with running suture. Conduct

a second count of the instrument, needle, sponge, and lap pad. Irrigate and approximate the subcutaneous tissues and close the skin.

Urinary System

Kidney

Incision

Nephrolithotomy is the surgical removal of stones from the kidney, and pyelolithotomy is the surgical removal of stones from the renal pelvis. This section of the guidelines refers to the removal of stones from the kidney or renal pelvis using a percutaneous antegrade approach. Breaking and removing stones is separate from accessing the kidney (ie, 50040, 50432, 50433, 52334), accessing the kidney with dilation of the tract to accommodate an endoscope used in an endourologic procedure (ie, 50437), or dilation of a previously established tract to accommodate an endoscope used in an endourologic procedure (ie, 50436). These procedures include the antegrade removal of stones in the calyces, renal pelvis, and/or ureter with the antegrade placement of catheters, stents, and tubes, but do not include retrograde placement of catheters, stents, and tubes.

Code 50080 describes nephrolithotomy or pyelolithotomy using a percutaneous antegrade approach with endoscopic instruments to break and remove kidney stones of 2 cm or smaller.

Code 50081 includes the elements of 50080, but it is reported for stones larger than 2 cm, branching, stones in multiple locations, ureteral stones, or in patients with complicated anatomy.

Creation of percutaneous access or dilation of the tract to accommodate large endoscopic instruments used in stone removals (50436, 50437) is not included in 50080, 50081, and may be reported separately, if performed. Codes 50080, 50081 include placement of any stents or drainage catheters that remain indwelling after the procedure.

Report one unit of 50080 or 50081 per side (ie, per kidney), regardless of the number of stones broken and/or removed or locations of the stones. For bilateral procedure, report 50080, 50081 with modifier 50. When 50080 is performed on one side and 50081 is performed on the contralateral side, modifier 50 is not applicable. Placement of additional accesses, if needed, into the kidney, and removal of stones through other approaches (eg, open or retrograde) may be reported separately, if performed.

Surgery / Urinary System 50010-53899

▶(For open retroperitoneal exploration, use 49010)◀

▶(For open drainage of retroperitoneal abscess, use 49060)◀

▶(For open excision or destruction of intra-abdominal [ie, peritoneal, mesenteric, retroperitoneal] primary or secondary tumor[s] or cyst[s], see 49186, 49187, 49188, 49189, 49190)◀

Rationale

Cross-reference parenthetical notes have been added in the Incision subsection of the Kidney section to direct users to the appropriate codes for open retroperitoneal exploration, open drainage of retroperitoneal abscess, and open excision or destruction of intra-abdominal primary or secondary tumor(s).

Refer to the codebook and the Rationale for codes 49186-49190 for a full discussion of these changes.

50120   Pyelotomy; with exploration

(For renal endoscopy performed in conjunction with this procedure, see 50570-50580)

50125   with drainage, pyelostomy

50130   with removal of calculus (pyelolithotomy, pelviolithotomy, including coagulum pyelolithotomy)

▶(50135 has been deleted)◀

Rationale

To ensure the CPT 2025 code set reflects current clinical practice, code 50135, *Pyelotomy; complicated (eg, secondary operation, congenital kidney abnormality)*, has been deleted due to low utilization. A parenthetical note has been added to indicate this deletion.

Excision

▶(For open excision or destruction of retroperitoneal tumor[s] or cyst[s] [other than endometriomas], see 49186, 49187, 49188, 49189, 49190)◀

(For laparoscopic ablation of renal mass lesion(s), use 50542)

▶(For excision or destruction of endometriomas, open method, use 58999)◀

Rationale

Parenthetical note cross-references have been added and revised in the Excision subsection of the Kidney section to accommodate the addition of codes 49186-49190 for open excision or destruction of retroperitoneal tumor(s).

Refer to the codebook and the Rationale for codes 49186-49190 for a full discussion of these changes.

Bladder

Incision

▲ 51020   Cystotomy or cystostomy, with fulguration and/or insertion of radioactive material

▶(51030 has been deleted)◀

Rationale

To ensure the CPT 2025 code set reflects current clinical practice, code 51030, *Cystotomy or cystostomy; with cryosurgical destruction of intravesical lesion*, has been deleted due to low utilization. A parenthetical note has been added to indicate this deletion. In accordance with the deletion of code 51030, code 51020 has been revised with the removal of the semicolon because it is no longer a parent code.

Introduction

51720   Bladder instillation of anticarcinogenic agent (including retention time)

● 51721   Insertion of transurethral ablation transducer for delivery of thermal ultrasound for prostate tissue ablation, including suprapubic tube placement during the same session and placement of an endorectal cooling device, when performed

▶(Do not report 51721 in conjunction with 51701, 51702, 55881, 55882, 72195, 72196, 72197, 77022)◀

▶(For insertion of transurethral ultrasound transducer and ablation of prostate tissue using thermal ultrasound transducer performed by the same physician, use 55882)◀

Rationale

Code 51721 and two parenthetical notes have been added to provide instruction and to report services for the insertion of a transurethral ablation transducer for the delivery of a thermal ultrasound for prostate tissue ablation.

Refer to the codebook and the Rationale for codes 55881 and 55882 for a full discussion of these changes.

Clinical Example (51721)

A 67-year-old male, who has prostate cancer, presents for a magnetic resonance imaging (MRI)-monitored transurethral thermal ultrasound ablation.

Description of Procedure (51721)

Prepare and drape the anterior pelvis, and place the suprapubic catheter. Transfer and position the patient appropriately in the MRI scanner to begin the process of placing the necessary applicators for the procedure. Perform a rectal examination to assess the adequacy of bowel preparation, and place an endorectal cooling device with balloon into the rectum. Prepare and drape the patient's anterior pelvis and penis in sterile fashion, and place a Foley catheter via the urethra into the bladder to empty it. Then partially fill the bladder with sterile fluid, and advance a guidewire through the catheter and coil it into the bladder. Remove the Foley catheter over the wire. Following anesthetization of the urethra with lidocaine gel, insert and position the transurethral ultrasound ablation transducer over the guidewire in the urethra with the catheter tip extending into the bladder. Remove the guidewire, and secure the transurethral ultrasound ablation transducer within the tested MRI-compatible robot. After MRI scout imaging is obtained, remove any air bubbles within the treatment field or endorectal cooling device by deflating, inflating, and twisting the endorectal device. Acquire a brief MRI scan again to ensure all air bubbles that could impede the cooling of the endorectal device have been removed. Next, acquire multiplanar MRI images to confirm the correct positioning of the ultrasound transurethral ablation transducer and endorectal cooling device by another physician on a separate workstation. Advance the patient back into the bore, and reacquire and review localizer images.

If needed, achieve more favorable urethral treatment device and rectal cooling device positioning in the MRI magnet room. This is achieved by backing the patient out of the bore and manually adjusting the ultrasound applicator positioning and angulation, as well as the endorectal cooling device positioning, lubrication, and balloon volume. The physician leaves the patient care area, the remainder of the MRI-guided ablation is performed, and the physician returns once the ablation is completed. Remove the transurethral transducer. If no suprapubic catheter was placed, place a wire through the transducer into the bladder and remove the transducer over the wire under sterile conditions. Advance a Foley

catheter over the wire, and remove the wire from the Foley catheter that is connected to a bag. Lastly, remove the endorectal device.

Endoscopy—Cystoscopy, Urethroscopy, Cystourethroscopy

52000 Cystourethroscopy (separate procedure)

▶(Do not report 52000 in conjunction with 52001, 52320, 52325, 52327, 52330, 52332, 52334, 52341, 52342, 52343, 52356, 57240, 57260, 57265, 0935T)◀

(Do not report 52000 in conjunction with 57240, 57260, 57265)

Rationale

In accordance with the establishment of code 0935T, an exclusionary parenthetical note following code 52000 has been revised with the addition of codes 57240, 57260, 57265, and 0935T, which should not be reported with code 52000.

Refer to the codebook and the Rationale for code 0935T for a full discussion of these changes.

52001 Cystourethroscopy with irrigation and evacuation of multiple obstructing clots

(Do not report 52001 in conjunction with 52000)

——— *Coding Tip* ———

Restrictions for Reporting Temporary Catheter Insertion and Removal with Cystourethroscopy

The insertion and removal of a temporary ureteral catheter (52005) during diagnostic or therapeutic cystourethroscopy with ureteroscopy and/or pyeloscopy is included in 52320-52356 and should not be reported separately.

CPT Coding Guidelines, Urinary System, Bladder Transurethral Surgery, Ureter and Pelvis

52005 Cystourethroscopy, with ureteral catheterization, with or without irrigation, instillation, or ureteropyelography, exclusive of radiologic service;

▶(Do not report 52005 in conjunction with 0935T)◀

52007 with brush biopsy of ureter and/or renal pelvis

(For image-guided biopsy of ureter and/or renal pelvis without endoscopic guidance, use 50606)

Rationale

In accordance with the establishment of code 0935T, an exclusionary parenthetical note has been added following code 52005 to restrict reporting code 52005 with code 0935T.

Refer to the codebook and the Rationale for code 0935T for a full discussion of these changes.

Transurethral Surgery

Urethra and Bladder

52282   Cystourethroscopy, with insertion of permanent urethral stent

(For placement of temporary prostatic urethral stent, use 53855)

▶(For insertion of prostatic urethral scaffold, use 0941T)◀

52310   Cystourethroscopy, with removal of foreign body, calculus, or ureteral stent from urethra or bladder (separate procedure); simple

52315   complicated

▶(For removal and replacement of prostatic urethral scaffold, use 0942T)◀

▶(For removal of prostatic urethral scaffold, use 0943T)◀

Rationale

In accordance with the establishment of codes 0941T-0943T, cross-reference parenthetical notes have been added following codes 52282 and 52315 directing users to the new codes.

Refer to the codebook and the Rationale for codes 0941T-0943T for a full discussion of these changes.

Vesical Neck and Prostate

52441   Cystourethroscopy, with insertion of permanent adjustable transprostatic implant; single implant

+ 52442   each additional permanent adjustable transprostatic implant (List separately in addition to code for primary procedure)

(Use 52442 in conjunction with 52441)

(To report removal of implant[s], use 52310)

▶(For insertion of a permanent urethral stent, use 52282. For insertion of a temporary prostatic urethral stent, use 53855. For insertion of prostatic urethral scaffold, use 0941T)◀

Rationale

In accordance with the establishment of codes 0941T-0943T, the cross-reference parenthetical note following code 52442 has been revised to direct users to code 0941T for the insertion of a prostatic urethral scaffold.

Refer to the codebook and the Rationale for codes 0941T-0943T for a full discussion of these changes.

Urethra

Other Procedures

53855   Insertion of a temporary prostatic urethral stent, including urethral measurement

(For insertion of permanent urethral stent, use 52282)

▶(For insertion of prostatic urethral scaffold, use 0941T)◀

Rationale

In accordance with the establishment of codes 0941T-0943T, a cross-reference parenthetical note has been added following code 53855 to direct users to code 0941T for the insertion of a prostatic urethral scaffold.

Refer to the codebook and the Rationale for codes 0941T-0943T for a full discussion of these changes.

53860   Transurethral radiofrequency micro-remodeling of the female bladder neck and proximal urethra for stress urinary incontinence

● **53865**   Cystourethroscopy with insertion of temporary device for ischemic remodeling (ie, pressure necrosis) of bladder neck and prostate

▶(For insertion of a permanent urethral stent, use 52282)◀

▶(For insertion of a temporary prostatic urethral stent without cystourethroscopy, including urethral measurement, use 53855)◀

▶(For catheterization with removal of temporary device for ischemic remodeling of bladder neck and prostate, use 53866)◀

● **53866** Catheterization with removal of temporary device for ischemic remodeling (ie, pressure necrosis) of bladder neck and prostate

▶(For cystourethroscopy with removal of temporary device for ischemic remodeling of bladder neck and prostate, use 52310)◀

▶(For insertion of temporary device for ischemic remodeling of bladder neck and prostate, use 53865)◀

Rationale

For the CPT 2025 code set, two new Category I codes have been established to report bladder and neck prostate procedures. Before 2025, there were no appropriate codes to report the insertion or removal of temporary devices used to remodel the bladder neck and prostate. Code 53865 was established to report cystourethroscopy with the insertion of a temporary device for ischemic remodeling of the bladder neck and prostate. Code 53866 was established to report the catheterization with the removal of a temporary device for ischemic remodeling of the bladder neck and prostate.

Several parenthetical notes have been added to instruct users on the appropriate use of the new codes. Three instructional parenthetical notes have been added following code 53865 to direct users to the appropriate codes for the insertion of a permanent urethral stent (52282), the insertion of a temporary prostatic urethral stent when performed without cystourethroscopy (53855), and the removal of a temporary device for ischemic remodeling of the bladder neck and prostate (53866). Two cross-reference parenthetical notes have been added following code 53866 to direct users to the appropriate codes for cystourethroscopy with the removal of a temporary device for ischemic remodeling (52310) and the insertion of a temporary device for ischemic remodeling of the bladder neck and prostate (53865). Note that if cystourethroscopy is used for the removal of the temporary device, users are directed to report code 52310 instead of code 53866.

Clinical Example (53865)

A 68-year-old male has a six-month history of lower urinary tract symptoms due to benign prostatic hyperplasia. The patient has an elevated International Prostate Symptom Score, a low-peak urinary flow rate, and an elevated post-void residual volume. Ultrasound shows the patient's prostate is greater than 25 grams. His symptoms have failed to improve with pharmacologic therapy.

Description of Procedure (53865)

Insert a rigid cystoscope into the meatus and advance into the bladder to completely assess the lower urinary tract, including the anterior urethra, prostatic urethra, and bladder. Leave the cystoscopic sheath in place, and remove the bridge and camera. Then place the temporary ischemic remodeling device through the cystoscopic sheath and deploy it into the bladder. Remove the cystoscope. Under direct vision, advance the cystoscope into the bladder in parallel to the ischemic remodeling device again. Carefully manipulate the device into the appropriate position under direct vision using the device guidewire. Once the device is appropriately positioned with the anchoring leaflet posterior and just distal to the bladder neck, remove the cystoscope. Remove the guidewire to expose the anchoring sutures and secure the sutures to the patient.

Clinical Example (53866)

A 68-year-old male, who previously underwent insertion of a temporary device for an ischemic remodeling of the bladder neck and prostate to treat his lower urinary tract symptoms because of benign prostatic hyperplasia, is scheduled to have the device removed via catheterization under local anesthetic.

Description of Procedure (53866)

Place a grasper through a urinary catheter to grip the retrieval suture. Pass the suture through the catheter. Then advance the catheter over the retrieval suture through the urethra until it contacts the temporary device for ischemic remodeling. Apply firm, steady pressure to the retrieval suture until the temporary remodeling device is brought securely into the urinary catheter. Then remove the catheter, temporary remodeling device, and retrieval suture completely.

Male Genital System

Penis

Repair

▶(54438 has been deleted)◀

Rationale

To ensure the CPT 2025 code set reflects current clinical practice, code 54438, *Replantation, penis, complete amputation including urethral repair*, has been deleted due to low utilization. A parenthetical note has been added to indicate this deletion.

Prostate

Other Procedures

55880   Ablation of malignant prostate tissue, transrectal, with high intensity–focused ultrasound (HIFU), including ultrasound guidance

● **55881**   Ablation of prostate tissue, transurethral, using thermal ultrasound, including magnetic resonance imaging guidance for, and monitoring of, tissue ablation;

►(Do not report 55881 in conjunction with 55882)◄

►(For insertion of transurethral ultrasound transducer and ablation of prostate tissue using thermal ultrasound transducer performed by the same physician, use 55882)◄

● **55882**   with insertion of transurethral ultrasound transducer for delivery of thermal ultrasound, including suprapubic tube placement and placement of an endorectal cooling device, when performed

►(Do not report 55882 in conjunction with 55881)◄

►(Do not report 55881, 55882 in conjunction with 51701, 51702, 51721, 72195, 72196, 72197, 77022)◄

Rationale

Three new Category I codes (51721, 55881, 55882) have been established to report thermal ultrasound prostate tissue ablation. Several parenthetical notes have been added following these new codes.

Codes 51721, 55881, and 55882 have been added to report transurethral ultrasound ablation of the prostate for the treatment of prostate cancer. These codes include guidance for accessing the tissue and for monitoring during the procedure and placement of the device. Code 51721 is reported for the insertion of transurethral ablation transducer for the delivery of a thermal ultrasound for prostate tissue ablation, including the placement of a suprapubic tube and a cooling device that actively protects the urethra and rectum for the preservation of a male patient's functional abilities. Code 55881 is reported for magnetic resonance imaging guidance for and monitoring of tissue ablation. Code 55882 is reported for the provision of both procedures, ie, the placement of the device and the treatment (including guidance to access the site and monitor the progress of the procedure). These three codes have been included to allow separate reporting when the insertion of transurethral ultrasound transducers for the thermal ultrasound delivery and the prostate tissue ablation are performed by separate physicians. Codes 51721 and 55881 are reported for separate provisions of each service by a different physician, and code 55882 is reported for the provision of

both services by the same physician. A parenthetical instruction following code 51721 directs users to code 55882 when both procedures are done by the same physician.

In accordance with the establishment of codes 51721, 55881, and 55882, exclusionary and cross-reference parenthetical notes have been added within the Urinary and Male Genital sections to clarify the appropriate reporting of this new service. This includes exclusionary parenthetical notes following codes 51721, 55881, and 55882, as well as cross-reference parenthetical notes following codes 51721 and 55881 to direct users to report code 55882.

Clinical Example (55881)

A 67-year-old male, who has prostate cancer, presents for a magnetic resonance imaging (MRI)-monitored transurethral thermal ultrasound ablation.

Description of Procedure (55881)

Transfer the patient to the MRI scanner, and the other physician places and secures the necessary catheters and applicators. Place an MRI surface coil over the patient's pelvis, check all straps and pressure points, and advance the patient head first into the MRI machine for imaging. Perform a brief MRI scout scan to determine if any air bubbles are in the rectum after the placement of the transurethral ultrasound ablation transducer and endorectal cooling tube. The other physician checks for any air bubbles and adjusts the applicators. Acquire a brief MRI scan again to ensure all air bubbles that could impede the cooling of the endorectal device have been removed. Next, acquire and use multiplanar MRI images to confirm the correct positioning of the ultrasound transurethral ablation transducer and endorectal cooling device. Create three-dimensional reformatted images in the treatment-planning software on a separate workstation and reviewed by the physician. Advance the patient back into the bore, and reacquire and review localizer images. Confirm satisfactory device positioning and register the position of the ultrasound transurethral ablation transducer by visualization of fiducial markers located within the applicator. Make any needed minor adjustments to the position of the applicator. Obtain and transfer the treatment-planning quality MRI images to the treatment-planning software within a separate workstation. If prostatic calcifications that would impede treatment are detected, shift the ultrasound applicator further, placing the calcification between transducer elements to reduce the ultrasound energy absorbed and reflected by the calcification. Generate a detailed treatment plan by manually contouring the target volume of the prostate tissue and outlining the boundary of the ablation zone where the treatment will be directed, while contouring the surrounding critical structures of the rectal wall, neurovascular bundles, external urinary sphincter, and internal urinary sphincter that are to be avoided from ablation. The treatment-planning system creates a report of the MRI temperature images to confirm whether the thermometry precision can be achieved or if any manual correction of geometric distortion in the images is needed. The physician reviews the report and makes any adjustments to the placement of the ultrasound transurethral ablation transducer. Any adjustments will require a new MRI dataset, new contouring of the target tissues, ablation zone, and critical structures, and a treatment plan regenerated. Review the new report from the treatment planning system again to confirm that the treatment plan can be achieved and no other adjustments are needed. Using the MRI-compatible robotic positioning system, advance the ultrasound transurethral ablation transducer for precise ablation of the prescribed, targeted volume and zone. The treating physician determines the rotational angle and direction of rotation for the ultrasound applicator. Additional MRI images may be acquired to confirm that the planned target volume of prostate tissue is within the prescribed ablation volume and that the normal tissue and critical structures are adequately spared prior to the ablation. Administer a second dose of anti-spasmodic drug, and the physician initiates the closed-loop MRI-guided ultrasound ablation treatment. Throughout the treatment, each ultrasound transurethral ablation transducer emits the planned intensity and frequency of the ultrasound energy, while also modulating the rotation rate of the transducer to achieve an optimal ablative temperature within the treatment target and ablation zone. Real-time MRI images and MRI thermometry images are acquired continuously throughout the treatment and displayed, as they are acquired for the physician to closely monitor the amount of energy delivered by each transducer. Based on the thermal feedback response of the target and ablation zone, modulate the treatment to pause or adjust the robotically driven ultrasound transducer. Any changes that require repositioning the patient or due to any changes in the surrounding environment affecting the position of the ultrasound transurethral ablation transducer, or if the patient requires stopping treatment, proceed with a 20-minute cool-down phase of the target tissues, subsequent new MRI images, and treatment plan. Once the prescribed treatment zone is ablated, acquire pre- and postcontrast-enhanced MRI images immediately following the treatment to confirm satisfactory ablation. The physician reviews the completion imaging to confirm no intraprocedural complication(s) occurred. Turn off the power to the system electronics. Remove the anterior MRI coil and positioning straps. Detach the ultrasound applicator from the robotic positioning system, system electronics,

and fluid tube sets. Remove the applicators, and the other physician manages the catheters.

Clinical Example (55882)

A 67-year-old male, who has prostate cancer, presents for a magnetic resonance imaging (MRI)-monitored transurethral thermal ultrasound ablation.

Description of Procedure (55882)

Prepare and drape the anterior pelvis and place the suprapubic catheter. Transfer and position the patient appropriately in the MRI scanner to begin the process of placing the necessary applicators for the procedure. Perform a rectal examination to assess the adequacy of bowel preparation, and place an endorectal cooling device with balloon into the rectum. Prepare and drape the patient's anterior pelvis and penis in sterile fashion and place a Foley catheter via the urethra into the bladder to empty it. Then partially fill the bladder with sterile fluid, and advance a guidewire through the catheter and coil it into the bladder. Remove the Foley catheter over the wire. Following anesthetization of the urethra with lidocaine gel, insert and position the transurethral ultrasound ablation transducer over the guidewire in the urethra with the tip extending into the bladder. Remove the guidewire, and secure and test the transurethral ultrasound ablation transducer within the MRI-compatible robot. Place an MRI surface coil over the patient's pelvis, check all straps and pressure points, and advance the patient head first into the MRI machine for imaging. Perform a brief, MRI scout scan to determine if any air bubbles are in the rectum after the placement of the transurethral ultrasound ablation transducer and endorectal cooling tube. Remove any air bubbles within the treatment field or endorectal cooling device by deflating, inflating, and twisting the endorectal device. Again, acquire a brief MRI scan to ensure that all air bubbles that could impede the cooling of the endorectal device have been removed. Next, acquire and use multiplanar MRI images to confirm the correct positioning of the ultrasound transurethral ablation transducer and endorectal cooling device. Create three-dimensional, reformatted images in the treatment-planning software on a separate workstation, which are reviewed by the physician. Then advance the patient back into the bore, and reacquire and review localizer images. If needed, achieve more favorable urethral treatment device and rectal cooling device positioning in the MRI magnet room. This is performed by backing the patient out of the bore and manually adjusting the ultrasound applicator positioning and angulation, as well as the endorectal cooling device positioning, lubrication, and balloon volume. Then advance the patient back into the bore, and reacquire and review the localizer images. After confirming the satisfactory device positioning, register the position of

★=Telemedicine ◀=Audio-only ✚=Add-on code 𝒩=FDA approval pending #=Resequenced code ⊘=Modifier 51 exempt

the ultrasound transurethral ablation transducer by visualization of fiducial markers located within the applicator. Make any needed minor adjustments to the position of the applicator. Obtain and transfer treatment-planning quality MRI images to the treatment-planning software within a separate workstation. If prostatic calcifications that would impede treatment are detected, shift the ultrasound applicator further, placing the calcification between transducer elements to reduce the ultrasound energy absorbed and reflected by the calcification. Generate a detailed treatment plan by manually contouring the target volume of prostate tissue and outlining the boundary of the ablation zone where the treatment will be directed, while contouring the surrounding critical structures of the rectal wall, neurovascular bundles, external urinary sphincter, and internal urinary sphincter that are to be avoided from ablation. The treatment-planning system creates a report of the MRI temperature images to confirm whether the thermometry precision can be achieved or if any manual correction of geometric distortion in the images is needed. The physician reviews the report and makes any adjustments to the placement of the ultrasound transurethral ablation transducer. Any adjustments will require a new MRI dataset, new contouring of the target tissues, ablation zone, and critical structures, and a treatment plan to be generated. The new report from the treatment-planning system is again reviewed to confirm that the treatment plan can be achieved and no other adjustments are needed. Using the MRI-compatible robotic positioning system, advance the ultrasound transurethral ablation transducer for precise ablation of the prescribed, targeted volume and zone. The treating physician determines the rotational angle and direction of rotation for the ultrasound applicator. Additional MRI images may be acquired to confirm that the planned target volume of prostate tissue is within the prescribed ablation volume and that the normal tissue and critical structures are adequately spared prior to the ablation. Administer a second dose of anti-spasmodic drug, and the physician initiates the closed-loop MRI-guided ultrasound ablation treatment. Throughout the treatment, each ultrasound transurethral ablation transducer emits the planned intensity and frequency of the ultrasound energy, while also modulating the rotation rate of the transducer to achieve an optimal ablative temperature within the treatment target and ablation zone. Real-time MRI images and MRI thermometry images are acquired continuously throughout the treatment and are displayed as they are acquired for the physician to closely monitor the amount of energy delivered by each transducer. Based on the thermal feedback response of the target and ablation zone, the treatment is modulated to pause or adjust the robotically driven ultrasound transducer. Any changes that require repositioning the patient or due to any changes in the surrounding environment affecting the

position of the ultrasound transurethral ablation transducer, or if the patient requires stopping treatment, proceed with a 20-minute cool-down phase of the target tissues, subsequent new MRI images, and treatment plan. Once the prescribed treatment zone is ablated, acquire pre- and postcontrast-enhanced MRI images immediately following the treatment to confirm satisfactory ablation. The physician reviews the completion imaging to confirm that no intraprocedural complication(s) occurred. Turn off the power to the system electronics. Remove the anterior MRI coil and positioning straps. Detach the ultrasound applicator from the robotic positioning system, system electronics, and fluid tube sets. Remove the transurethral transducer. If no suprapubic catheter was placed, place a wire under sterile conditions through the transducer into the bladder and remove the transducer over the wire. Advance a Foley catheter over the wire and remove the wire from the Foley catheter that is connected to a bag. Lastly, remove the endorectal device.

Female Genital System

(For pelvic laparotomy, use 49000)

(For paracentesis, see 49082, 49083, 49084)

(For secondary closure of abdominal wall evisceration or disruption, use 49900)

(For fulguration or excision of lesions, laparoscopic approach, use 58662)

▶(For excision or destruction of endometriomas, open method, use 58999)◀

(For chemotherapy, see 96401-96549)

Rationale

A cross-reference parenthetical note in the Female Genital System section has been revised by deleting codes 49203, 49205, 58957, and 58958, directing users to code 58999 to report the excision or destruction of endometriomas via an open method.

Refer to the codebook and the Rationale for codes 49186-49190 for a full discussion of these changes.

Oviduct/Ovary

Repair

58740   Lysis of adhesions (salpingolysis, ovariolysis)

(For laparoscopic approach, use 58660)

(For fulguration or excision of lesions, laparoscopic approach, use 58662)

▶(For excision or destruction of endometriomas, open method, use 58999)◀

Rationale

A cross-reference parenthetical note has been revised in the Repair subsection of the Oviduct/Ovary section to direct users to code 58999 to report the excision or destruction of endometriomas via an open method.

Refer to the codebook and the Rationale for codes 49186-49190 for a full discussion of this change.

Ovary

Excision

58940   Oophorectomy, partial or total, unilateral or bilateral;

(For oophorectomy with concomitant debulking for ovarian malignancy, use 58952)

58943   for ovarian, tubal or primary peritoneal malignancy, with para-aortic and pelvic lymph node biopsies, peritoneal washings, peritoneal biopsies, diaphragmatic assessments, with or without salpingectomy(s), with or without omentectomy

▶(Do not report 58943 in conjunction with 49186, 49187, 49188, 49189, 49190)◀

58950   Resection (initial) of ovarian, tubal or primary peritoneal malignancy with bilateral salpingo-oophorectomy and omentectomy;

58951   with total abdominal hysterectomy, pelvic and limited para-aortic lymphadenectomy

58952   with radical dissection for debulking (ie, radical excision or destruction, intra-abdominal or retroperitoneal tumors)

▶(Do not report 58950, 58951, 58952 in conjunction with 49186, 49187, 49188, 49189, 49190)◀

▶(For resection of recurrent ovarian, tubal, primary peritoneal, or uterine malignancy, use 58958)◀

58953   Bilateral salpingo-oophorectomy with omentectomy, total abdominal hysterectomy and radical dissection for debulking;

58954   with pelvic lymphadenectomy and limited para-aortic lymphadenectomy

▶(Do not report 58953, 58954 in conjunction with 49186, 49187, 49188, 49189, 49190)◀

58956   Bilateral salpingo-oophorectomy with total omentectomy, total abdominal hysterectomy for malignancy

▶(Do not report 58956 in conjunction with 49186, 49187, 49188, 49189, 49190, 49255, 58150, 58180, 58262, 58263, 58550, 58661, 58700, 58720, 58900, 58925, 58940, 58958)◀

▶(58957 has been deleted. For resection [tumor debulking] of recurrent ovarian, endometrial, tubal, or primary peritoneal gynecological malignancies, with omentectomy, if performed, without lymphadenectomy, see 49186, 49187, 49188, 49189, 49190)◀

▲ **58958**   Resection (tumor debulking) of recurrent ovarian, tubal, primary peritoneal, uterine malignancy (intra-abdominal, retroperitoneal tumors), with omentectomy, if performed, with pelvic lymphadenectomy and limited para-aortic lymphadenectomy

▶(Do not report 58958 in conjunction with 38770, 38780, 44005, 49000, 49186, 49187, 49188, 49189, 49190, 49215, 49255, 58900-58960)◀

58960   Laparotomy, for staging or restaging of ovarian, tubal, or primary peritoneal malignancy (second look), with or without omentectomy, peritoneal washing, biopsy of abdominal and pelvic peritoneum, diaphragmatic assessment with pelvic and limited para-aortic lymphadenectomy

▶(Do not report 58960 in conjunction with 49186, 49187, 49188, 49189, 49190, 58958)◀

Rationale

Code 58957 has been deleted to accommodate the addition of codes 49186-49190 for the open excision or destruction of retroperitoneal tumor(s). Code 58958 has been revised with the removal of the semicolon because it is no longer a child code to code 58957. Parenthetical notes have also been added and revised within the Excision subsection of the Ovary section.

Refer to the codebook and the Rationale for codes 49186-49190 for a full discussion of these changes.

Endocrine System

Parathyroid, Thymus, Adrenal Glands, Pancreas, and Carotid Body

Excision

60540   Adrenalectomy, partial or complete, or exploration of adrenal gland with or without biopsy, transabdominal, lumbar or dorsal (separate procedure);

60545   with excision of adjacent retroperitoneal tumor

(Do not report 60540, 60545 in conjunction with 50323)

▶(For open excision or destruction of remote or disseminated pheochromocytoma, see 49186, 49187, 49188, 49189, 49190)◀

(For laparoscopic approach, use 60650)

(For bilateral procedure, report 60540 with modifier 50)

Rationale

A parenthetical note has been revised within the Parathyroid, Thymus, Adrenal Glands, Pancreas, and Carotid Body subsection of the Endocrine System section to accommodate the addition of codes 49186-49190 for the open excision or destruction of retroperitoneal tumor(s).

Refer to the codebook and the Rationale for codes 49186-49190 for a full discussion of these changes.

Other Procedures

● **60660** Ablation of 1 or more thyroid nodule(s), one lobe or the isthmus, percutaneous, including imaging guidance, radiofrequency

▶(Do not report 60660 in conjunction with 76940, 76942, 77013, 77022)◀

▶(For laser ablation of benign thyroid nodule[s], use 0673T)◀

+● **60661** Ablation of 1 or more thyroid nodule(s), additional lobe, percutaneous, including imaging guidance, radiofrequency (List separately in addition to code for primary procedure)

▶(Use 60661 in conjunction with 60660)◀

▶(Do not report 60661 in conjunction with 76940, 76942, 77013, 77022)◀

Rationale

A new Category I code (60660) has been established to report percutaneous radiofrequency ablation of one or more thyroid nodules in one lobe or the isthmus and includes imaging guidance for the procedure. In addition, a new add-on code (60661) has been established to report percutaneous radiofrequency ablation of one or more thyroid nodules in an additional lobe with the necessary imaging guidance.

In accordance with the establishment of codes 60660 and 60661, several parenthetical notes have been added to provide guidance for the appropriate reporting of these new codes. In addition, a parenthetical note instructs users on how to report laser ablation of benign thyroid nodules.

Clinical Example (60660)

A 45-year-old female presents with dysphagia and has a benign thyroid nodule in the lower pole of the right lobe. The patient is seeking treatment for symptom relief.

Description of Procedure (60660)

Using an in-plane oblique approach, advance the ablation probe into the target lesion under continuous ultrasound guidance. Using a thyroid-specific ablation technique, perform repetitive small-volume overlapping ablations with intermittent probe repositioning. Perform this technique with continuous monitoring using ultrasound by leaving the probe in place until the surrounding tissue is hyperechoic by ultrasound and then move the probe into a new position for further ablation. Continue this from deep to superficial until the lesion is treated, preserving an untreated margin of 3 to 5 mm to avoid damage to other neck structures. Then remove the probe and achieve hemostasis with light manual compression for an extended period of time. The physician performs post-ablation ultrasound to evaluate for color Doppler signal in the treated nodule to evaluate for treatment completion and that there is no undertreatment or complicating feature and records the permanent ultrasound images.

Clinical Example (60661)

A 45-year-old female presents with dysphagia and has a benign thyroid nodule in the lower pole of the right lobe and a benign thyroid nodule in the midpole of the left lobe. The patient is seeking treatment for symptom relief. [**Note:** This is an add-on code for the additional work related to ablating an additional nodule in the additional thyroid lobe. The work related to the first ablation is reported separately as the primary procedure and not included in the work of this add-on code.]

Description of Procedure (60661)

Following the ablation of a known benign thyroid nodule in one lobe, perform an ultrasound evaluation of the contralateral lobe to locate the new benign target lesion. Overlying gas from the previous ablation may obstruct the view of the lesion, which may make locating the second lesion more difficult. Anesthetize the overlying soft tissues with local anesthesia. Using an in-plane oblique approach, advance the ablation probe into the lesion under continuous ultrasound guidance. Using a thyroid-specific ablation technique, perform repetitive small-volume overlapping ablations with intermittent electrode repositioning. Perform this technique with continuous monitoring using ultrasound by leaving the probe in place until the surrounding tissue is hyperechoic by ultrasound, and then move the probe into a new position for further ablation. Continue from deep to superficial until the lesion is treated, preserving an untreated margin of 3 to 5 mm to avoid damage to other structures. The physician performs post-ablation ultrasound to evaluate for color Doppler signal in the additionally treated nodule to ensure the treatment is complete and that there is no undertreatment or complicating feature and records the permanent ultrasound images.

60699   Unlisted procedure, endocrine system

Nervous System

Skull, Meninges, and Brain

Stereotaxis

● **61715**   Magnetic resonance image guided high intensity focused ultrasound (MRgFUS), stereotactic ablation of target, intracranial, including stereotactic navigation and frame placement, when performed

▶(Do not report 61715 in conjunction with 61781, 61800)◀

▶(Do not report 61715 in conjunction with 70540, 70542, 70543, 70544, 70545, 70546, 70551, 70552, 70553, when performed in the same session)◀

Rationale

One new Category I code (61715) has been established to report intracranial stereotactic target ablation using magnetic resonance image-guided high intensity–focused ultrasound. To support the addition of this new code, two exclusionary parenthetical notes have been added to clarify the appropriate reporting of this code. Several existing parenthetical notes have been revised with the removal of code 0398T.

Code 61715 describes a noninvasive method to ablate tissue within the skull without open surgery. It may be used to treat medically refractory movement disorders, such as essential tremors, with a noninvasive thalamotomy. The method involves performing an ultrasound to ablate tissue at the focal point of the beams. The code descriptor lists all services inherently included as part of the procedure. In addition, to accommodate the addition of the new code, Category III code 0398T and its cross-reference parenthetical note have been deleted. Parenthetical notes following the code have been added to note the deletion of code 0398T and to direct users to code 61715.

An exclusionary parenthetical note restricts reporting code 61715 in conjunction with cranial stereotactic computer–assisted (navigational) procedure (61781) or the application of a stereotactic headframe (61800). In addition, an exclusionary parenthetical note following code 61715 has been added to restrict reporting code 61715 in conjunction with various imaging procedures (70540-70546, 70551-70553) when performed during the same session.

Clinical Example (61715)

A 73-year-old male presents with a 21-year history of essential tremor that has progressed to disabling action tremor in both upper extremities, despite repeated trials of several anti-tremor medications. The patient has age-typical comorbidities with significant disabilities due to essential tremor despite medical treatment. At this stage, he was referred for magnetic resonance (MR)-guided, focused ultrasound for intracranial ablation (thalamotomy).

Description of Procedure (61715)

Import the previous high-resolution MR and computed tomography (CT) images into the workstation, and the treating physician reviews them to identify and mark any calcifications within the brain that can interfere with the ultrasound beam paths that must be excluded from treatment. Mark the sinuses and disable any beams that potentially traverse those spaces. Acquire initial planning images of the patient and fuse pre-treatment CT and real-time MR images. Identify the target on the MR images and compare to the focal point of the transducer. Realign the stereotactic frame to the transducer to place the target within 5 mm of the transducer focal point. Evaluate the patient's tremor symptoms as a baseline for comparison throughout the procedure. Initiate low-intensity (nontreatment level) sonications to align the focal point of the transducer to the anatomic target. Apply sonications to raise tissue temperature by 2° to 5°C. Measure the heat with real-time MR imaging (MRI) and re-aim the transducer to align the actual heat spot in the patient with the intended target. Repeat this process until the actual heat spot coincides with the anatomic target. Next, increase the energy of the transducer to heat the target by 8° to 14°C. During this phase, the physician evaluates the response of the patient's tremor and the emergence of any potential unwanted side effects. Based on the patient's physiologic response, the physician evaluates the likely structure being heated and adjusts the treatment accordingly. Repeat the process as needed and re-aim the transducer until the treatment is applied at the proper physiologic location. Once the treatment location is precisely identified, apply sonication(s) to raise the temperature to approximately 60°C. Perform continuous patient monitoring to evaluate symptom relief and any potential side effects. Repeat sonications until the desired treatment effect is noted.

| 61720 | Creation of lesion by stereotactic method, including burr hole(s) and localizing and recording techniques, single or multiple stages; globus pallidus or thalamus |
| 61735 | subcortical structure(s) other than globus pallidus or thalamus |

Extracranial Nerves, Peripheral Nerves, and Autonomic Nervous System

Introduction/Injection of Anesthetic Agent (Nerve Block), Diagnostic or Therapeutic

Somatic Nerves

Codes 64400-64489 describe the introduction/injection of an anesthetic agent and/or steroid into the somatic nervous system for diagnostic or therapeutic purposes. For injection or destruction of genicular nerve branches, see 64454, 64624, respectively.

Codes 64400-64450, 64454 describe the injection of an anesthetic agent(s) and/or steroid into a nerve plexus, nerve, or branch. These codes are reported once per nerve plexus, nerve, or branch as described in the descriptor regardless of the number of injections performed along the nerve plexus, nerve, or branch described by the code.

Imaging guidance and localization may be reported separately for 64400, 64405, 64408, 64420, 64421, 64425, 64430, 64435, 64449, 64450. Imaging guidance and any injection of contrast are inclusive components of 64415, 64416, 64417, 64445, 64446, 64447, 64448, 64451, 64454.

Codes 64455, 64479, 64480, 64483, 64484 are reported for single or multiple injections on the same site. For 64479, 64480, 64483, 64484, imaging guidance (fluoroscopy or CT) and any injection of contrast are inclusive components and are not reported separately. For 64455, imaging guidance (ultrasound, fluoroscopy, CT) and localization may be reported separately.

▶Codes 64461, 64462, 64463 describe injection of a paravertebral block (PVB). Codes 64486, 64487, 64488, 64489 describe injection of an abdominal fascial plane block. Imaging guidance and any injection of contrast are inclusive components of 64461, 64462, 64463, 64486, 64487, 64488, 64489 and are not reported separately.◀

64400	Injection(s), anesthetic agent(s) and/or steroid; trigeminal nerve, each branch (ie, ophthalmic, maxillary, mandibular)
64466	Code is out of numerical sequence. See 64483-64487
64467	Code is out of numerical sequence. See 64483-64487
64468	Code is out of numerical sequence. See 64483-64487
64469	Code is out of numerical sequence. See 64483-64487

64473	Code is out of numerical sequence. See 64483-64487
64474	Code is out of numerical sequence. See 64483-64487
# 64461	Paravertebral block (PVB) (paraspinous block), thoracic; single injection site (includes imaging guidance, when performed)
#+ 64462	second and any additional injection site(s) (includes imaging guidance, when performed) (List separately in addition to code for primary procedure)

(Use 64462 in conjunction with 64461)

(Do not report 64462 more than once per day)

| # 64463 | continuous infusion by catheter (includes imaging guidance, when performed) |

(Do not report 64461, 64462, 64463 in conjunction with 62320, 62324, 64420, 64421, 64479, 64480, 64490, 64491, 64492, 76942, 77002, 77003)

| #● 64466 | Thoracic fascial plane block, unilateral; by injection(s), including imaging guidance, when performed |
| #● 64467 | by continuous infusion(s), including imaging guidance, when performed |

▶(Do not report 64466, 64467 in conjunction with 76942, 77001, 77002, 77012, 77021)◀

| #● 64468 | Thoracic fascial plane block, bilateral; by injection(s), including imaging guidance, when performed |
| #● 64469 | by continuous infusion(s), including imaging guidance, when performed |

▶(Do not report 64468, 64469 in conjunction with 76942, 77001, 77002, 77012, 77021)◀

| #● 64473 | Lower extremity fascial plane block, unilateral; by injection(s), including imaging guidance, when performed |
| #● 64474 | by continuous infusion(s), including imaging guidance, when performed |

▶(Do not report 64473, 64474 in conjunction with 76942, 77001, 77002, 77012, 77021)◀

Rationale

Codes 64466-64474 have been established to report unilateral (64466, 64467) and bilateral (64468, 64469) thoracic and unilateral lower extremity (LE) (64473, 64474) fascial plane blocks. Guidelines and parenthetical notes have been revised and added throughout the CPT 2025 code set to accommodate the addition of the new codes.

Fascial plane blocks are regional anesthesia techniques that administer local anesthetics for postoperative pain control and analgesia. For these procedures, the space (or "plane") between two discrete fascial layers is the target of needle insertion and injection. Local anesthetic spreads to the nerves and travels within this plane to adjacent tissues to achieve analgesic pain control. Codes

Surgery / Nervous System 61000-64999

64486-64489 are reported for abdominal level blocks performed on the transverse abdominal plane (TAP). The descriptors for codes 64466-64469 identify thoracic blocks and include language that designates (1) where the injections are performed (ie, thoracic), (2) laterality of the injection (ie, unilateral or bilateral), and (3) how the anesthetic is administered (ie, injection vs continuous infusion[s]). Codes 64473 and 64474 have been established to report these same services for LE fascial block and pain management services and include the same differentiations as previously noted for thoracic blocks (ie, location, laterality, and administration type).

Guidelines and parenthetical notes in the code set have been added and updated to accommodate the addition of the new codes, where appropriate. This includes the addition of new exclusionary parenthetical notes and the addition of codes 64466-64474 to certain existing, exclusionary parenthetical notes throughout the code set. These exclusionary parenthetical notes list imaging guidance services that are inherently included as part of the new fascial block procedures, such as certain ultrasound, fluoroscopy, and computed tomography guidance procedures.

The changes to guidelines and parenthetical notes also include the updated guidelines to reflect "abdominal fascial plane" instead of "TAP" to provide terminology within instructions that aligns with the language of the new codes and the appropriate codes to report abdominal fascial plane block procedures (64486-64489).

Clinical Example (64466)

A 45-year-old female undergoes breast surgery under general anesthesia. To provide postoperative pain control and minimize opioid usage, a thoracic fascial plane block is placed.

Description of Procedure (64466)

Place an ultrasound transducer over the target area for the thoracic fascial plane block. Using continuous ultrasound guidance, identify the thoracic wall layers. Visualize correct needle location by hydrodissection. After identifying the appropriate anatomic structures, advance a needle into the interfascial plane. Inject local anesthetic (eg, 0.25% bupivacaine).

Clinical Example (64467)

A 59-year-old female undergoes cardiac surgery via a minimally invasive approach and limited right thoracotomy under general anesthesia. To provide postoperative pain control and minimize opioid usage, a thoracic fascial plane block with catheter placement for continuous infusion is placed.

Description of Procedure (64467)

Place an ultrasound transducer over the target area for the thoracic fascial plane block. Using continuous ultrasound guidance, identify the thoracic wall layers. Then insert the placement needle deep into the erector spinae muscle. Visualize the correct needle location by hydrodissection. After identifying the appropriate anatomic structures, insert a catheter through the placement needle and remove the needle. Secure the catheter and then apply a sterile occlusive dressing. Infuse local anesthetic (eg, 0.25% bupivacaine) unilaterally into the fascial plane.

Clinical Example (64468)

A 65-year-old female undergoes bilateral breast surgery under general anesthesia. To provide postoperative pain control and minimize opioid usage, a bilateral thoracic fascial plane block is placed.

Description of Procedure (64468)

Place an ultrasound transducer over the target area for the thoracic fascial plane block. Using continuous ultrasound guidance, identify the thoracic wall layers. Visualize correct needle location by hydrodissection. After identifying the appropriate anatomic structures, advance a needle into the interfascial plane. Inject local anesthetic (eg, 0.25% bupivacaine). Then carry out a repeat procedure in an identical fashion on the opposite side.

Clinical Example (64469)

A 75-year-old female undergoes cardiac surgery by median sternotomy under general anesthesia. To provide postoperative pain control and minimize opioid usage, a bilateral thoracic fascial plane block with catheter placement for continuous infusion is placed.

Description of Procedure (64469)

Place an ultrasound transducer over the target area for the thoracic fascial plane block. Using continuous ultrasound guidance, identify the thoracic wall layers. Then insert the placement needle deep into the erector spinae muscle. Visualize correct needle location by hydrodissection. After identifying the appropriate anatomic structures, insert a catheter through the placement needle and remove the needle. Secure the catheter and then apply a sterile occlusive dressing. Perform a repeat procedure in an identical fashion on the opposite side. Deliver local anesthetic (eg, 0.25% bupivacaine) via two separate infusion pumps.

Clinical Example (64473)

A 55-year-old female undergoes elective total hip arthroplasty under general anesthesia. To provide postoperative pain control and minimize opioid usage, a lower extremity fascial plane block is placed.

Description of Procedure (64473)

Place an ultrasound transducer over the target area for the lower extremity fascial plane block. Using continuous ultrasound guidance, identify the appropriate tissue plane for the fascia iliaca block. Visualize correct needle location by hydrodissection. After identifying the appropriate anatomic structures, insert a needle between the fascia iliaca and iliacus muscle. Inject local anesthetic (eg, 0.25% bupivacaine).

Clinical Example (64474)

An 81-year-old female undergoes hip fracture repair under general anesthesia. To provide postoperative pain control and minimize opioid usage, a lower extremity fascial plane block with catheter placement for continuous infusion is placed.

Description of Procedure (64474)

Place an ultrasound transducer in an axial (transverse) plane over the target area for the lower extremity fascial plane block. Using continuous ultrasound guidance, identify the appropriate tissue plane for the fascia iliaca block. Then insert the placement needle between the fascia iliaca and the iliacus muscle. Visualize correct needle location by hydrodissection. After identifying the appropriate anatomic structures, insert a catheter through the placement needle and remove the needle. Secure the catheter and then apply a sterile occlusive dressing. Infuse local anesthetic (eg, 0.25% bupivacaine) unilaterally into the fascial plane.

Neurostimulators (Peripheral Nerve)

64553 Percutaneous implantation of neurostimulator electrode array; cranial nerve

(For percutaneous electrical stimulation of a cranial nerve using needle[s] or needle electrode[s] [eg, PENS, PNT], use 64999)

(For open placement of cranial nerve (eg, vagus, trigeminal) neurostimulator pulse generator or receiver, see 61885, 61886, as appropriate)

▶(For open implantation of vagus nerve integrated neurostimulation system, see 0908T, 0909T)◀

64568 Open implantation of cranial nerve (eg, vagus nerve) neurostimulator electrode array and pulse generator

(Do not report 64568 in conjunction with 61885, 61886, 64570)

▶(For open implantation of vagus nerve integrated neurostimulation system, see 0908T, 0909T)◀

64569 Revision or replacement of cranial nerve (eg, vagus nerve) neurostimulator electrode array, including connection to existing pulse generator

(Do not report 64569 in conjunction with 64570 or 61888)

(For replacement of pulse generator, use 61885)

64570 Removal of cranial nerve (eg, vagus nerve) neurostimulator electrode array and pulse generator

(Do not report 64570 in conjunction with 61888)

▶(For removal of vagus nerve integrated neurostimulation system, use 0910T)◀

Rationale

New parenthetical notes have been added in the Neurostimulators (Peripheral Nerve) subsection of the Extracranial Nerves, Peripheral Nerves, and Autonomic Nervous System section to direct users to the appropriate codes for vagus nerve-integrated neurostimulation system procedures.

Refer to the codebook and the Rationale for codes 0908T-0912T for a full discussion of the changes.

64595 Revision or removal of peripheral, sacral, or gastric neurostimulator pulse generator or receiver, with detachable connection to electrode array

(For revision or removal of percutaneous electrode array with integrated neurostimulator, use 64598)

Eye and Ocular Adnexa

Anterior Segment

Iris, Ciliary Body

Repair

66680 Repair of iris, ciliary body (as for iridodialysis)

(For reposition or resection of uveal tissue with perforating wound of cornea or sclera, use 65285)

66682 Suture of iris, ciliary body (separate procedure) with retrieval of suture through small incision (eg, McCannel suture)

● **66683**   Implantation of iris prosthesis, including suture fixation and repair or removal of iris, when performed

▶(Use 66683 in conjunction with 66825, 66830, 66840, 66850, 66852, 66920, 66930, 66940, 66982, 66983, 66984, 66985, 66986, 66987, 66988, 66989, 66991, for lens or intraocular lens surgery[ies] performed concurrently)◀

▶(Do not report 66683 in conjunction with 65800, 65810, 65815, 65865, 65870, 65875, 66020, 66030, 66500, 66505, 66600, 66625, 66630, 66635, 66680, 66682, 66770, 67500, 67515, 69990, for the same eye, same surgeon, or same operative session)◀

▶(For severing adhesions of anterior segment, incisional technique, without concurrent iris prosthesis implantation, see 65865, 65870, 65875, 65880)◀

▶(For removal of iris tissue without concurrent iris prosthesis implantation, see 66600, 66605, 66625, 66630, 66635)◀

▶(For repair of iris without concurrent iris prosthesis implantation, see 66680, 66682)◀

Rationale

Category I code 66683 has been established to report the implantation of an iris prosthesis, including suture fixation and repair or removal of the iris when performed. In addition, a number of parenthetical notes have been established to accommodate the addition of the new code.

Insertion of an iris prosthesis is performed for patients with conditions such as aniridia (absence of the iris) or traumatic injury to the iris. Damage to the iris may cause visual function deficiencies such as photophobia and disabling glare. This ophthalmic surgery treats diseases of the eye such as acquired aniridia.

In support of the establishment of code 66683, Category III codes 0616T-0618T have been deleted. These codes have been deleted and converted to Category I code 66683, consolidating all three procedures formerly described in the three deleted codes.

Inclusionary, exclusionary, and cross-reference parenthetical notes have been added following code 66683 to instruct users on the appropriate reporting of code 66683, as well as to direct users to other codes. This includes parenthetical notes that provide guidance for other services that may be additionally reported and services that are excluded from reporting in conjunction with the new procedure.

Clinical Example (66683)

A 44-year-old male patient presents with acquired aniridia from a penetrating injury to the left eyelid, cornea, iris, and lens. Emergency treatment at the time of the injury stabilized the left eye; however, the patient has persistent debilitating glare from partial aniridia. The surgeon implants an artificial iris in front of the previously implanted intraocular lens (IOL).

Description of Procedure (66683)

Perform a paracentesis into the anterior chamber superiorly. Make a self-sealing, clear corneal incision temporally. Insert a vitrectomy handpiece through the corneal incision and place a chamber maintainer in the paracentesis. Remove the vitreous present in the anterior chamber with the high-speed vitreous cutter and aspiration. Inject a viscoelastic agent to deepen the anterior chamber. Use a viscoelastic and sharp dissection to release synechiae between the remaining iris anteriorly and the lens capsule and intraocular lens posteriorly. Excise necrotic iris tissue. Control bleeding with intraocular epinephrine and injection of viscoelastic. Test the centration and stability of the IOL with hooks. Center the IOL/capsular bag complex and stabilize with a capsular tension ring. Place a scleral pocket and polypropylene scleral sutures as needed. Place radial incisions in areas of the fibrotic anterior capsule to relieve capsular phimosis.

Use a 27-gauge needle attached to a viscoelastic syringe to dissect the anterior lens capsule from the surface of the previously implanted IOL. Use calipers to measure the white-to-white distance to size the artificial iris implant. Trephine the implant to the appropriate diameter. Use microscissors to create two peripheral iridotomies in the implant. Load the iris implant into an injection cartridge lined with viscoelastic. Insert the cartridge tip through the corneal incision and advance the implant into the anterior chamber. Use hooks to position the implant in the capsular bag if the capsule has been fully freed from the IOL surface. Otherwise, place the implant in the sulcus anterior to the IOL/capsular bag complex. Use polypropylene sutures as needed to stabilize the implant when there are peripheral defects in the zonular support system. Aspirate the remaining viscoelastic with an irrigation/aspiration/cutter handpiece. Remove any residual vitreous from the anterior chamber with the vitrectomy handpiece. Adjust the pressure in the eye by injecting intraocular balanced salt solution. Test the incisions for integrity and place corneoscleral sutures as needed. Remove the lid speculum and drapes. Patch the eye and shield with antibiotic ointment.

★ = Telemedicine   ◀ = Audio-only   ✚ = Add-on code   ⁄ᴎ = FDA approval pending   # = Resequenced code   ⊘ = Modifier 51 exempt

Posterior Segment

Retina or Choroid

Destruction

67229   Treatment of extensive or progressive retinopathy, 1 or more sessions, preterm infant (less than 37 weeks gestation at birth), performed from birth up to 1 year of age (eg, retinopathy of prematurity), photocoagulation or cryotherapy

(For bilateral procedure, use modifier 50 with 67208, 67210, 67218, 67220, 67227, 67228, 67229)

(For unlisted procedures on retina, use 67299)

▶(For photobiomodulation therapy of retina, single session, use 0936T)◀

Rationale

In accordance with the addition of Category III code 0936T, a cross-reference parenthetical note has been added following code 67229.

Refer to the codebook and the Rationale for code 0936T for a full discussion of these changes.

Notes

Radiology

Summary of Additions, Deletions, and Revisions

The summary of changes shows the actual changes that have been made to the code descriptors.

New codes appear with a bullet (●) and are indicated as "Code added." Revised codes are preceded with a triangle (▲). Within revised codes, or if a code symbol has been deleted, the deleted language and code symbol appear with a ~~strikethrough~~, while new text appears <u>underlined</u>.

The ∕ symbol is used to identify codes for vaccines that are pending FDA approval. The # symbol is used to identify codes that have been resequenced. CPT add-on codes are annotated by the + symbol. The ⊘ symbol is used to identify codes that are exempt from the use of modifier 51. The ★ symbol is used to identify codes that may be used for reporting telemedicine services. The ✣ symbol is used to identify a proprietary laboratory analyses (PLA) test that has an identical descriptor as another PLA test. A PLA code that satisfies Category I code criteria and has been accepted by the CPT Editorial Panel is annotated with the ↕ symbol. The ◀ symbol is used to identify codes that may be used to report audio-only telemedicine services when appended by modifier 93 **(see Appendix T)**.

Code	Description
#●76014	Code added
#+●76015	Code added
#●76016	Code added
#⊘●76017	Code added
#⊘●76018	Code added
#⊘●76019	Code added

Radiology

Diagnostic Radiology (Diagnostic Imaging)

Head and Neck

70551   Magnetic resonance (eg, proton) imaging, brain (including brain stem); without contrast material

70552   with contrast material(s)

70553   without contrast material, followed by contrast material(s) and further sequences

     (For magnetic spectroscopy, use 76390)

▶Functional MRI involves identification and mapping of stimulation of brain function. When neurofunctional tests are administered by a technologist or other non-physician or non-psychologist, use 70554. When neurofunctional tests are entirely administered by a physician or other qualified health care professional or psychologist, use 70555.◀

Rationale

In accordance with efforts to standardize references to "nonphysician qualified health care professional" throughout the Current Procedural Terminology (CPT) 2025 code set, the guidelines following code 70553 have been revised to include "or other qualified health care professional."

Refer to the codebook and the Rationale for the Medical Team Conferences subsection guidelines for a full discussion of these changes.

Heart

Cardiac magnetic imaging differs from traditional magnetic resonance imaging (MRI) in its ability to provide a physiologic evaluation of cardiac function. Traditional MRI relies on static images to obtain clinical diagnoses based upon anatomic information. Improvement in spatial and temporal resolution has expanded the application from an anatomic test and includes physiologic evaluation of cardiac function. Flow and velocity assessment for valves and intracardiac shunts is performed in addition to a function and morphologic evaluation. Use 75559 with 75565 to report flow with pharmacologic wall motion stress evaluation without contrast. Use 75563 with 75565 to report flow with pharmacologic perfusion stress with contrast.

Cardiac MRI for velocity flow mapping can be reported in conjunction with 75557, 75559, 75561, or 75563.

▶Listed procedures may be performed independently or in the course of overall medical care. If the individual providing these services is also responsible for diagnostic workup and/or follow-up care of the patient, also see appropriate sections. Only one procedure in the series 75557-75563 is appropriately reported per session.

To report absolute quantitation of myocardial blood flow (AQMBF), cardiac magnetic resonance (CMR), see 0899T, 0900T. Report 0899T, 0900T in conjunction with code for primary procedure.◀

Rationale

The introductory guidelines for the Heart subsection in the Diagnostic Radiology (Diagnostic Imaging) subsection have been revised by removing the sentence "Only one add-on code for flow velocity can be reported per session" and adding new introductory guideline language to clarify when it is appropriate to report codes 0899T and 0900T for absolute quantitation of myocardial blood flow (AQMBF) and cardiac magnetic resonance (CMR) in conjunction with the codes for primary procedures.

Refer to the codebook and the Rationale for codes 0899T and 0900T for a full discussion of these changes.

Cardiac MRI studies may be performed at rest and/or during pharmacologic stress. Therefore, the appropriate stress testing code from the 93015-93018 series should be reported in addition to 75559 or 75563.

Cardiac computed tomography (CT) and coronary computed tomographic angiography (CTA) include the axial source images of the pre-contrast, arterial phase sequence, and venous phase sequence (if performed), as well as the two-dimensional and three-dimensional reformatted images resulting from the study, including cine review. Each of the contrast enhanced cardiac CT and coronary CTA codes (75572, 75573, 75574) includes conventional quantitative assessment(s) intrinsic to the service listed in the code descriptor (ie, quantification of coronary percentage stenosis, ventricular volume[s], ejection fraction[s], and stroke volume[s]), when performed. Report only one computed tomography heart service per encounter (75571, 75572, 75573, 75574).

     (For separate injection procedures for vascular radiology, see **Surgery** section, 36000-36299)

     (For cardiac catheterization procedures, see 93451-93572)

   ★ = Telemedicine   ◀ = Audio-only   ✚ = Add-on code   ⁄ = FDA approval pending   # = Resequenced code   ⊘ = Modifier 51 exempt

75561 Cardiac magnetic resonance imaging for morphology and function without contrast material(s), followed by contrast material(s) and further sequences;

75563 with stress imaging

▶(Use 75563 in conjunction with 0899T, 0900T for absolute quantification of myocardial blood flow [AQMBF] with cardiac magnetic resonance [CMR])◀

Rationale

In accordance with the establishment of Category III codes 0899T and 0900T, an instructional parenthetical note following code 75563 has been added to direct users to add-on codes 0899T and 0900T for AQMBF with CMR.

Refer to the codebook and the Rationale for codes 0899T and 0900T for a full discussion of these changes.

Vascular Procedures

Aorta and Arteries

Selective vascular catheterizations should be coded to include introduction and all lesser order selective catheterizations used in the approach (eg, the description for a selective right middle cerebral artery catheterization includes the introduction and placement catheterization of the right common and internal carotid arteries).

Additional second and/or third order arterial catheterizations within the same family of arteries supplied by a single first order artery should be expressed by 36218 or 36248. Additional first order or higher catheterizations in vascular families supplied by a first order vessel different from a previously selected and coded family should be separately coded using the conventions described above.

The lower extremity endovascular revascularization codes describing services performed for occlusive disease (37220-37235) include catheterization (36200, 36140, 36245-36248) in the work described by the codes. Catheterization codes are not additionally reported for diagnostic lower extremity angiography when performed through the same access site as the therapy (37220-37235) performed in the same session. However, catheterization for the diagnostic lower extremity angiogram may be reported separately if a different arterial puncture site is necessary.

For angiography performed in conjunction with therapeutic transcatheter radiological supervision and interpretation services, see the radiology **Transcatheter Procedures** guidelines.

Diagnostic angiography (radiological supervision and interpretation) codes should NOT be used with interventional procedures for:

1. Contrast injections, angiography, roadmapping, and/or fluoroscopic guidance for the intervention,

2. Vessel measurement, and

3. Post-angioplasty/stent/atherectomy angiography, as this work is captured in the radiological supervision and interpretation code(s). In those therapeutic codes that include radiological supervision and interpretation, this work is captured in the therapeutic code.

Diagnostic angiography performed at the time of an interventional procedure is separately reportable if:

1. No prior catheter-based angiographic study is available and a full diagnostic study is performed, and the decision to intervene is based on the diagnostic study, OR

2. A prior study is available, but as documented in the medical record:

   a. The patient's condition with respect to the clinical indication has changed since the prior study, OR

   b. There is inadequate visualization of the anatomy and/or pathology, OR

   c. There is a clinical change during the procedure that requires new evaluation outside the target area of intervention.

▶Diagnostic angiography performed at a separate session from an interventional procedure is separately reported.◀

If diagnostic angiography is necessary, is performed at the same session as the interventional procedure and meets the above criteria, modifier 59 must be appended to the diagnostic radiological supervision and interpretation code(s) to denote that diagnostic work has been done following these guidelines.

Diagnostic angiography performed at the time of an interventional procedure is NOT separately reportable if it is specifically included in the interventional code descriptor.

▶Add-on code 75774 may be used with both arteries and veins for each additional vessel.◀

(For intravenous procedure, see 36000, 36005-36015, and for intra-arterial procedure, see 36100-36248)

(For radiological supervision and interpretation, see 75600-75893)

Rationale

The aorta and arteries guidelines in the Vascular Procedures subsection have been revised for clarification by including a sentence stating that add-on code 75774

Radiology 70010-79999

(angiography) may be used with both arteries and veins for each additional vessel, ending any possible confusion over the use of the code.

75600   Aortography, thoracic, without serialography, radiological supervision and interpretation

(For supravalvular aortography performed at the time of cardiac catheterization, use 93567, which includes imaging supervision, interpretation, and report)

+ 75774   Angiography, selective, each additional vessel studied after basic examination, radiological supervision and interpretation (List separately in addition to code for primary procedure)

(Use 75774 in addition to code for specific initial vessel studied)

(Do not report 75774 as part of diagnostic angiography of the extracranial and intracranial cervicocerebral vessels. It may be appropriate to report 75774 for diagnostic angiography of upper extremities and other vascular beds performed in the same session)

(For cardiac catheterization procedures, see 93452-93462, 93563, 93564, 93565, 93566, 93567, 93568, 93569, 93573, 93574, 93575, 93593, 93594, 93595, 93596, 93597)

(For radiological supervision and interpretation of dialysis circuit angiography performed through existing access[es] or catheter-based arterial access, use 36901 with modifier 52)

Transcatheter Procedures

75989   Radiological guidance (ie, fluoroscopy, ultrasound, or computed tomography), for percutaneous drainage (eg, abscess, specimen collection), with placement of catheter, radiological supervision and interpretation

(Do not report 75989 in conjunction with 10030, 32554, 32555, 32556, 32557, 33017, 33018, 33019, 47490, 49405, 49406, 49407)

▶Magnetic Resonance Safety Implant/Foreign Body Procedures◀

▶Implanted medical devices or foreign bodies can increase the risk of injury or death for a patient entering the magnetic resonance (MR) environment, either for diagnostic MR procedures or for procedures performed under MR imaging guidance.

Implants may have FDA-approved labeling specifying conditions under which an MR examination could be safely performed. These conditions can specify the type of MR equipment to use, preparation of the implant before the MR procedure, anatomical regions that should be excluded from MR examination, limitations on MR scan time and energy deposition, and/or implant components that may contraindicate MR examination.

Codes 76014, 76015, 76016 describe MR safety-planning services performed in advance of the date of the MR procedure. For 76014, implant-safety conditions and additional procedures required to safely perform the requested MR examination are documented for inclusion in the medical record by a technologist or other MR safety-trained clinical staff. Contraindications to MR are also documented. For patients with complex, multiple, or incompletely documented implants, use 76015 to report prolonged MR safety implant/foreign body assessment by clinical staff. For an implant and/or foreign body that lacks MR conditional labeling, is contraindicated for MR, or may result in a limited MR examination, use 76016 to report the performance of an MR safety determination by a physician or other qualified health care professional (QHP) responsible for the safe performance of the MR procedure, with a written report.

Codes 76017, 76018, 76019 describe MR safety services performed on the day of the MR examination under supervision of the physician or other QHP responsible for the safe performance of the MR procedure. The need for these services depends on the design of the medical implant, and the MR conditional labeling of the implant, if available. Use 76017 to report medical physics services provided during the MR examination, with a written report. Use 76018 to report the preparation and documentation of an electronic implant into an MR-protective mode. Use 76019 to report specified positioning and/or immobilization of an implant during the MR examination, with documentation for inclusion in the medical record.

Cardiac devices (eg, pacemakers and defibrillators) may require interrogation or programming services before or after the performance of the MR examination to put them in a mode safe for the MR scan. For cardiac device interrogation or programming, see the appropriate cardiac device evaluation code. Similarly, neurostimulation devices may require analysis-programming before being placed into an MR-protective mode, or after the performance of the MR examination. For electronic analysis-programming of neurostimulation devices, see the appropriate analysis-programming code. If cardiac device evaluation or neurostimulator analysis-programming is performed on the same day, report 76018 only if a separate individual performs additional preparation of the electronic implant into an MR-protective mode immediately before patient entry to the MR environment. For reprogramming of programmable cerebrospinal shunt after the performance of the MR examination, use 62252.◀

#● **76014**   MR safety implant and/or foreign body assessment by trained clinical staff, including identification and verification of implant components from appropriate sources (eg, surgical reports, imaging reports, medical device databases, device vendors, review of prior imaging), analyzing current MR conditional status of individual components and systems, and consulting published professional guidance with written report; initial 15 minutes

#+● **76015**   each additional 30 minutes (List separately in addition to code for primary procedure)

▶(Use 76015 in conjunction with 76014)◀

▶(Do not report 76015 more than three times per encounter)◀

#● **76016**   MR safety determination by a physician or other qualified health care professional responsible for the safety of the MR procedure, including review of implant MR conditions for indicated MR examination, analysis of risk vs clinical benefit of performing MR examination, and determination of MR equipment, accessory equipment, and expertise required to perform examination, with written report

#⊘● **76017**   MR safety medical physics examination customization, planning and performance monitoring by medical physicist or MR safety expert, with review and analysis by physician or other qualified health care professional to prioritize and select views and imaging sequences, to tailor MR acquisition specific to restrictive requirements or artifacts associated with MR conditional implants or to mitigate risk of non-conditional implants or foreign bodies, with written report

▶(Use 76017 in conjunction with 76018, 76019, when implant requires electronics preparation or positioning and/or immobilization before MR)◀

#⊘● **76018**   MR safety implant electronics preparation under supervision of physician or other qualified health care professional, including MR-specific programming of pulse generator and/or transmitter to verify device integrity, protection of device internal circuitry from MR electromagnetic fields, and protection of patient from risks of unintended stimulation or heating while in the MR room, with written report

▶(Use 76018 in conjunction with 76017, when implant also requires medical physics examination customization)◀

#⊘● **76019**   MR safety implant positioning and/or immobilization under supervision of physician or other qualified health care professional, including application of physical protections to secure implanted medical device from MR-induced translational or vibrational forces, magnetically induced functional changes, and/or prevention of radiofrequency burns from inadvertent tissue contact while in the MR room, with written report

▶(Use 76019 in conjunction with 76017, when implant also requires medical physics examination customization)◀

Rationale

Six new codes (76014-76019) have been established to report magnetic resonance (MR) safety implant or foreign body assessment, MR safety determination, MR safety medical physics examination customization, MR safety implant electronics preparation, and MR safety implant positioning or immobilization. A new subsection with instructional guidelines and parenthetical notes has been established in the Radiology section.

This new subsection describes the work of reviewing records and decision-making when assessing implanted medical devices in patients who may require an MR examination for either diagnostic or interventional reasons. These services differ from evaluation and management (E/M) services because the work performed for an E/M service is not specific to MR safety. While the patient's history may be reviewed, complete MR safety information may not be available.

The new guidelines outline the importance and specific use of these services. Codes 76014-76016 describe MR safety–planning services performed in advance of the date of the MR procedure. Codes 76014 and 76015 include documenting MR conditions, contraindications, and following instructions for equipment and personnel scheduling and do not include independent decision-making. Code 76015 is an add-on code for each additional 30 minutes and should be reported only in conjunction with code 76014. Code 76015 may not be reported more than three times per encounter. Codes 76014 and 76015 are reported when the assessment is performed by trained clinical staff.

Report code 76016 for an MR safety determination and a written report by a physician or other qualified health care professional (QHP) who is responsible for the safe performance of the MR procedure.

Codes 76017-76019 describe MR safety services performed on the day of the MR examination under the supervision of the physician or other QHP responsible for the safe performance of the MR procedure. Parentheticals have been added following each of these codes to provide further guidance on how the codes may be used together.

Report code 76017 for medical physics services provided during the MR examination, including a written report. Codes 76018 and 76019 may be reported in conjunction with code 76017 if an implant requires medical physics examination customization.

Report code 76018 for the preparation and documentation of an electronic implant into an MR-protective mode. Code 76018 may be reported in conjunction with code 76017, when the implant also requires medical physics examination customization.

Radiology 70010-79999

Report code 76019 for the specified positioning and/or immobilization of an implant during the MR examination and the documentation for inclusion in the medical record. Code 76017 may be reported in conjunction with code 76019, when the implant also requires medical physics examination customization.

Codes 76017-76019 are modifier 51-exempt because although these procedures are typically performed with another procedure, they may be reported as stand-alone procedures.

Clinical Example (76014)

A 36-year-old female, who has a vagus nerve neurostimulator to control drug-resistant epilepsy, presents with neck pain after a fall. A magnetic resonance (MR) of the cervical spine is ordered. Eligibility for MR examination of the cervical spine depends on implant model.

Description of Procedure (76014)

N/A

Clinical Example (76015)

A 72-year-old male, who has a spinal cord neurostimulator for pain management, presents with radiculopathy. Magnetic resonance imaging (MRI) of the lumbar spine is ordered. Model information for implanted leads is missing from the local medical record. Magnetic resonance (MR) conditions for the implant are dependent on the lead model, and certain lead models have anatomical exclusion zones over the implant. [**Note:** This is an add-on code for the additional prolonged work when multiple implants, implant components, surgical revisions to the implant, or undocumented implants must be assessed for MR conditional status. The work associated with the first 15 minutes of MR safety implant/foreign body assessment is reported separately with the primary procedure and not included in the work of this add-on code. The work associated with each additional 30 minutes of MR safety implant/foreign body assessment is reported with this add-on code. This add-on code may be reported a maximum of three times per encounter.]

Description of Procedure (76015)

N/A

Clinical Example (76016)

A 70-year-old male, who is on anticoagulation with a pacemaker, presents with elevated prostate-specific antigen and suspected prostate cancer. A 3 Tesla prostate magnetic resonance imaging (MRI) or a 1.5 Tesla

prostate MRI with an endorectal coil is considered as an alternative to standard prostate biopsy. Magnetic resonance (MR) safety assessment demonstrates a pacemaker that is not a complete MR conditional pacemaker system, lacking MR conditional labeling and programming modes.

Description of Procedure (76016)

Review the MR examination parameters for conformance with implanted-device safety instructions, and if they do not, the radiologist decides whether informed consent should be obtained before the MR examination. Consider alternative diagnostic tests for appropriateness and relative risk. The radiologist may make recommendations for alternate diagnostic tests or procedures or MR requirements, including MR equipment, accessory equipment, and the required expertise of qualified health care professionals or clinical staff supervising the preparations or execution of the MR examination, which should be provided in a written report.

Clinical Example (76017)

A 67-year-old female, who has a fully implanted deep brain stimulation (DBS) system for treatment of Parkinson disease, presents with new, onset seizures and right-sided weakness. Magnetic resonance imaging (MRI) is ordered. Magnetic resonance (MR) safety assessment demonstrates all DBS components are part of a complete MR conditional DBS system, with MR conditions restricting scan time and energy deposition. DBS analysis and programming are performed by the patient's neurologist before reporting for the MR examination. The patient's tremor returns with the system programmed to MR mode. A medical physicist is scheduled to interactively customize and monitor the performance of the MR examination to meet restrictive MR conditions of the DBS system.

Description of Procedure (76017)

The radiologist reviews images in real time during examination acquisition for diagnostic quality. Provide feedback to the technologist and medical physicist on whether the image contrast looks correct and if scan parameter adjustments or additional views are necessary. Confirm patient compliance with prolonged scan times and scanner idle times for implant cooling, and revise technique for patient noncompliance or motion artifact. The radiologist will consider additional views to cut from protocol to avoid exceeding the total scan time restrictions of the implant. Dictate implant-related limitations to diagnostic quality and interpretation of performed examination.

Clinical Example (76018)

A 55-year-old female, who has a neurostimulation system, complains of new symptoms of low-back pain, with persistent symptoms following 6 weeks of conservative treatment. A diagnostic magnetic resonance (MR) examination of the lumbar spine is ordered. The patient reports to the MR department with the fully charged patient controller for her sacral nerve modulation system.

Description of Procedure (76018)

Supervise MR-specific programming, monitoring patient tolerance, and side effects of modified therapies. If available, review interrogation results for battery voltage and lead impedances. Assess patient's condition and whether it is appropriate to proceed with the MR examination. Verify MR conditional status and implant programming before patient entrance to the MR scan room. Confirm the lack of complication from implant exposure to MR environment. Evaluate out-of-range parameters.

Clinical Example (76019)

A 26-year-old male, who is diagnosed with neurofibromatosis type 2 with an auditory brainstem implant (ABI), requires a magnetic resonance imaging (MRI) of the brain and the entire spine for annual surveillance of central nervous system (CNS) tumors. Magnetic resonance (MR) safety assessment demonstrates all internal ABI components are part of a complete MR conditional system, with MR conditions requiring the application of a head-wrap immobilization kit to secure an internal magnet within the ABI or the surgical resection of the internal magnet.

Description of Procedure (76019)

For implants requiring immobilization, apply a secure compression bandage over the implant, with a bracing splint directly over the components, a Kerlix bandage, and a self-adherent elastic wrap. The physician or other qualified health care professional monitors the patient's condition during positioning and introduction to the MR scan room. Position the patient on the MR scanner bed outside of the MR scan room, with attention to the implant manufacturer's MR conditional positioning instructions and exclusion zones. Slowly wheel the scanner bed into the MR scan room, dock to the scanner, and advance the imaging volume with slow table speed to reduce translational forces and discomfort at the site of the implant. If the patient cannot tolerate the pain, slowly remove the patient from the MR scanner on the MR scanner bed and remove patient from the MR scan room. After exiting the MR scan room, whether it is from MR examination discontinuation or

completion, remove the compression wrap. Inspect the implant location for evidence of implant migration, malfunction, or tissue damage. Provide the patient with educational materials for when to seek follow-up for their implant if pain persists. Document implant positioning and immobilization precautions in a written report along with positioning/immobilization recommendations for future MR examination orders.

Other Procedures

76010	Radiologic examination from nose to rectum for foreign body, single view, child
76014	Code is out of numerical sequence. See 75984-76010
76015	Code is out of numerical sequence. See 75984-76010
76016	Code is out of numerical sequence. See 75984-76010
76017	Code is out of numerical sequence. See 75984-76010
76018	Code is out of numerical sequence. See 75984-76010
76019	Code is out of numerical sequence. See 75984-76010
76376	3D rendering with interpretation and reporting of computed tomography, magnetic resonance imaging, ultrasound, or other tomographic modality with image postprocessing under concurrent supervision; not requiring image postprocessing on an independent workstation

(Use 76376 in conjunction with code[s] for base imaging procedure[s])

▶(Do not report 76376 in conjunction with 31627, 34839, 70496, 70498, 70544, 70545, 70546, 70547, 70548, 70549, 71275, 71555, 72159, 72191, 72198, 73206, 73225, 73706, 73725, 74174, 74175, 74185, 74261, 74262, 74263, 75557, 75559, 75561, 75563, 75565, 75571, 75572, 75573, 75574, 75635, 76377, 77046, 77047, 77048, 77049, 77061, 77062, 77063, 78012-78999, 93319, 93355, 0523T, 0559T, 0560T, 0561T, 0562T, 0623T, 0624T, 0625T, 0626T, 0633T, 0634T, 0635T, 0636T, 0637T, 0638T, 0710T, 0711T, 0712T, 0713T, 0876T)◀

(For noninvasive arterial plaque analysis using software processing of data from computerized tomography angiography to quantify structure and composition of the vessel wall, including assessment for lipid-rich necrotic core plaque, see 0710T, 0711T, 0712T, 0713T)

76377	requiring image postprocessing on an independent workstation

(Use 76377 in conjunction with code[s] for base imaging procedure[s])

Radiology 70010-79999

Radiology 70010-79999

▶(Do not report 76377 in conjunction with 34839, 70496, 70498, 70544, 70545, 70546, 70547, 70548, 70549, 71275, 71555, 72159, 72191, 72198, 73206, 73225, 73706, 73725, 74174, 74175, 74185, 74261, 74262, 74263, 75557, 75559, 75561, 75563, 75565, 75571, 75572, 75573, 75574, 75635, 76376, 77046, 77047, 77048, 77049, 77061, 77062, 77063, 78012-78999, 93319, 93355, 0523T, 0559T, 0560T, 0561T, 0562T, 0623T, 0624T, 0625T, 0626T, 0633T, 0634T, 0635T, 0636T, 0637T, 0638T, 0710T, 0711T, 0712T, 0713T, 0876T)◀

(76376, 76377 require concurrent supervision of image postprocessing 3D manipulation of volumetric data set and image rendering)

(For noninvasive arterial plaque analysis using software processing of data from computerized tomography angiography to quantify structure and composition of the vessel wall, including assessment for lipid-rich necrotic core plaque, see 0710T, 0711T, 0712T, 0713T)

Rationale

In accordance with the establishment of Category III code 0876T, the exclusionary parenthetical notes following codes 76376 and 76377 have been revised with the addition of code 0876T.

Refer to the codebook and the Rationale for code 0876T for a full discussion of these changes.

Diagnostic Ultrasound

Head and Neck

76510   Ophthalmic ultrasound, diagnostic; B-scan and quantitative A-scan performed during the same patient encounter

76511   quantitative A-scan only

76512   B-scan (with or without superimposed non-quantitative A-scan)

76513   anterior segment ultrasound, immersion (water bath) B-scan or high resolution biomicroscopy, unilateral or bilateral

▶(For computerized ophthalmic diagnostic imaging of the anterior and posterior segments using technology other than ultrasound, see 92132, 92133, 92134, 92137)◀

Rationale

In support of the addition of code 92137, the cross-reference note following code 76513 has been revised to include code 92137 and delete the term "scanning" in congruence with other changes in the CPT 2025 code set.

Refer to the codebook and the Rationale for code 92137 for a full discussion of these changes.

Ultrasonic Guidance Procedures

76942   Ultrasonic guidance for needle placement (eg, biopsy, aspiration, injection, localization device), imaging supervision and interpretation

▶(Do not report 76942 in conjunction with 10004, 10005, 10006, 10021, 10030, 19083, 19285, 20604, 20606, 20611, 27096, 32408, 32554, 32555, 32556, 32557, 37760, 37761, 43232, 43237, 43242, 45341, 45342, 46948, 55874, 64415, 64416, 64417, 64445, 64446, 64447, 64448, 64466, 64467, 64468, 64469, 64473, 64474, 64479, 64480, 64483, 64484, 64490, 64491, 64493, 64494, 64495, 76975, 0213T, 0214T, 0215T, 0216T, 0217T, 0218T, 0232T, 0481T, 0582T)◀

(For harvesting, preparation, and injection[s] of platelet rich plasma, use 0232T)

Rationale

Codes 64466-64469, 64473, and 64474 have been added to the exclusionary parenthetical note within the Ultrasonic Guidance Procedures subsection to accommodate the addition of new codes for reporting thoracic and lower extremity fascial plane blocks.

Refer to the codebook and the Rationale for codes 64466-64469, 64473, and 64474 for a full discussion of these changes.

Radiologic Guidance

Fluoroscopic Guidance

(Do not report guidance codes 77001, 77002, 77003 for services in which fluoroscopic guidance is included in the descriptor)

+ 77001 Fluoroscopic guidance for central venous access device placement, replacement (catheter only or complete), or removal (includes fluoroscopic guidance for vascular access and catheter manipulation, any necessary contrast injections through access site or catheter with related venography radiologic supervision and interpretation, and radiographic documentation of final catheter position) (List separately in addition to code for primary procedure)

▶(Do not report 77001 in conjunction with 33957, 33958, 33959, 33962, 33963, 33964, 36568, 36569, 36572, 36573, 36584, 36836, 36837, 64466, 64467, 64468, 64469, 64473, 64474, 77002)◀

(If formal extremity venography is performed from separate venous access and separately interpreted, use 36005 and 75820, 75822, 75825, or 75827)

Rationale

Codes 64466-64469, 64473, and 64474 have been added to the exclusionary parenthetical note following code 77001 to accommodate the addition of new codes for reporting thoracic and lower extremity fascial plane blocks.

Refer to the codebook and the Rationale for codes 64466-64469, 64473, and 64474 for a full discussion of these changes.

Computed Tomography Guidance

77012 Computed tomography guidance for needle placement (eg, biopsy, aspiration, injection, localization device), radiological supervision and interpretation

(Do not report 77011, 77012 in conjunction with 22586)

▶(Do not report 77012 in conjunction with 10009, 10010, 10030, 27096, 32408, 32554, 32555, 32556, 32557, 62270, 62272, 62328, 62329, 64466, 64467, 64468, 64469, 64473, 64474, 64479, 64480, 64483, 64484, 64490, 64491, 64492, 64493, 64494, 64495, 64633, 64634, 64635, 64636, 0232T, 0481T, 0629T, 0630T)◀

(For harvesting, preparation, and injection[s] of platelet-rich plasma, use 0232T)

Rationale

Codes 64466-64469, 64473, and 64474 have been added to an exclusionary parenthetical note following code 77012 to accommodate the addition of new codes for reporting thoracic and lower extremity fascial plane blocks.

Refer to the codebook and the Rationale for codes 64466-64469, 64473, and 64474 for a full discussion of these changes.

Magnetic Resonance Imaging Guidance

77021 Magnetic resonance imaging guidance for needle placement (eg, for biopsy, needle aspiration, injection, or placement of localization device) radiological supervision and interpretation

(For procedure, see appropriate organ or site)

▶(Do not report 77021 in conjunction with 10011, 10012, 10030, 19085, 19287, 32408, 32554, 32555, 32556, 32557, 64466, 64467, 64468, 64469, 64473, 64474, 0232T, 0481T)◀

(For harvesting, preparation, and injection[s] of platelet-rich plasma, use 0232T)

Rationale

Codes 64466-64469, 64473, and 64474 have been added to the exclusionary parenthetical note following code 77021 to accommodate the addition of new codes for reporting thoracic and lower extremity fascial plane blocks.

Refer to the codebook and the Rationale for codes 64466-64469, 64473, and 64474 for a full discussion of these changes.

Notes

Pathology and Laboratory

Summary of Additions, Deletions, and Revisions

The summary of changes shows the actual changes that have been made to the code descriptors.

New codes appear with a bullet (●) and are indicated as "Code added." Revised codes are preceded with a triangle (▲). Within revised codes, or if a code symbol has been deleted, the deleted language and code symbol appear with a ~~strikethrough~~, while new text appears <u>underlined</u>.

The ⚡ symbol is used to identify codes for vaccines that are pending FDA approval. The **#** symbol is used to identify codes that have been resequenced. CPT add-on codes are annotated by the **+** symbol. The ⊘ symbol is used to identify codes that are exempt from the use of modifier 51. The ★ symbol is used to identify codes that may be used for reporting telemedicine services. The ✕ symbol is used to identify a proprietary laboratory analyses (PLA) test that has an identical descriptor as another PLA test. A PLA code that satisfies Category I code criteria and has been accepted by the CPT Editorial Panel is annotated with the ↕ symbol. The ◀ symbol is used to identify codes that may be used to report audio-only telemedicine services when appended by modifier 93 **(see Appendix T)**.

Code	Description
#●81195	Code added
▲81432	Hereditary breast cancer-related disorders (eg, hereditary breast cancer, hereditary ovarian cancer, hereditary endometrial cancer, <u>hereditary pancreatic cancer, hereditary prostate cancer), genomic sequence analysis panel, 5 or more genes, interrogation for sequence variants and copy number variants</u>; ~~genomic sequence analysis panel, must include sequencing of at least 10 genes, always including BRCA1, BRCA2, CDH1, MLH1, MSH2, MSH6, PALB2, PTEN, STK11, and TP53~~
~~81433~~	~~Hereditary breast cancer-related disorders (eg, hereditary breast cancer, hereditary ovarian cancer, hereditary endometrial cancer); duplication/deletion analysis panel, must include analyses for BRCA1, BRCA2, MLH1, MSH2, and STK11~~
▲81435	Hereditary colon cancer<u>-related</u> disorders (eg, Lynch syndrome, PTEN hamartoma syndrome, Cowden syndrome, familial adenomatosis polyposis)<u>, genomic sequence analysis panel, 5 or more genes, interrogation for sequence variants and copy number variants</u>; ~~genomic sequence analysis panel, must include sequencing of at least 10 genes, including APC, BMPR1A, CDH1, MLH1, MSH2, MSH6, MUTYH, PTEN, SMAD4, and STK11~~
~~81436~~	~~Hereditary colon cancer disorders (eg, Lynch syndrome, PTEN hamartoma syndrome, Cowden syndrome, familial adenomatosis polyposis); duplication/deletion analysis panel, must include analysis of at least 5 genes, including MLH1, MSH2, EPCAM, SMAD4, and STK11~~
▲81437	Hereditary neuroendocrine tumor<u>-related</u> disorders (eg, medullary thyroid carcinoma, parathyroid carcinoma, malignant pheochromocytoma or paraganglioma)<u>, genomic sequence analysis panel, 5 or more genes, interrogation for sequence variants and copy number variants</u>; ~~genomic sequence analysis panel, must include sequencing of at least 6 genes, including MAX, SDHB, SDHC, SDHD, TMEM127, and VHL~~
~~81438~~	~~Hereditary neuroendocrine tumor disorders (eg, medullary thyroid carcinoma, parathyroid carcinoma, malignant pheochromocytoma or paraganglioma); duplication/deletion analysis panel, must include analyses for SDHB, SDHC, SDHD, and VHL~~
●81515	Code added
●81558	Code added
●82233	Code added

Code	Description
●82234	Code added
●83884	Code added
●84393	Code added
●84394	Code added
86327	~~crossed (2-dimensional assay)~~
86490	~~coccidioidomycosis~~
●86581	Code added
●87513	Code added
# ▲87624	Human Papillomavirus (HPV), high-risk types (eg, 16, 18, 31, 33, 35, 39, 45, 51, 52, 56, 58, 59, 68)<u>, pooled result</u>
# ●87626	Code added
# ●87564	Code added
●87594	Code added
▲88387	Macroscopic examination, dissection, and preparation of tissue for non-microscopic analytical studies (eg, nucleic acid-based molecular studies)<u>, each tissue preparation (eg, a single lymph node)</u>; ~~each tissue preparation (eg, a single lymph node)~~
88388	~~Macroscopic examination, dissection, and preparation of tissue for non-microscopic analytical studies (eg, nucleic acid-based molecular studies); in conjunction with a touch imprint, intraoperative consultation, or frozen section, each tissue preparation (eg, a single lymph node) (List separately in addition to code for primary procedure)~~
0078U	~~Pain management (opioid-use disorder) genotyping panel, 16 common variants (ie, *ABCB1, COMT, DAT1, DBH, DOR, DRD1, DRD2, DRD4, GABA, GAL, HTR2A, HTTLPR, MTHFR, MUOR, OPRK1, OPRM1*), buccal swab or other germline tissue sample, algorithm reported as positive or negative risk of opioid-use disorder~~
0167U	~~Gonadotropin, chorionic (hCG), immunoassay with direct optical observation, blood~~
0204U	~~Oncology (thyroid), mRNA, gene expression analysis of 593 genes (including *BRAF, RAS, RET, PAX8,* and *NTRK*) for sequence variants and rearrangements, utilizing fine needle aspirate, reported as detected or not detected~~
▲0248U	Oncology ~~(brain)~~, spheroid cell culture in ~~a~~ 3D microenvironment, 12<u>-</u>drug panel, ~~tumor~~ <u>brain- or brain metastasis–</u>response prediction for each drug
▲0351U	Infectious disease (bacterial or viral), biochemical assays, tumor necrosis factor-related apoptosis-inducing ligand (TRAIL), interferon gamma-induced protein-10 (IP-10), and C-reactive protein, serum, <u>or venous whole blood,</u> algorithm reported as likelihood of bacterial infection
0352U	~~Infectious disease (bacterial vaginosis and vaginitis), multiplex amplified probe technique, for detection of bacterial vaginosis–associated bacteria (BVAB-2, Atopobium vaginae, and Megasphera type 1), algorithm reported as detected or not detected and separate detection of Candida species (C. albicans, C. tropicalis, C. parapsilosis, C. dubliniensis), Candida glabrata/Candida krusei, and trichomonas vaginalis, vaginal-fluid specimen, each result reported as detected or not detected~~
0353U	~~Infectious agent detection by nucleic acid (DNA), Chlamydia trachomatis and Neisseria gonorrhoeae, multiplex amplified probe technique, urine, vaginal, pharyngeal, or rectal, each pathogen reported as detected or not detected~~
0354U	~~Human papilloma virus (HPV), high-risk types (ie, 16, 18, 31, 33, 45, 52 and 58) qualitative mRNA expression of E6/E7 by quantitative polymerase chain reaction (qPCR)~~
▲0356U	Oncology (oropharyngeal <u>or anal</u>), evaluation of 17 DNA biomarkers using droplet digital PCR (ddPCR), cell-free DNA, algorithm reported as a prognostic risk score for cancer recurrence

★=Telemedicine   ◀=Audio-only   ✚=Add-on code   ✗=FDA approval pending   #=Resequenced code   ⊘=Modifier 51 exempt

Code	Description
0396U	~~Obstetrics (pre-implantation genetic testing), evaluation of 300000 DNA single-nucleotide polymorphisms (SNPs) by microarray, embryonic tissue, algorithm reported as a probability for single-gene germline conditions~~
▲0403U	Oncology (prostate), mRNA, gene expression profiling of 18 genes, first-catch ~~post-digital rectal examination~~ urine ~~(or processed first-catch urine)~~, algorithm reported as percentage of likelihood of detecting clinically significant prostate cancer
0416U	~~Infectious agent detection by nucleic acid (DNA), genitourinary pathogens, identification of 20 bacterial and fungal organisms, including identification of 20 associated antibiotic-resistance genes, if performed, multiplex amplified probe technique, urine~~
●0420U	Code added
●0421U	Code added
●0422U	Code added
●0423U	Code added
●0424U	Code added
●0425U	Code added
●0426U	Code added
+●0427U	Code added
●0428U	Code added
●0429U	Code added
●0430U	Code added
●0431U	Code added
●0432U	Code added
●0433U	Code added
●0434U	Code added
●0435U	Code added
●0436U	Code added
●0437U	Code added
●0438U	Code added
●0439U	Code added
●0440U	Code added
●0441U	Code added
●0442U	Code added
●0443U	Code added
●0444U	Code added
●0445U	Code added
●0446U	Code added

▲ = Revised code   ● = New code   ▶ ◀ = Contains new or revised text   ✕ = Duplicate PLA test   ↑↓ = Category I PLA

Code	Description
●0447U	Code added
●0448U	Code added
●0449U	Code added
●0450U	Code added
●0451U	Code added
●0452U	Code added
●0453U	Code added
✕●0454U	Code added
●0455U	Code added
●0456U	Code added
●0457U	Code added
●0458U	Code added
●0459U	Code added
●0460U	Code added
●0461U	Code added
●0462U	Code added
●0463U	Code added
●0464U	Code added
●0465U	Code added
●0466U	Code added
●0467U	Code added
●0468U	Code added
●0469U	Code added
●0470U	Code added
●0471U	Code added
●0472U	Code added
●0473U	Code added
●0474U	Code added
●0475U	Code added
●0476U	Code added
●0477U	Code added
●0478U	Code added
●0479U	Code added

★=Telemedicine   ◀=Audio-only   ✛=Add-on code   ✗=FDA approval pending   #=Resequenced code   ⊘=Modifier 51 exempt

Code	Description
●0480U	Code added
●0481U	Code added
●0482U	Code added
●0483U	Code added
●0484U	Code added
●0485U	Code added
●0486U	Code added
●0487U	Code added
●0488U	Code added
●0489U	Code added
●0490U	Code added
●0491U	Code added
●0492U	Code added
●0493U	Code added
●0494U	Code added
●0495U	Code added
●0496U	Code added
●0497U	Code added
●0498U	Code added
●0499U	Code added
●0500U	Code added
●0501U	Code added
●0502U	Code added
●0503U	Code added
●0504U	Code added
●0505U	Code added
●0506U	Code added
●0507U	Code added
●0508U	Code added
●0509U	Code added
●0510U	Code added
●0511U	Code added
●0512U	Code added

Code	Description
●0513U	Code added
●0514U	Code added
●0515U	Code added
●0516U	Code added
●0517U	Code added
●0518U	Code added
●0519U	Code added
●0520U	Code added

★=Telemedicine   ◀=Audio-only   ✚=Add-on code   ✗=FDA approval pending   #=Resequenced code   ⊘=Modifier 51 exempt

Pathology and Laboratory

Molecular Pathology

Definitions

For purposes of CPT reporting, the following definitions apply:

Copy number variants (CNVs): structural changes in the genome composed of large deletions or duplications. CNVs can be found in the germline, but can also occur in somatic cells. See also Duplication/Deletion (Dup/Del).

▶***Cytogenomic:*** a comprehensive genome-wide analysis of chromosomal and genetic abnormalities using molecular-based technologies.◀

DNA methylation: the process of adding methyl groups to a DNA sequence, specifically adenine and cytosine nucleotides, thereby affecting transcription of that sequence. DNA hyper-methylation in a gene promoter typically represses gene transcription. DNA methylation serves as a regulatory mechanism in numerous scenarios including development, chromosome inactivation, and carcinogenesis.

Rationale

In support of the establishment of code 81195 in the Molecular Pathology subsection, the cytogenomic definition has been revised for reporting a comprehensive genome-wide analysis of chromosomal and genetic abnormalities using molecular-based technologies. The revised definition assists users in understanding how to report the new code.

Refer to the codebook and the Rationale for code 81195 for a full discussion of these changes.

Tier 1 Molecular Pathology Procedures

81195   Code is out of numerical sequence. See 81228-81235

 # 81277   Cytogenomic neoplasia (genome-wide) microarray analysis, interrogation of genomic regions for copy number and loss-of-heterozygosity variants for chromosomal abnormalities

(Do not report analyte-specific molecular pathology procedures separately when the specific analytes are included as part of the cytogenomic microarray analysis for neoplasia)

(Do not report 88271 when performing cytogenomic microarray analysis)

#● 81195   Cytogenomic (genome-wide) analysis, hematologic malignancy, structural variants and copy number variants, optical genome mapping (OGM)

81230   Code is out of numerical sequence. See 81225-81229

81231   Code is out of numerical sequence. See 81225-81229

 # 81161   *DMD (dystrophin)* (eg, Duchenne/Becker muscular dystrophy) deletion analysis, and duplication analysis, if performed

Rationale

A new Category I code (81195) has been established in the Tier 1 Molecular Pathology Procedures subsection to report optical genome mapping (OGM) methods for cytogenomic chromosomal abnormalities.

Code 81195 is reported for the identification of OGM, which is a non-sequencing, DNA-based technology that provides a comprehensive assessment of cytogenomic analysis by enabling the detection of both structural variants and copy number variants. It does this by integrating the functionalities of conventional cytogenetics (karyotyping), fluorescence in situ hybridization, and chromosomal microarray into a single assay. Specifically, this procedure makes up for the anomalies that occur when these testing methods are used individually (eg, "cryptic karyotyping"—an absence of a certain type of cell necessary for leukemia, lymphoma, or myeloma analysis; low resolution of the targeted cells; or other anomalies).

The definition of cytogenomic has been revised in the guidelines for the Molecular Pathology subsection to clarify what is being tested (chromosomal and genetic abnormalities) and how the test is performed (comprehensive genome-wide analysis using molecular-based technologies).

Clinical Example (81195)

A 45-year-old female was diagnosed with B-cell acute lymphoblastic leukemia. Bone marrow aspirate was sent for optical genome mapping (OGM) testing.

Description of Procedure (81195)

Label and load the extracted genomic DNA from bone marrow into a flowcell. Use an OGM system to untangle, linearize, and image the DNA, and then assemble the DNA into a genome and analyze it. Send the report to the ordering clinician.

Genomic Sequencing Procedures and Other Molecular Multianalyte Assays

▲ **81432**   Hereditary breast cancer-related disorders (eg, hereditary breast cancer, hereditary ovarian cancer, hereditary endometrial cancer, hereditary pancreatic cancer, hereditary prostate cancer), genomic sequence analysis panel, 5 or more genes, interrogation for sequence variants and copy number variants

▶(Do not report 81432 in conjunction with 81435, 81437)◀

▶(81433 has been deleted. To report only a duplication/deletion analysis panel for hereditary breast cancer-related disorders, use 81479)◀

81434   Hereditary retinal disorders (eg, retinitis pigmentosa, Leber congenital amaurosis, cone-rod dystrophy), genomic sequence analysis panel, must include sequencing of at least 15 genes, including *ABCA4, CNGA1, CRB1, EYS, PDE6A, PDE6B, PRPF31, PRPH2, RDH12, RHO, RP1, RP2, RPE65, RPGR,* and *USH2A*

▲ **81435**   Hereditary colon cancer-related disorders (eg, Lynch syndrome, PTEN hamartoma syndrome, Cowden syndrome, familial adenomatosis polyposis), genomic sequence analysis panel, 5 or more genes, interrogation for sequence variants and copy number variants

▶(Do not report 81435 in conjunction with 81432, 81437)◀

▶(81436 has been deleted. To report only a duplication/deletion analysis panel for hereditary colon cancer-related disorders, use 81479)◀

▲ **81437**   Hereditary neuroendocrine tumor-related disorders (eg, medullary thyroid carcinoma, parathyroid carcinoma, malignant pheochromocytoma or paraganglioma), genomic sequence analysis panel, 5 or more genes, interrogation for sequence variants and copy number variants

▶(Do not report 81437 in conjunction with 81432, 81435)◀

▶(81438 has been deleted. To report only a duplication/deletion analysis panel for hereditary neuroendocrine tumor-related disorders, use 81479)◀

Rationale

Changes have been made to the genomic sequencing procedure codes for hereditary cancer and tumor disorders. Codes 81432, 81435, and 81437 have been editorially revised; and codes 81433, 81436, and 81438 have been deleted.

Before 2025, codes 81432 and 81435 included the sequencing of at least 10 genes, and at least six genes for code 81437. Each code descriptor listed specific genes, but did not specify interrogation for sequence variants and copy-number variants. For the Current Procedural Terminology (CPT) 2025 code set, the required list of specific genes has been removed from all three codes so their descriptors describe the sequencing of five or more genes. Interrogation for sequence variants and copy number variants have been added to the descriptors. These changes have been made to codes 81432, 81435, and 81437 to accurately reflect current practice. Code 81432 has been further revised with the addition of hereditary pancreatic cancer and hereditary prostate cancer to the list of disorder examples. Codes 81435 and 81437 have been further revised by replacing "cancer disorders" and "tumor disorders" with "cancer-related disorders" and "tumor-related disorders," respectively, for consistency with the descriptor (ie, as a "related" disorder) of code 81432. Exclusionary parenthetical notes have been added to restrict reporting codes 81432, 81435, and 81437 together.

Codes 81433, 81436, and 81438 have been deleted due to low utilization. Cross-reference parenthetical notes have been added directing users to code 81479 to report a duplication or deletion analysis panel.

Clinical Example (81432)

A 36-year-old female, who has breast cancer and a family history of breast and ovarian cancer, is evaluated for mutations in genes known to be involved in hereditary breast cancer-related disorders. A whole-blood sample is submitted for hereditary breast cancer-related disorder panel testing.

Description of Procedure (81432)

Isolate high-quality DNA from the patient's blood sample. Enrich DNA targets with hybrid capture for at least five genes associated with hereditary breast cancer-related disorders. The products undergo massively parallel DNA sequencing of the coding regions and intron/exon boundaries. The pathologist or other qualified health care professional evaluates the results to identify nucleotide sequence variants. The pathologist or other qualified health care professional composes a report that specifies the patient's mutation status. Generate a report and communicate the results to the appropriate caregivers.

Clinical Example (81435)

A 24-year-old male, who has a strong family history of colorectal cancer, is evaluated for a suspected hereditary colon cancer disorder. A whole-blood sample is submitted for hereditary colon cancer disorder panel testing.

Description of Procedure (81435)

Isolate and subject high-quality DNA from the patient's blood sample to polymerase chain reaction (PCR) amplification for at least five genes associated with Lynch syndrome and/or hereditary colon cancer. The PCR products undergo massively parallel DNA sequencing. The pathologist or other qualified health care professional evaluates the results to identify nucleotide sequence variants. The pathologist or other qualified health care professional composes a report that specifies the patient's mutation status. Generate a report and communicate the results to appropriate caregivers.

Clinical Example (81437)

A 30-year-old female, who has sporadic paraganglioma and a negative family history, is evaluated for hereditary neuroendocrine tumor disorders. A whole-blood sample is submitted for hereditary neuroendocrine tumor disorder genomic sequence testing.

Description of Procedure (81437)

Isolate high-quality DNA from the patient's blood sample. Enrich DNA targets with hybrid capture for at least five genes associated with hereditary neuroendocrine tumors. The products undergo massively parallel DNA sequencing of the coding regions and intron/exon boundaries. The pathologist or other qualified health care professional evaluates the results to identify nucleotide sequence variants. The pathologist or other qualified health care professional composes a report that specifies the patient's mutation status. Generate a report and communicate the results to the appropriate caregivers.

Multianalyte Assays with Algorithmic Analyses

81514   Infectious disease, bacterial vaginosis and vaginitis, quantitative real-time amplification of DNA markers for Gardnerella vaginalis, Atopobium vaginae, Megasphaera type 1, Bacterial Vaginosis Associated Bacteria-2 (BVAB-2), and Lactobacillus species (L. crispatus and L. jensenii), utilizing vaginal-fluid specimens, algorithm reported as a positive or negative for high likelihood of bacterial vaginosis, includes separate detection of Trichomonas vaginalis and/or Candida species (C. albicans, C. tropicalis, C. parapsilosis, C. dubliniensis), Candida glabrata, Candida krusei, when reported

(Do not report 81514 in conjunction with 87480, 87481, 87482, 87510, 87511, 87512, 87660, 87661)

● 81515   Infectious disease, bacterial vaginosis and vaginitis, real-time PCR amplification of DNA markers for Atopobium vaginae, Atopobium species, Megasphaera type 1, and Bacterial Vaginosis Associated Bacteria-2 (BVAB-2), utilizing vaginal-fluid specimens, algorithm reported as positive or negative for high likelihood of bacterial vaginosis, includes separate detection of Trichomonas vaginalis and Candida species (C. albicans, C. tropicalis, C. parapsilosis, C. dubliniensis), Candida glabrata/ Candida krusei, when reported

Rationale

A new Category I multianalyte assay with algorithmic analysis (MAAA) code (81515) has been established to report the detection of bacterial vaginosis and vaginitis-associated diseases. In addition, a cross-reference parenthetical note following code 0352U has been added to direct users to code 81515 for the new testing procedure.

Code 81515 describes a polymerase chain reaction assay used to facilitate the diagnosis of vaginal infections in female patients with a clinical presentation consistent with bacterial vaginosis, vulvovaginal candidiasis, or trichomoniasis. The test uses an algorithm for organisms associated with bacterial vaginosis combined with the detection of Candida species associated with vulvovaginal candidiasis and Trichomonas vaginalis to obtain results.

To accommodate code 81515, proprietary laboratory analyses (PLA) code 0352U has been deleted. A cross-reference parenthetical note has been established to direct users to the new code.

A separate listing of this code that includes the proprietary test name has been added to Appendix O of the CPT 2025 code set.

Clinical Example (81515)

A 26-year-old female presents with symptoms suggestive of vaginitis (eg, bacterial vaginosis, vulvovaginal candidiasis, and/or trichomoniasis). A vaginal swab is collected for a molecular vaginitis panel.

Description of Procedure (81515)

The clinician collects a vaginal swab sample with the specimen-collection kit provided with the test. Extract and submit nucleic acids to quantitative real-time polymerase chain reaction for the detection of various pathogens associated with vaginitis. Test results are generated as positive or negative for bacterial vaginosis, Candida species, Candida glabrata/Candida krusei, and Trichomonas vaginalis. Send the report to the ordering clinician.

▲ = Revised code   ● = New code   ▶ ◀ = Contains new or revised text   ✕ = Duplicate PLA test   ↕ = Category I PLA   American Medical Association   85

Pathology and Laboratory 80047-89398, 0001U-0520U

81554 Pulmonary disease (idiopathic pulmonary fibrosis [IPF]), mRNA, gene expression analysis of 190 genes, utilizing transbronchial biopsies, diagnostic algorithm reported as categorical result (eg, positive or negative for high probability of usual interstitial pneumonia [UIP])

● **81558** Transplantation medicine (allograft rejection, kidney), mRNA, gene expression profiling by quantitative polymerase chain reaction (qPCR) of 139 genes, utilizing whole blood, algorithm reported as a binary categorization as transplant excellence, which indicates immune quiescence, or not transplant excellence, indicating subclinical rejection

Rationale

Code 81558 has been established to report a gene expression profile and algorithmic analysis for the identification of quiescence (dormancy) of kidney transplant rejection in kidney transplant patients.

Code 81558 identifies an MAAA that is a gene expression profile test that determines immune quiescence status. This is important for ascertaining the likelihood of a transplanted kidney being rejected by the patient. An analysis of immune quiescence status is used following kidney transplantation to determine the risk of subclinical rejection. Analyzing immune quiescence status can help avoid the need for a surveillance biopsy. As a result, this test may determine if a transplanted kidney is "transplant excellence" (which indicates immune quiescence) or "not transplant excellence" (which indicates subclinical rejection of the organ).

Clinical Example (81558)

A 56-year-old female presents to her physician for a follow-up after her kidney transplant. A blood sample is submitted for testing.

Description of Procedure (81558)

Subject RNA extracted from whole blood to downstream complementary DNA (cDNA) synthesis. Amplify and subject the cDNA to quantitative polymerase chain reaction analysis for the relevant gene set. Feed the data into a custom bioinformatics pipeline that algorithmically transforms the expression of the relevant genes to create a binary categorization as transplant excellence, which indicates immune quiescence or not transplant excellence, indicating subclinical rejection.

Chemistry

82150 Amylase

▶(For amyloid, beta, see 82233, 82234)◀

Rationale

In accordance with the establishment of codes 82233 and 82234, a cross-reference parenthetical note has been added following code 82150 to refer users to codes 82233 and 82234 for amyloid beta testing.

Refer to the codebook and the Rationale for codes 82233 and 82234 for a full discussion of these changes.

82232 Beta-2 microglobulin

(Bicarbonate, use 82374)

● **82233** Beta-amyloid; 1-40 (Abeta 40)

● **82234** 1-42 (Abeta 42)

Rationale

Two new Category I codes (82233, 82234) have been established in the Chemistry subsection to report testing for amyloid beta 1-40 (Abeta 40) and 1-42 (Abeta 42).

Code 82233 is reported for Abeta 40 protein by quantitative immunoassay, and code 82234 is reported for Abeta 42 protein by quantitative immunoassay.

Codes 82233 and 82234 are analyte-specific codes that describe the detection of Abeta-40 and Abeta-42, which result from enzymatic cleavage of the amyloid precursor protein (APP). The analysis for major beta-amyloid metabolic products is useful for identifying amyloid plaques. Reporting Abeta 40 and 42 as a ratio enables the detection of diseases, such as Alzheimer disease, because a low ratio is associated with patients who have clinical diagnoses of these diseases.

Clinical Example (82233)

A 65-year-old female presents for neurologic evaluation of gradual cognitive decline. Measurement of beta-amyloid 1-40 is requested to assess cognitive decline.

Description of Procedure (82233)

Test the sample for beta-amyloid 1-40 protein by quantitative immunoassay and report the results.

Clinical Example (82234)

A 65-year-old female presents for neurologic evaluation of gradual cognitive decline. Measurement of beta-amyloid 1-42 is requested to assess cognitive decline.

Description of Procedure (82234)

Test the sample for beta-amyloid 1-42 by quantitative immunoassay and report the results.

83883	Nephelometry, each analyte not elsewhere specified
● 83884	Neurofilament light chain (NfL)

Rationale

A new Category I code (83884) has been established in the Chemistry subsection to report neurofilament light chain (NfL) testing. Code 83884 describes the specific measurement of NfL, a test for multiple sclerosis prognostication, as well as monitoring disease activity in response to treatment.

Clinical Example (83884)

A 38-year-old female, who has an established diagnosis of multiple sclerosis, is referred to a neurologist to monitor disease activity. A blood sample is obtained for neurofilament light chain (NfL) testing.

Description of Procedure (83884)

Test sample for NfL chain by quantitative immunoassay. Report results.

84392	Sulfate, urine
	(Sulfhemoglobin, use hemoglobin, 83060)
	(T-3, see 84479-84481)
	(T-4, see 84436-84439)
● 84393	Tau, phosphorylated (eg, pTau 181, pTau 217), each
● 84394	Tau, total (tTau)

Rationale

Two new Category I codes (84393, 84394) have been established in the Chemistry subsection to report testing for phosphorylated Tau (pTau) (84393) for the early detection of diseases such as Alzheimer disease and testing for total Tau (tTau) (84394) to identify several types of dementia.

Newly developed technology enables testing for tau proteins to determine a number of dementia-related disorders of the brain, including Alzheimer disease in various stages of development and Creutzfeldt-Jakob disease. These conditions can be identified by an analysis of tau proteins, which are intracellular proteins released after neuronal cell death. Tau proteins are involved in microtubule assembly and stabilization, which are important for nerve cell structure and function. Hyperphosphorylation of tau proteins results in less effective microtubule assembly because this causes neurofibrillary tangles.

Code 84393 is reported for testing for pTau for the early detection of Alzheimer disease. It does this by testing for pTau in cerebrospinal spinal fluid and blood plasma. The amount of pTau correlates to the progression of the disease (ie, detection can begin at the earliest stages of dementia).

Code 84394 is reported for testing for tTau. The tTau assay measures all the isoforms that Tau presents and is considered a general marker for neurodegeneration and its association in the pathology of various types of dementia. A measure of the ratios of existing Tau proteins enables the determination of different diseases.

Clinical Example (84393)

A 65-year-old female presents for neurologic evaluation of gradual cognitive decline. Measurement of phosphorylated Tau is requested.

Description of Procedure (84393)

Test the patient's sample for phosphorylated Tau by quantitative immunoassay and report the results.

Clinical Example (84394)

A 65-year-old female presents for neurologic evaluation of gradual cognitive decline. Measurement of total Tau is requested.

Description of Procedure (84394)

Test the patient's sample for total Tau by quantitative immunoassay and report the results.

Immunology

86003   Allergen specific IgE; quantitative or semiquantitative, crude allergen extract, each

(For total quantitative IgE, use 82785)

86005   qualitative, multiallergen screen (eg, disk, sponge, card)

86008   quantitative or semiquantitative, recombinant or purified component, each

▶(For amyloid, beta, see 82233, 82234)◀

(For total qualitative IgE, use 83518)

(Alpha-1 antitrypsin, see 82103, 82104)

(Alpha-1 feto-protein, see 82105, 82106)

(Anti-AChR [acetylcholine receptor] antibody, see 86041, 86042, 86043)

(Anticardiolipin antibody, use 86147)

(Anti-DNA, use 86225)

(Anti-deoxyribonuclease titer, use 86215)

Rationale

In accordance with the establishment of codes 82233 and 82234, a cross-reference parenthetical note has been added following code 86008 to refer users to codes 82233 and 82234 for amyloid beta testing.

Refer to the codebook and the Rationale for codes 82233 and 82234 for a full discussion of these changes.

86155   Chemotaxis assay, specify method

(Clostridium difficile toxin, use 87230)

▶(Coccidioides, antibodies to, use 86635)◀

Rationale

In accordance with the deletion of code 86490, the second cross-reference parenthetical note following code 86155 has been revised to reflect this change.

Refer to the codebook and the Rationale for code 86490 for a full discussion of this change.

86320   Immunoelectrophoresis; serum

86325   other fluids (eg, urine, cerebrospinal fluid) with concentration

▶(86327 has been deleted)◀

Rationale

To ensure the CPT 2025 code set reflects current clinical practice, code 86327, *Immunoelectrophoresis; crossed (2-dimensional assay),* has been deleted due to low utilization. A parenthetical note has been added to indicate this deletion.

86485   Skin test; candida

(For antibody, candida, use 86628)

86486   unlisted antigen, each

▶(86490 has been deleted)◀

Rationale

To ensure the CPT 2025 code set reflects current clinical practice, code 86490, *Skin test; coccidioidomycosis,* has been deleted due to low utilization. A parenthetical note has been added to indicate this deletion.

86510   histoplasmosis

(For histoplasma, antibody, use 86698)

86580   tuberculosis, intradermal

(For tuberculosis test, cell mediated immunity measurement of gamma interferon antigen response, use 86480)

(For skin tests for allergy, see 95012-95199)

(Smooth muscle antibody, use 86015)

(Sporothrix, antibodies to, see code for specific method)

● **86581**   Streptococcus pneumoniae antibody (IgG), serotypes, multiplex immunoassay, quantitative

86590   Streptokinase, antibody

(For antibodies to infectious agents, see 86602-86804)

(Streptolysin O antibody, see antistreptolysin O, 86060, 86063)

Rationale

A new Category I code (86581) has been added in the Immunology subsection to report testing for Streptococcus pneumoniae. This new code describes (1) what is being tested and (2) the complexity of the immunoassay, which is a multiplex assay. Testing for Streptococcus pneumoniae serotypes enables specificity to report how Streptococcus pneumoniae antibody testing is performed.

Clinical Example (86581)

A 6-year-old female presents with a history of recurrent ear infections, bronchitis, and pneumonia. A pneumococcal vaccine is administered and follow-up levels of Streptococcus pneumoniae antibody (IgG) serotypes are requested to assess for potential immunodeficiency.

Description of Procedure (86581)

Test the patient's serum by multiplex immunoassay. Report the quantitative results.

Microbiology

87468	Infectious agent detection by nucleic acid (DNA or RNA); Anaplasma phagocytophilum, amplified probe technique
87512	Gardnerella vaginalis, quantification
● 87513	Helicobacter pylori (H. pylori), clarithromycin resistance, amplified probe technique

▶(For H. pylori, stool, use 87338)◀

▶(For H. pylori, immunoassay, use 87339)◀

▶(For assays that detect clarithromycin resistance and identify H. pylori using a single procedure, use 87513)◀

▶(For H. pylori, without clarithromycin resistance by amplified probe nucleic acid testing, use 87798)◀

Rationale

Infectious agent detection code 87513 has been added to the Microbiology subsection to identify a new procedure for clarithromycin resistance testing for H. pylori. In addition, new parenthetical notes have been added to direct users to the appropriate codes for testing for specific bacteria.

Code 87513 provides specificity for the organism detected and the resistance target performed in a single procedure. Before 2025, the existing codes were analyte-specific and therefore not applicable to other primary source organisms or antibiotic-resistance testing.

Code 87513 describes assays that detect clarithromycin resistance and identify H. pylori using a single procedure. Four cross-reference parenthetical notes following code 87513 have been added to direct users to various H. pylori testing procedures.

Clinical Example (87513)

A 45-year-old female presents to her physician with dyspepsia suggestive of chronic active gastritis or peptic ulcer disease. A fecal sample is collected for Helicobacter pylori (H. pylori) detection and clarithromycin resistance testing.

Description of Procedure (87513)

Process the fecal sample and run a polymerase chain reaction assay to detect the presence of H. pylori and clarithromycin resistance. Report the results.

# ▲ 87624	Human Papillomavirus (HPV), high-risk types (eg, 16, 18, 31, 33, 35, 39, 45, 51, 52, 56, 58, 59, 68), pooled result

(When both low-risk and high-risk HPV types are performed in a single assay, use only 87624)

# ● 87626	Human Papillomavirus (HPV), separately reported high-risk types (eg, 16, 18, 31, 45, 51, 52) and high-risk pooled result(s)

▶(Do not report 87626 in conjunction with 87624, 87625, for the same procedure)◀

▶(For singular pooled result of high-risk HPV types [eg, 16, 18, 31, 33, 35, 39, 45, 51, 52, 58, 59, 68], use 87624)◀

▶(For separately reported high-risk HPV types 16 and 18 only, including type 45, if performed, use 87625)◀

# 87625	Human Papillomavirus (HPV), types 16 and 18 only, includes type 45, if performed

▶(For Human Papillomavirus [HPV] detection of five or greater separately reported high-risk HPV types [ie, genotyping], use 87626)◀

Rationale

Code 87626 has been established in the Microbiology subsection to report testing for high-risk types of human papillomavirus (HPV). Code 87624 has been revised to include pooled results, and Category III code 0500T has been deleted. Parenthetical notes have been added or revised to accommodate the changes.

Code 87626 describes separately reported high-risk genotypes and pooled results in a single test. An exclusionary parenthetical note has been added to preclude the reporting of code 87626 in conjunction with codes 87624 and 87625 for the same procedure. Two parenthetical notes have been added following code 87626 to direct users to the appropriate codes for reporting either singular-pooled results of high-risk HPV types (87624) or separately reported specific high-risk HPV types (87625).

Code 87624 has been revised to include pooled results of high-risk HPV types. Category III code 0500T has been deleted. The parenthetical notes following codes 87625 and 87910 have been revised to reflect the deleted code and to direct users to the appropriate code for high-risk HPV types (eg, 16, 18, 31, 45, 51, 52) individually and in high-risk pooled result(s) in a single test (87626). In addition, cross-reference parenthetical notes direct users to the appropriate codes to report: (1) singular-pooled results of high-risk HPV types (87624); (2) separately reported high-risk HPV types 16 and 18 only, and 45, if performed (87625); or (3) separately reported high-risk genotypes and pooled results in a single test (87626).

The existing Category I codes (87624, 87625) differ from code 87626 because they lack the necessary level of specificity to differentiate between qualitative testing of HPV as pooled results of high-risk types and genotyping for high-risk types in a single analysis.

Clinical Example (87626)

A 35-year-old female presents for her routine gynecologic examination. The clinician orders a primary human papillomavirus (HPV) screening test to evaluate individual high-risk genotypes.

Description of Procedure (87626)

Subject an aliquot from the cytology preservation vial to amplification of target DNA by polymerase chain reaction for the detection of 14 high-risk HPV. Generate a report, including the individual genotype results. The laboratory director reviews and signs the report and sends the report to the ordering clinician.

87562	Mycobacteria avium-intracellulare, quantification
#● 87564	Mycobacterium tuberculosis, rifampin resistance, amplified probe technique

▶(For assays that detect rifampin resistance and identify Mycobacterium tuberculosis using a single procedure, use 87564)◀

Rationale

Infectious agent detection code 87564 has been added to the Microbiology subsection to identify a new procedure for rifampin resistance testing for Mycobacterium tuberculosis. In addition, a new parenthetical note has been added to direct users to the appropriate code for testing for this specific bacteria.

Code 87564 provides specificity for the organism detected and the resistance target performed in a single procedure. Before 2025, the existing codes were analyte-specific and

therefore not applicable to other primary source organisms or antibiotic-resistance testing.

Code 87564 describes assays that detect rifampin resistance and identify Mycobacterium tuberculosis using a single procedure. A cross-reference parenthetical note following code 87564 has been added to direct users to code 87564 when performing a single procedure assay to detect rifampin resistance and identify Mycobacterium tuberculosis.

Clinical Example (87564)

A 45-year-old male with a known human immunodeficiency virus infection presents to his physician with symptoms suggestive of pulmonary tuberculosis. A sputum sample is collected for Mycobacterium tuberculosis detection and resistance to rifampin testing.

Description of Procedure (87564)

Transfer the sputum sample to the test cartridge. Assay amplifies Mycobacterium tuberculosis complex-specific sequences for detection and identification and rpoB gene for detection of rifampin resistance–associated mutations. Report the results.

87563	Mycoplasma genitalium, amplified probe technique
87564	Code is out of numerical sequence. See 87561-87580
87580	Mycoplasma pneumoniae, direct probe technique
87593	Orthopoxvirus (eg, monkeypox virus, cowpox virus, vaccinia virus), amplified probe technique, each
● 87594	Pneumocystis jirovecii, amplified probe technique

Rationale

Code 87594 has been established in the Microbiology subsection to report testing of Pneumocystis jirovecii by amplified probe technique. The addition of this new code may help detect life-threatening infections caused by Pneumocystis jirovecii in patients who are immunocompromised.

Clinical Example (87594)

A 35-year-old male, who is immunosuppressed, presents with shortness of breath, nonproductive cough, and fever. His chest radiograph showed bilateral, diffuse interstitial infiltrates. Bronchoalveolar lavage fluid specimen was obtained and submitted for Pneumocystis jirovecii polymerase chain reaction (PCR) testing.

Description of Procedure (87594)

Test the patient's bronchoalveolar lavage specimen for Pneumocystis jirovecii DNA by real-time PCR. Report qualitative results.

87623	Code is out of numerical sequence. See 87538-87541
87624	Code is out of numerical sequence. See 87538-87541
87625	Code is out of numerical sequence. See 87538-87541
87626	Code is out of numerical sequence. See 87538-87541

87631 respiratory virus (eg, adenovirus, influenza virus, coronavirus, metapneumovirus, parainfluenza virus, respiratory syncytial virus, rhinovirus), includes multiplex reverse transcription, when performed, and multiplex amplified probe technique, multiple types or subtypes, 3-5 targets

87910 Infectious agent genotype analysis by nucleic acid (DNA or RNA); cytomegalovirus

(For infectious agent drug susceptibility phenotype prediction for HIV-1, use 87900)

▶(For Human Papillomavirus [HPV] for high-risk types [ie, genotyping] of five or greater separately reported HPV types, use 87626)◀

Rationale

In accordance with the deletion of code 0500T, the parenthetical note following code 87910 has been revised to reflect the deleted code and to direct users to the appropriate code for high-risk HPV types (eg, 16, 18, 31, 45, 51, 52) individually and as high-risk pooled result(s) in a single test.

Refer to the codebook and the Rationale for codes 87624 and 87626 for a full discussion of these changes.

Cytogenetic Studies

▶Cytogenetic study procedures that are not specified in 88230-88291 and are not in the Surgical Pathology (88300-88387) subsection may be reported using the unlisted cytogenetic study code 88299.◀

Molecular pathology procedures should be reported using the appropriate code from Tier 1 (81161, 81200-81383), Tier 2 (81400-81408), Genomic Sequencing Procedures and Other Molecular Multianalyte Assays (81410-81471), or Multianalyte Assays with Algorithmic Analyses (81500-81512) sections. If no specific code exists, one of the unlisted codes (81479 or 81599) should be used.

(For acetylcholinesterase, use 82013)

(For alpha-fetoprotein, serum or amniotic fluid, see 82105, 82106)

(For laser microdissection of cells from tissue sample, see 88380)

88230 Tissue culture for non-neoplastic disorders; lymphocyte

Rationale

In accordance with the deletion of code 88388, the Cytogenetic Studies guidelines have been revised to reflect this change.

Refer to the codebook and the Rationale for code 88388 for a full discussion of this change.

Surgical Pathology

▶Services 88300 through 88309 include accession, examination, and reporting. They do not include the services designated in codes 88311 through 88387 and 88399, which are coded in addition when provided.◀

The unit of service for codes 88300 through 88309 is the specimen.

A specimen is defined as tissue or tissues that is (are) submitted for individual and separate attention, requiring individual examination and pathologic diagnosis. Two or more such specimens from the same patient (eg, separately identified endoscopic biopsies, skin lesions) are each appropriately assigned an individual code reflective of its proper level of service.

Service code 88300 is used for any specimen that in the opinion of the examining pathologist can be accurately diagnosed without microscopic examination. Service code 88302 is used when gross and microscopic examination is performed on a specimen to confirm identification and the absence of disease. Service codes 88304 through 88309 describe all other specimens requiring gross and microscopic examination, and represent additional ascending levels of physician work. Levels 88302 through 88309 are specifically defined by the assigned specimens.

Any unlisted specimen should be assigned to the code which most closely reflects the physician work involved when compared to other specimens assigned to that code.

▶Surgical pathology procedures that are not specified in 88300-88387 may be reported using the unlisted surgical pathology procedure code 88399.◀

(Do not report 88302-88309 on the same specimen as part of Mohs surgery)

88300 **Level I** - Surgical pathology, gross examination only

Pathology and Laboratory 80047-89398, 0001U-0520U

▲ **88387** Macroscopic examination, dissection, and preparation of tissue for non-microscopic analytical studies (eg, nucleic acid-based molecular studies), each tissue preparation (eg, a single lymph node)

(Do not report 88387 for tissue preparation for microbiologic cultures or flow cytometric studies)

▶(Do not report 88387 in conjunction with 88329-88334)◀

▶(88388 has been deleted)◀

Rationale

To ensure the CPT 2025 code set reflects current clinical practice, add-on code 88388, *Macroscopic examination, dissection, and preparation of tissue for non-microscopic analytical studies (eg, nucleic acid-based molecular studies); in conjunction with a touch imprint, intraoperative consultation, or frozen section, each tissue preparation (eg, a single lymph node) (List separately in addition to code for primary procedure)*, has been deleted due to low utilization. A parenthetical note has been added to indicate this deletion. In accordance with this deletion, code 88387 has been revised with the removal of the semicolon because it is no longer a parent code. The Surgical Pathology subsection guidelines have been revised to reflect the deletion of code 88388.

Proprietary Laboratory Analyses

▶(0078U has been deleted)◀

▶(0167U has been deleted)◀

▶(0204U has been deleted)◀

▲ **0248U** Oncology, spheroid cell culture in 3D microenvironment, 12-drug panel, brain- or brain metastasis–response prediction for each drug

⌘ **0260U** Rare diseases (constitutional/heritable disorders), identification of copy number variations, inversions, insertions, translocations, and other structural variants by optical genome mapping

▶(For additional PLA codes with identical clinical descriptor, see 0264U, 0454U. See Appendix O or the most current listing on the AMA CPT website to determine appropriate code assignment)◀

⌘ **0264U** Rare diseases (constitutional/heritable disorders), identification of copy number variations, inversions, insertions, translocations, and other structural variants by optical genome mapping

▶(For additional PLA codes with identical clinical descriptor, see 0260U, 0454U. See Appendix O or the most current listing on the AMA CPT website to determine appropriate code assignment)◀

▲ **0351U** Infectious disease (bacterial or viral), biochemical assays, tumor necrosis factor-related apoptosis-inducing ligand (TRAIL), interferon gamma-induced protein-10 (IP-10), and C-reactive protein, serum, or venous whole blood, algorithm reported as likelihood of bacterial infection

▶(0352U has been deleted. To report infectious disease, bacterial vaginosis and vaginitis, real-time PCR amplification of DNA markers for algorithm reported as high likelihood of bacterial vaginosis, use 81515)◀

▶(0353U has been deleted)◀

▶(0354U has been deleted)◀

▲ **0356U** Oncology (oropharyngeal or anal), evaluation of 17 DNA biomarkers using droplet digital PCR (ddPCR), cell-free DNA, algorithm reported as a prognostic risk score for cancer recurrence

▶(0396U has been deleted)◀

▲ **0403U** Oncology (prostate), mRNA, gene expression profiling of 18 genes, first-catch urine, algorithm reported as percentage of likelihood of detecting clinically significant prostate cancer

▶(0416U has been deleted)◀

● **0420U** Oncology (urothelial), mRNA expression profiling by real-time quantitative PCR of *MDK, HOXA13, CDC2, IGFBP5,* and *CXCR2* in combination with droplet digital PCR (ddPCR) analysis of 6 single-nucleotide polymorphisms (SNPs) of genes *TERT* and *FGFR3*, urine, algorithm reported as a risk score for urothelial carcinoma

● **0421U** Oncology (colorectal) screening, quantitative real-time target and signal amplification of 8 RNA markers *(GAPDH, SMAD4, ACY1, AREG, CDH1, KRAS, TNFRSF10B, EGLN2)* and fecal hemoglobin, algorithm reported as a positive or negative for colorectal cancer risk

● **0422U** Oncology (pan-solid tumor), analysis of DNA biomarker response to anti-cancer therapy using cell-free circulating DNA, biomarker comparison to a previous baseline pre-treatment cell-free circulating DNA analysis using next-generation sequencing, algorithm reported as a quantitative change from baseline, including specific alterations, if appropriate

● **0423U** Psychiatry (eg, depression, anxiety), genomic analysis panel, including variant analysis of 26 genes, buccal swab, report including metabolizer status and risk of drug toxicity by condition

★=Telemedicine ◀=Audio-only ✦=Add-on code ⊘=FDA approval pending #=Resequenced code ⊘=Modifier 51 exempt

● **0424U** Oncology (prostate), exosome-based analysis of 53 small noncoding RNAs (sncRNAs) by quantitative reverse transcription polymerase chain reaction (RT-qPCR), urine, reported as no molecular evidence, low-, moderate-, or elevated-risk of prostate cancer

● **0425U** Genome (eg, unexplained constitutional or heritable disorder or syndrome), rapid sequence analysis, each comparator genome (eg, parents, siblings)

● **0426U** Genome (eg, unexplained constitutional or heritable disorder or syndrome), ultra-rapid sequence analysis

+● **0427U** Monocyte distribution width, whole blood (List separately in addition to code for primary procedure)

▶(Use 0427U in conjunction with 85004, 85025)◀

● **0428U** Oncology (breast), targeted hybrid-capture genomic sequence analysis panel, circulating tumor DNA (ctDNA) analysis of 56 or more genes, interrogation for sequence variants, gene copy number amplifications, gene rearrangements, microsatellite instability, and tumor mutation burden

● **0429U** Human papillomavirus (HPV), oropharyngeal swab, 14 high-risk types (ie, 16, 18, 31, 33, 35, 39, 45, 51, 52, 56, 58, 59, 66, and 68)

● **0430U** Gastroenterology, malabsorption evaluation of alpha-1-antitrypsin, calprotectin, pancreatic elastase and reducing substances, feces, quantitative

● **0431U** Glycine receptor alpha1 IgG, serum or cerebrospinal fluid (CSF), live cell-binding assay (LCBA), qualitative

● **0432U** Kelch-like protein 11 (KLHL11) antibody, serum or cerebrospinal fluid (CSF), cell-binding assay, qualitative

● **0433U** Oncology (prostate), 5 DNA regulatory markers by quantitative PCR, whole blood, algorithm, including prostate-specific antigen, reported as likelihood of cancer

● **0434U** Drug metabolism (adverse drug reactions and drug response), genomic analysis panel, variant analysis of 25 genes with reported phenotypes

● **0435U** Oncology, chemotherapeutic drug cytotoxicity assay of cancer stem cells (CSCs), from cultured CSCs and primary tumor cells, categorical drug response reported based on cytotoxicity percentage observed, minimum of 14 drugs or drug combinations

● **0436U** Oncology (lung), plasma analysis of 388 proteins, using aptamer-based proteomics technology, predictive algorithm reported as clinical benefit from immune checkpoint inhibitor therapy

● **0437U** Psychiatry (anxiety disorders), mRNA, gene expression profiling by RNA sequencing of 15 biomarkers, whole blood, algorithm reported as predictive risk score

● **0438U** Drug metabolism (adverse drug reactions and drug response), buccal specimen, gene-drug interactions, variant analysis of 33 genes, including deletion/duplication analysis of *CYP2D6*, including reported phenotypes and impacted gene-drug interactions

● **0439U** Cardiology (coronary heart disease [CHD]), DNA, analysis of 5 single-nucleotide polymorphisms (SNPs) (rs11716050 [LOC105376934], rs6560711 [WDR37], rs3735222 [SCIN/LOC107986769], rs6820447 [intergenic], and rs9638144 [ESYT2]) and 3 DNA methylation markers (cg00300879 [transcription start site {TSS200} of CNKSR1], cg09552548 [intergenic], and cg14789911 [body of SPATC1L]), qPCR and digital PCR, whole blood, algorithm reported as a 4-tiered risk score for a 3-year risk of symptomatic CHD

● **0440U** Cardiology (coronary heart disease [CHD]), DNA, analysis of 10 single-nucleotide polymorphisms (SNPs) (rs710987 [LINC010019], rs1333048 [CDKN2B-AS1], rs12129789 [KCND3], rs942317 [KTN1-AS1], rs1441433 [PPP3CA], rs2869675 [PREX1], rs4639796 [ZBTB41], rs4376434 [LINC00972], rs12714414 [TMEM18], and rs7585056 [TMEM18]) and 6 DNA methylation markers (cg03725309 [SARS1], cg12586707 [CXCL1], cg04988978 [MPO], cg17901584 [DHCR24-DT], cg21161138 [AHRR], and cg12655112 [EHD4]), qPCR and digital PCR, whole blood, algorithm reported as detected or not detected for CHD

● **0441U** Infectious disease (bacterial, fungal, or viral infection), semiquantitative biomechanical assessment (via deformability cytometry), whole blood, with algorithmic analysis and result reported as an index

● **0442U** Infectious disease (respiratory infection), Myxovirus resistance protein A (MxA) and C-reactive protein (CRP), fingerstick whole blood specimen, each biomarker reported as present or absent

● **0443U** Neurofilament light chain (NfL), ultra-sensitive immunoassay, serum or cerebrospinal fluid

● **0444U** Oncology (solid organ neoplasia), targeted genomic sequence analysis panel of 361 genes, interrogation for gene fusions, translocations, or other rearrangements, using DNA from formalin-fixed paraffin-embedded (FFPE) tumor tissue, report of clinically significant variant(s)

● **0445U** β-amyloid (Abeta42) and phospho tau (181P) (pTau181), electrochemiluminescent immunoassay (ECLIA), cerebral spinal fluid, ratio reported as positive or negative for amyloid pathology

● **0446U** Autoimmune diseases (systemic lupus erythematosus [SLE]), analysis of 10 cytokine soluble mediator biomarkers by immunoassay, plasma, individual components reported with an algorithmic risk score for current disease activity

Pathology and Laboratory 80047-89398, 0001U-0520U

● **0447U** Autoimmune diseases (systemic lupus erythematosus [SLE]), analysis of 11 cytokine soluble mediator biomarkers by immunoassay, plasma, individual components reported with an algorithmic prognostic risk score for developing a clinical flare

● **0448U** Oncology (lung and colon cancer), DNA, qualitative, next-generation sequencing detection of single-nucleotide variants and deletions in *EGFR* and *KRAS* genes, formalin-fixed paraffin-embedded (FFPE) solid tumor samples, reported as presence or absence of targeted mutation(s), with recommended therapeutic options

● **0449U** Carrier screening for severe inherited conditions (eg, cystic fibrosis, spinal muscular atrophy, beta hemoglobinopathies [including sickle cell disease], alpha thalassemia), regardless of race or self-identified ancestry, genomic sequence analysis panel, must include analysis of 5 genes *(CFTR, SMN1, HBB, HBA1, HBA2)*

● **0450U** Oncology (multiple myeloma), liquid chromatography with tandem mass spectrometry (LC-MS/MS), monoclonal paraprotein sequencing analysis, serum, results reported as baseline presence or absence of detectable clonotypic peptides

● **0451U** Oncology (multiple myeloma), LC-MS/MS, peptide ion quantification, serum, results compared with baseline to determine monoclonal paraprotein abundance

● **0452U** Oncology (bladder), methylated *PENK* DNA detection by linear target enrichment-quantitative methylation-specific real-time PCR (LTE-qMSP), urine, reported as likelihood of bladder cancer

● **0453U** Oncology (colorectal cancer), cell-free DNA (cfDNA), methylation-based quantitative PCR assay *(SEPTIN9, IKZF1, BCAT1,* Septin9-2, *VAV3, BCAN)*, plasma, reported as presence or absence of circulating tumor DNA (ctDNA)

⌘● **0454U** Rare diseases (constitutional/heritable disorders), identification of copy number variations, inversions, insertions, translocations, and other structural variants by optical genome mapping

▶(For additional PLA codes with identical clinical descriptor, see 0260U, 0264U. See Appendix O or the most current listing on the AMA CPT website to determine appropriate code assignment)◀

● **0455U** Infectious agents (sexually transmitted infection), Chlamydia trachomatis, Neisseria gonorrhoeae, and Trichomonas vaginalis, multiplex amplified probe technique, vaginal, endocervical, gynecological specimens, oropharyngeal swabs, rectal swabs, female or male urine, each pathogen reported as detected or not detected

● **0456U** Autoimmune (rheumatoid arthritis), next-generation sequencing (NGS), gene expression testing of 19 genes, whole blood, with analysis of anti-cyclic citrullinated peptides (CCP) levels, combined with sex, patient global assessment, and body mass index (BMI), algorithm reported as a score that predicts nonresponse to tumor necrosis factor inhibitor (TNFi) therapy

● **0457U** Perfluoroalkyl substances (PFAS) (eg, perfluorooctanoic acid, perfluorooctane sulfonic acid), 9 PFAS compounds by LC-MS/MS, plasma or serum, quantitative

● **0458U** Oncology (breast cancer), S100A8 and S100A9, by enzyme-linked immunosorbent assay (ELISA), tear fluid with age, algorithm reported as a risk score

● **0459U** β-amyloid (Abeta42) and total tau (tTau), electrochemiluminescent immunoassay (ECLIA), cerebral spinal fluid, ratio reported as positive or negative for amyloid pathology

● **0460U** Oncology, whole blood or buccal, DNA single-nucleotide polymorphism (SNP) genotyping by real-time PCR of 24 genes, with variant analysis and reported phenotypes

● **0461U** Oncology, pharmacogenomic analysis of single-nucleotide polymorphism (SNP) genotyping by real-time PCR of 24 genes, whole blood or buccal swab, with variant analysis, including impacted gene-drug interactions and reported phenotypes

● **0462U** Melatonin levels test, sleep study, 7 or 9 sample melatonin profile (cortisol optional), enzyme-linked immunosorbent assay (ELISA), saliva, screening/preliminary

● **0463U** Oncology (cervix), mRNA gene expression profiling of 14 biomarkers (E6 and E7 of the highest-risk human papillomavirus [HPV] types 16, 18, 31, 33, 45, 52, 58), by real-time nucleic acid sequence-based amplification (NASBA), exo- or endocervical epithelial cells, algorithm reported as positive or negative for increased risk of cervical dysplasia or cancer for each biomarker

● **0464U** Oncology (colorectal) screening, quantitative real-time target and signal amplification, methylated DNA markers, including LASS4, LRRC4 and PPP2R5C, a reference marker ZDHHC1, and a protein marker (fecal hemoglobin), utilizing stool, algorithm reported as a positive or negative result

● **0465U** Oncology (urothelial carcinoma), DNA, quantitative methylation-specific PCR of 2 genes *(ONECUT2, VIM)*, algorithmic analysis reported as positive or negative

● **0466U** Cardiology (coronary artery disease [CAD]), DNA, genome-wide association studies (564856 single-nucleotide polymorphisms [SNPs], targeted variant genotyping), patient lifestyle and clinical data, buccal swab, algorithm reported as polygenic risk to acquired heart disease

● **0467U** Oncology (bladder), DNA, next-generation sequencing (NGS) of 60 genes and whole genome aneuploidy, urine, algorithms reported as minimal residual disease (MRD) status positive or negative and quantitative disease burden

★ = Telemedicine ◀ = Audio-only ✛ = Add-on code ✎ = FDA approval pending # = Resequenced code ⊘ = Modifier 51 exempt

● **0468U** Hepatology (nonalcoholic steatohepatitis [NASH]), miR-34a-5p, alpha 2-macroglobulin, YKL40, HbA1c, serum and whole blood, algorithm reported as a single score for NASH activity and fibrosis

● **0469U** Rare diseases (constitutional/heritable disorders), whole genome sequence analysis for chromosomal abnormalities, copy number variants, duplications/ deletions, inversions, unbalanced translocations, regions of homozygosity (ROH), inheritance pattern that indicate uniparental disomy (UPD), and aneuploidy, fetal sample (amniotic fluid, chorionic villus sample, or products of conception), identification and categorization of genetic variants, diagnostic report of fetal results based on phenotype with maternal sample and paternal sample, if performed, as comparators and/or maternal cell contamination

● **0470U** Oncology (oropharyngeal), detection of minimal residual disease by next-generation sequencing (NGS) based quantitative evaluation of 8 DNA targets, cell-free HPV 16 and 18 DNA from plasma

● **0471U** Oncology (colorectal cancer), qualitative real-time PCR of 35 variants of *KRAS* and *NRAS* genes (exons 2, 3, 4), formalin-fixed paraffin-embedded (FFPE), predictive, identification of detected mutations

● **0472U** Carbonic anhydrase VI (CA VI), parotid specific/secretory protein (PSP) and salivary protein (SP1) IgG, IgM, and IgA antibodies, enzyme-linked immunosorbent assay (ELISA), semiqualitative, blood, reported as predictive evidence of early Sjögren's syndrome

● **0473U** Oncology (solid tumor), next-generation sequencing (NGS) of DNA from formalin-fixed paraffin-embedded (FFPE) tissue with comparative sequence analysis from a matched normal specimen (blood or saliva), 648 genes, interrogation for sequence variants, insertion and deletion alterations, copy number variants, rearrangements, microsatellite instability, and tumor-mutation burden

● **0474U** Hereditary pan-cancer (eg, hereditary sarcomas, hereditary endocrine tumors, hereditary neuroendocrine tumors, hereditary cutaneous melanoma), genomic sequence analysis panel of 88 genes with 20 duplications/deletions using next-generation sequencing (NGS), Sanger sequencing, blood or saliva, reported as positive or negative for germline variants, each gene

● **0475U** Hereditary prostate cancer-related disorders, genomic sequence analysis panel using next-generation sequencing (NGS), Sanger sequencing, multiplex ligation-dependent probe amplification (MLPA), and array comparative genomic hybridization (CGH), evaluation of 23 genes and duplications/deletions when indicated, pathologic mutations reported with a genetic risk score for prostate cancer

● **0476U** Drug metabolism, psychiatry (eg, major depressive disorder, general anxiety disorder, attention deficit hyperactivity disorder [ADHD], schizophrenia), whole blood, buccal swab, and pharmacogenomic genotyping of 14 genes and *CYP2D6* copy number variant analysis and reported phenotypes

● **0477U** Drug metabolism, psychiatry (eg, major depressive disorder, general anxiety disorder, attention deficit hyperactivity disorder [ADHD], schizophrenia), whole blood, buccal swab, and pharmacogenomic genotyping of 14 genes and *CYP2D6* copy number variant analysis, including impacted gene-drug interactions and reported phenotypes

● **0478U** Oncology (non-small cell lung cancer), DNA and RNA, digital PCR analysis of 9 genes (*EGFR, KRAS, BRAF, ALK, ROS1, RET, NTRK 1/2/3, ERBB2,* and *MET*) in formalin-fixed paraffin-embedded (FFPE) tissue, interrogation for single-nucleotide variants, insertions/deletions, gene rearrangements, and reported as actionable detected variants for therapy selection

● **0479U** Tau, phosphorylated, pTau217

● **0480U** Infectious disease (bacteria, viruses, fungi, and parasites), cerebrospinal fluid (CSF), metagenomic next-generation sequencing (DNA and RNA), bioinformatic analysis, with positive pathogen identification

● **0481U** *IDH1 (isocitrate dehydrogenase 1 [NADP+]), IDH2 (isocitrate dehydrogenase 2 [NADP+]),* and *TERT (telomerase reverse transcriptase)* promoter (eg, central nervous system [CNS] tumors), next-generation sequencing (single-nucleotide variants [SNV], deletions, and insertions)

● **0482U** Obstetrics (preeclampsia), biochemical assay of soluble fms-like tyrosine kinase 1 (sFlt-1) and placental growth factor (PlGF), serum, ratio reported for sFlt-1/PlGF, with risk of progression for preeclampsia with severe features within 2 weeks

● **0483U** Infectious disease (Neisseria gonorrhoeae), sensitivity, ciprofloxacin resistance (gyrA S91F point mutation), oral, rectal, or vaginal swab, algorithm reported as probability of fluoroquinolone resistance

● **0484U** Infectious disease (Mycoplasma genitalium), macrolide sensitivity (23S rRNA point mutation), oral, rectal, or vaginal swab, algorithm reported as probability of macrolide resistance

● **0485U** Oncology (solid tumor), cell-free DNA and RNA by next-generation sequencing, interpretative report for germline mutations, clonal hematopoiesis of indeterminate potential, and tumor-derived single-nucleotide variants, small insertions/deletions, copy number alterations, fusions, microsatellite instability, and tumor mutational burden

Pathology and Laboratory 80047-89398, 0001U-0520U

● **0486U**   Oncology (pan-solid tumor), next-generation sequencing analysis of tumor methylation markers present in cell-free circulating tumor DNA, algorithm reported as quantitative measurement of methylation as a correlate of tumor fraction

● **0487U**   Oncology (solid tumor), cell-free circulating DNA, targeted genomic sequence analysis panel of 84 genes, interrogation for sequence variants, aneuploidy corrected gene copy number amplifications and losses, gene rearrangements, and microsatellite instability

● **0488U**   Obstetrics (fetal antigen noninvasive prenatal test), cell-free DNA sequence analysis for detection of fetal presence or absence of 1 or more of the Rh, C, c, D, E, Duffy (Fya), or Kell (K) antigen in alloimmunized pregnancies, reported as selected antigen(s) detected or not detected

● **0489U**   Obstetrics (single-gene noninvasive prenatal test), cell-free DNA sequence analysis of 1 or more targets (eg, *CFTR, SMN1, HBB, HBA1, HBA2*) to identify paternally inherited pathogenic variants, and relative mutation-dosage analysis based on molecular counts to determine fetal inheritance of maternal mutation, algorithm reported as a fetal risk score for the condition (eg, cystic fibrosis, spinal muscular atrophy, beta hemoglobinopathies [including sickle cell disease], alpha thalassemia)

● **0490U**   Oncology (cutaneous or uveal melanoma), circulating tumor cell selection, morphological characterization and enumeration based on differential CD146, high molecular–weight melanoma-associated antigen, CD34 and CD45 protein biomarkers, peripheral blood

● **0491U**   Oncology (solid tumor), circulating tumor cell selection, morphological characterization and enumeration based on differential epithelial cell adhesion molecule (EpCAM), cytokeratins 8, 18, and 19, CD45 protein biomarkers, and quantification of estrogen receptor (ER) protein biomarker–expressing cells, peripheral blood

● **0492U**   Oncology (solid tumor), circulating tumor cell selection, morphological characterization and enumeration based on differential epithelial cell adhesion molecule (EpCAM), cytokeratins 8, 18, and 19, CD45 protein biomarkers, and quantification of PD-L1 protein biomarker–expressing cells, peripheral blood

● **0493U**   Transplantation medicine, quantification of donor-derived cell-free DNA (cfDNA) using next-generation sequencing, plasma, reported as percentage of donor-derived cell-free DNA

● **0494U**   Red blood cell antigen (fetal RhD gene analysis), next-generation sequencing of circulating cell-free DNA (cfDNA) of blood in pregnant individuals known to be RhD negative, reported as positive or negative

● **0495U**   Oncology (prostate), analysis of circulating plasma proteins (tPSA, fPSA, KLK2, PSP94, and GDF15), germline polygenic risk score (60 variants), clinical information (age, family history of prostate cancer, prior negative prostate biopsy), algorithm reported as risk of likelihood of detecting clinically significant prostate cancer

● **0496U**   Oncology (colorectal), cell-free DNA, 8 genes for mutations, 7 genes for methylation by real-time RT-PCR, and 4 proteins by enzyme-linked immunosorbent assay, blood, reported positive or negative for colorectal cancer or advanced adenoma risk

● **0497U**   Oncology (prostate), mRNA gene-expression profiling by real-time RT-PCR of 6 genes (*FOXM1, MCM3, MTUS1, TTC21B, ALAS1,* and *PPP2CA*), utilizing formalin-fixed paraffin-embedded (FFPE) tissue, algorithm reported as a risk score for prostate cancer

● **0498U**   Oncology (colorectal), next-generation sequencing for mutation detection in 43 genes and methylation pattern in 45 genes, blood, and formalin-fixed paraffin-embedded (FFPE) tissue, report of variants and methylation pattern with interpretation

● **0499U**   Oncology (colorectal and lung), DNA from formalin-fixed paraffin-embedded (FFPE) tissue, next-generation sequencing of 8 genes (*NRAS, EGFR, CTNNB1, PIK3CA, APC, BRAF, KRAS,* and *TP53*), mutation detection

● **0500U**   Autoinflammatory disease (VEXAS syndrome), DNA, *UBA1* gene mutations, targeted variant analysis (M41T, M41V, M41L, c.118-2A>C, c.118-1G>C, c.118-9_118-2del, S56F, S621C)

● **0501U**   Oncology (colorectal), blood, quantitative measurement of cell-free DNA (cfDNA)

● **0502U**   Human papillomavirus (HPV), E6/E7 markers for high-risk types (16, 18, 31, 33, 35, 39, 45, 51, 52, 56, 58, 59, 66, and 68), cervical cells, branched-chain capture hybridization, reported as negative or positive for high risk for HPV

● **0503U**   Neurology (Alzheimer disease), beta amyloid (Aβ40, Aβ42, Aβ42/40 ratio) and tau-protein (ptau217, np-tau217, ptau217/np-tau217 ratio), blood, immunoprecipitation with quantitation by liquid chromatography with tandem mass spectrometry (LC-MS/MS), algorithm score reported as likelihood of positive or negative for amyloid plaques

● **0504U**   Infectious disease (urinary tract infection), identification of 17 pathologic organisms, urine, real-time PCR, reported as positive or negative for each organism

● **0505U**   Infectious disease (vaginal infection), identification of 32 pathogenic organisms, swab, real-time PCR, reported as positive or negative for each organism

● **0506U**   Gastroenterology (Barrett's esophagus), esophageal cells, DNA methylation analysis by next-generation sequencing of at least 89 differentially methylated genomic regions, algorithm reported as likelihood for Barrett's esophagus

● **0507U** Oncology (ovarian), DNA, whole-genome sequencing with 5-hydroxymethylcytosine (5hmC) enrichment, using whole blood or plasma, algorithm reported as cancer detected or not detected

● **0508U** Transplantation medicine, quantification of donor-derived cell-free DNA using 40 single-nucleotide polymorphisms (SNPs), plasma, and urine, initial evaluation reported as percentage of donor-derived cell-free DNA with risk for active rejection

● **0509U** Transplantation medicine, quantification of donor-derived cell-free DNA using up to 12 single-nucleotide polymorphisms (SNPs) previously identified, plasma, reported as percentage of donor-derived cell-free DNA with risk for active rejection

● **0510U** Oncology (pancreatic cancer), augmentative algorithmic analysis of 16 genes from previously sequenced RNA whole-transcriptome data, reported as probability of predicted molecular subtype

● **0511U** Oncology (solid tumor), tumor cell culture in 3D microenvironment, 36 or more drug panel, reported as tumor-response prediction for each drug

● **0512U** Oncology (prostate), augmentative algorithmic analysis of digitized whole-slide imaging of histologic features for microsatellite instability (MSI) status, formalin-fixed paraffin-embedded (FFPE) tissue, reported as increased or decreased probability of MSI-high (MSI-H)

● **0513U** Oncology (prostate), augmentative algorithmic analysis of digitized whole-slide imaging of histologic features for microsatellite instability (MSI) and homologous recombination deficiency (HRD) status, formalin-fixed paraffin-embedded (FFPE) tissue, reported as increased or decreased probability of each biomarker

● **0514U** Gastroenterology (irritable bowel disease [IBD]), immunoassay for quantitative determination of adalimumab (ADL) levels in venous serum in patients undergoing adalimumab therapy, results reported as a numerical value as micrograms per milliliter (μg/mL)

● **0515U** Gastroenterology (irritable bowel disease [IBD]), immunoassay for quantitative determination of infliximab (IFX) levels in venous serum in patients undergoing infliximab therapy, results reported as a numerical value as micrograms per milliliter (μg/mL)

● **0516U** Drug metabolism, whole blood, pharmacogenomic genotyping of 40 genes and *CYP2D6* copy number variant analysis, reported as metabolizer status

● **0517U** Therapeutic drug monitoring, 80 or more psychoactive drugs or substances, LC-MS/MS, plasma, qualitative and quantitative therapeutic minimally and maximally effective dose of prescribed and non-prescribed medications

● **0518U** Therapeutic drug monitoring, 90 or more pain and mental health drugs or substances, LC-MS/MS, plasma, qualitative and quantitative therapeutic minimally effective range of prescribed and non-prescribed medications

● **0519U** Therapeutic drug monitoring, medications specific to pain, depression, and anxiety, LC-MS/MS, plasma, 110 or more drugs or substances, qualitative and quantitative therapeutic minimally effective range of prescribed, non-prescribed, and illicit medications in circulation

● **0520U** Therapeutic drug monitoring, 200 or more drugs or substances, LC-MS/MS, plasma, qualitative and quantitative therapeutic minimally effective range of prescribed and non-prescribed medications

Rationale

A total of 101 new PLA codes have been established for the CPT 2025 code set. PLA codes are released and published on a quarterly basis (fall, winter, spring, and summer) at https://www.ama-assn.org/practice-management/cpt/cpt-pla-codes. New codes are effective the quarter following their online publication. Other changes include the deletion of eight codes (0078U, 0167U, 0204U, 0352U, 0353U, 0354U, 0396U, 0416U); the revision of four codes (0248U, 0351U, 0356U, 0403U); the editorial revision of one test name (0407U); and the revision of the test, laboratory, and manufacturer names for codes 0047U and 0118U.

To accommodate the addition of new code 81515, PLA code 0352U has been deleted. A cross-reference parenthetical note has been established to direct users to the new code.

Refer to the codebook and the Rationale for code 81515 for a full discussion of these changes.

Clinical Example (0248U)

A 55-year-old female, who has suspected metastatic lung cancer to the brain, was observed via magnetic resonance imaging. A fresh tumor is sent to assess the tumor response to therapy.

Description of Procedure (0248U)

Receive tumor and dissociate and count cells. Grow cells in three-dimensional culture as spheroids, expose them to potential therapeutic agents, and assess by luminescence for cell viability. A qualified laboratory professional reviews the data and issues a report indicating tumor-specific drug responses.

Clinical Example (0403U)

A 65-year-old male presents to his urologist with a recent elevated prostate-specific antigen level of 9.3 ng/mL. Urine is submitted for analysis to determine the risk of having high-grade, clinically actionable prostate cancer.

Description of Procedure (0403U)

Subject the urine specimen to quantitative polymerase chain reaction to analyze 18 prostate cancer biomarkers. Calculate a score using a proprietary algorithm that reports a percent risk of detecting Gleason grade 7 prostate cancer on biopsy. A qualified laboratory professional prepares a report and sends the report to the ordering physician.

Clinical Example (0420U)

A 60-year-old male who smokes presents with microscopic hematuria. A urine sample is submitted to evaluate him for urothelial carcinoma.

Description of Procedure (0420U)

Isolate and subject messenger RNA from urine to real-time quantitative polymerase chain reaction of five genes (MDK, HOXA13, CDC2, IGFBP5, CXCR2) and droplet digital polymerase chain reaction DNA analysis of six single-nucleotide polymorphisms for genes FGFR3 and TERT. Incorporate the mRNA and DNA results using an algorithm to calculate a risk score for urothelial carcinoma. A qualified laboratory professional prepares a report specifying the risk status and communicates the results to the ordering provider.

Clinical Example (0421U)

A 45-year-old male presents for an initial routine colorectal cancer screening. A stool specimen is submitted to assess colorectal cancer risk.

Description of Procedure (0421U)

Assess a stool swab for fecal hemoglobin. Assess a stool sample for fecal RNA by droplet digital polymerase chain reaction. Use the software to evaluate these findings using an algorithm that generates a result (positive or negative) for colorectal cancer or advanced adenoma. A qualified health care professional composes a report and communicates the results to the ordering provider.

Clinical Example (0422U)

A 65-year-old female was recently diagnosed with stage IV lung adenocarcinoma. A baseline cell-free therapy selection test was performed. Nine weeks into therapy, blood is submitted to determine the alteration response to therapy.

Description of Procedure (0422U)

Isolate cell-free DNA from anticoagulated, stabilized peripheral whole blood, label with nonredundant oligonucleotides, use hybridization capture, and sequence using next-generation sequencing. Interrogate sequencing data for the presence of different genetic alterations and then compare them to a baseline sample and report as a percentage change from the baseline.

Clinical Example (0423U)

A 61-year-old female presents with intractable pain and anxiety due to metastatic colon cancer. Prior medications have not provided adequate relief. A buccal specimen is submitted for genomic analysis to assist with optimizing pharmacotherapy.

Description of Procedure (0423U)

Extract and genotype DNA from the buccal swab using real-time polymerase chain reaction to detect single-nucleotide polymorphisms variants in 26 genes (ABCB1, ABCB1 C3435T, CYP1A2, CYP2B6, CYP2C19, CYP2C9, CYP2D6, CYP3A4, CYP3A5, UGT1A4, UGT2B15, BDNF, HTR2A, MTHFR, SLC6A4, ADRA2A, COMT, DRD2, HTR2C, MC4R, ANK3, CACNA1C, GRIK1, HLA A*31:01, HLA A*15:02, OPRM1). A qualified laboratory professional prepares a report specifying the gene, genotype, phenotype, patient impact, and the metabolic enzyme and communicates the results to the ordering provider.

Clinical Example (0424U)

A 50-year-old male presents with clinical suspicion of prostate cancer.

Description of Procedure (0424U)

Isolate and assay exosomal RNA from non-digital rectal exam urine using high-density real-time quantitative polymerase chain reaction. Summarize and analyze fluorescent signal outputs for 53 exosomal RNA sequences for the absence or presence of low-, moderate-, or elevated-risk prostate cancer. A qualified laboratory professional assesses test quality, composes a report with the patient's classification, and sends it to appropriate licensed health care professionals.

Clinical Example (0425U)

An acutely ill infant presents with a severe congenital heart defect, malformed ears, and a cleft palate. Samples are submitted from comparators (eg, patients, siblings) for an evaluation to determine whether the findings occur from de novo or inherited.

★ = Telemedicine   ◀ = Audio-only   ✚ = Add-on code   ✒ = FDA approval pending   # = Resequenced code   ⊘ = Modifier 51 exempt

Description of Procedure (0425U)

Isolate genomic DNA from the whole blood of comparator family members. Perform polymerase chain reaction–free whole genome sequencing on comparators to accompany and inform proband (patient) analysis. Process genomic data in a bioinformatics pipeline and compare with a human reference genome for alignment and variant calling. Prioritize variants using the patient's phenotype and inheritance information from comparators to determine pathogenicity. A qualified laboratory professional curates the findings, prepares a report, and provides the findings to the ordering provider.

Clinical Example (0426U)

A six-day-old male was admitted to the neonatal intensive care unit with worsening seizures. Standard anti-epileptic treatment was not successful. A blood sample was submitted to identify potential actionable mutations.

Description of Procedure (0426U)

Isolate and prepare genomic DNA from whole blood drawn from the proband (patient) and the comparators (as available) with polymerase chain reaction–free libraries, followed by an ultrarapid workflow for whole genome sequencing. Compare variants using a bioinformatics software that uses a reference-genome curated by a qualified laboratory professional. Report the preliminary and final results to the ordering provider, when available (3 and 14 days, respectively).

Clinical Example (0427U)

A 66-year-old female presents to the emergency department with generalized weakness, elevated heart rate, chills, and agitation. A venous whole-blood sample is submitted for a monocyte distribution width (MDW) to evaluate whether the patient has sepsis. [**Note:** This is an add-on code. Only consider the additional work related to the primary procedure.]

Description of Procedure (0427U)

Analyze venous whole-blood sample collected in ethylenediaminetetraacetic acid to determine the MDW within 2 hours of collection. MDW values greater than 20.0 aid in determining sepsis risk. Report the results and other laboratory findings to the ordering provider.

Clinical Example (0428U)

A 65-year-old female, who has metastatic breast cancer, presents to her oncologist with disease progression. A tissue biopsy is infeasible. Plasma from whole blood is submitted for circulating tumor DNA (ctDNA) mutation analysis.

Description of Procedure (0428U)

Isolate plasma from whole blood and perform the ctDNA test using next-generation sequencing to assess for somatic mutations, including sequence variants, gene copy-number amplifications, gene rearrangements, microsatellite instability, and tumor mutational burden. A qualified laboratory professional reviews the findings and reports them to the ordering provider.

Clinical Example (0429U)

A 42-year-old patient presents with a recent history of high-risk oral sex. The physician collects a throat swab to look for high-risk human papillomavirus (HPV).

Description of Procedure (0429U)

Extract and test DNA from an oropharyngeal swab for 14 high-risk HPV types (ie, 16, 18, 31, 33, 35, 39, 45, 51, 52, 56, 58, 59, 66, and 68) using real-time polymerase chain reaction. A qualified laboratory professional reviews the results and reports them to the ordering provider.

Clinical Example (0430U)

A 4-year-old male presents to his physician with a history of persistent loose, mushy stools and weight loss over the past 9 months. Stool studies for malabsorption are ordered.

Description of Procedure (0430U)

Submit a fecal sample to test for calprotectin, reducing substances, alpha-1-antitrypsin, and elastase. Perform each test separately and report the quantitative results.

Clinical Example (0431U)

A 50-year-old female presents with 6 months of diffuse body stiffness and superimposed spasms resulting in injurious falls. After other evaluations are negative, given a suspected diagnosis of stiff person syndrome, glycine receptor antibody testing is ordered.

Description of Procedure (0431U)

Test cerebrospinal fluid using a live-cell binding assay to express the glycine receptor. If antibodies against the glycine receptor are present, only the induced cells will demonstrate antibody binding. Report a qualitative result to the qualified health care professional.

Clinical Example (0432U)

A 54-year-old male presents to his physician with difficulty walking and double vision. He has a recent history of testicular cancer. After other evaluations are negative and KLHL11 encephalitis is suspected, KLHL11 antibody testing is ordered.

Description of Procedure (0432U)

Test cerebrospinal fluid using a live-cell binding assay to express the recombinant KLHL11 protein. Then reflex the reactive samples on the screening assay to a confirmatory tissue immunofluorescence titer assay to identify a tissue-specific staining pattern characteristic of the presence of KLHL11 immunoglobulin G. If positive, provide a titer with a positive interpretation to the qualified health care professional.

Clinical Example (0433U)

A 58-year-old male has a raised prostate-specific antigen level of 3.0 ng/mL. The primary care physician sends a blood sample for DNA analysis to further refine his risk for prostate cancer.

Description of Procedure (0433U)

Extract and amplify DNA from whole blood using specific primers and probes using quantitative polymerase chain reaction for five DNA regulatory (epigenetic) markers called chromosome conformation signatures. An algorithm assigns a probability score defining the patient's likelihood of prostate cancer as "low probability" or "high probability." Issue a report to the ordering provider.

Clinical Example (0434U)

A 45-year-old male, who has major depressive disorder, presents to his physician after antidepressant medications were unsuccessful. A buccal swab is submitted for a pharmacogenomic panel.

Description of Procedure (0434U)

Extract and subject DNA from whole blood or buccal sample to polymerase chain reaction amplification of variants for 25 different genes (CYP1A2, CYP2B6, CYP2C9, CYP2C19, CYP2C cluster, CYP2D6 including copy-number, CPP3A4, CYP3A5, CYP4F2, COMT, DPYD, DRD2, GRIK4, HLA-A, HLA-B, HTR2A, HTR2C, IFNL4, NUDT15, OPRM1, SLC6A4, SLCO1B1, TMPT, UGT1A1, VKORC1). Generate a report with genotype results, phenotypic interpretation, and likely effects of the genetic variants on drug metabolism. Provide the report to the ordering physician.

Clinical Example (0435U)

A 55-year-old female, who has a headache, disorientation, and double vision, is diagnosed with a glioblastoma. A fresh sample of live, sterile tissue is submitted for chemotherapeutic drug-cytotoxicity testing.

Description of Procedure (0435U)

Submit and subject a fresh sample of live, sterile tumor tissue to cytotoxicity testing and individual chemotherapeutics. Report the assessment of toxicity in cancer stem cells and primary tumor cells relative to untreated controls as a percentage of cells killed. Issue a report to the ordering provider.

Clinical Example (0436U)

A 68-year-old male, who has metastatic non-small cell lung cancer, submitted blood to assess for the probability of clinical benefit from PD-1/PD-L1 inhibitors as a single agent or in combination with chemotherapy.

Description of Procedure (0436U)

Plasma undergoes proteomics profiling of 388 human proteins using an aptamer-based proteomics platform that measures protein expression levels in relative fluorescence units. Use an algorithm that uses findings to generate a predictive score (0 to 10) of clinical benefit and a result (positive/negative) combined with the PD-L1 category to guide treatment.

Clinical Example (0437U)

A 24-year-old female presents with panic attacks, feeling chronically on the edge, and avoids certain locations and situations. Blood is obtained to assess her risk of anxiety disorder and guide treatment.

Description of Procedure (0437U)

Isolate RNA from blood and sequence 15 biomarkers associated with anxiety to determine biomarker gene-expression levels. Apply a proprietary algorithm. A qualified laboratory professional compiles the report detailing risk and medication suggestions and communicates the report to the ordering provider.

Clinical Example (0438U)

A 68-year-old male, who is on antidepressants, started to experience bouts of drowsiness, insomnia, anxiety, and other reactions after failing multiple selective serotonin reuptake inhibitor medications was recently diagnosed with atrial fibrillation. A buccal swab is submitted for genomic testing to assess the patient's gene/variant mutation status.

Description of Procedure (0438U)

Isolate and analyze DNA from a buccal swab for 33 genes (ABCB1 [rs1045642], ABCG2, ADRA2A [1252G>C], ANKK1, ApoE, COMT[Val158Met], CYP1A2, CYP2B6, CYP2C8, CYP2C9, CYP2D6, CYP3A4, CYP3A5, CYP2C19, DBH[-1021T>C],

★ = Telemedicine   ◀ = Audio-only   ✚ = Add-on code   ✔ = FDA approval pending   # = Resequenced code   ⊘ = Modifier 51 exempt

DPYD, F2, F5, GRIK4, HLA-A*3101, HLA-B*1502, HTR2 A[rs6313], HTR2A [rs7997012], HTR2C [rs6318], IFNL3, ITGB3, MTHFR [(A1298C], MTHFR [C677T], OPRK1 [rs1051660], OPRM1 [118A>G], SLCO1B1, UGT1A1, UGT2B15, VKORC1, SLC6A4) using real-time polymerase chain reaction/fluorescence to detect clinically relevant genes with variant mutations from wild type. A qualified laboratory professional provides results. A pharmacist reviews and prepares a report that communicates a pharmacogenomic analysis for the ordering provider.

Clinical Example (0439U)

A 65-year-old-female presents with high blood pressure and elevated cholesterol and reports a smoking history. She does not have a history of atherosclerotic cardiovascular disease. Whole blood is submitted for genetic and epigenetic analysis to determine the patient's risk of developing symptomatic coronary heart disease (CHD) within 3 years.

Description of Procedure (0439U)

Isolate and subject DNA from whole blood to quantitative polymerase chain reaction (qPCR)/digital PCR (dPCR) (qPCR/dPCR) to analyze five single-nucleotide polymorphisms genotypes and three DNA methylation biomarkers. A qualified laboratory professional reviews the results and issues a report specifying the patient's 3-year CHD risk score to the ordering provider.

Clinical Example (0440U)

A 66-year-old female, who is obese with hypercholesterolemia, reports periodic chest pain with exertion. Blood is submitted for genetic and epigenetic analysis to determine the presence of coronary heart disease (CHD).

Description of Procedure (0440U)

Isolate and subject DNA from whole blood to quantitative polymerase chain reaction (qPCR)/digital PCR (dPCR) (qPCR/dPCR) to analyze 10 single-nucleotide polymorphisms genotypes and six DNA methylation biomarkers. A qualified laboratory professional reviews the results and generates a report indicating whether CHD is detected or not detected to the ordering provider.

Clinical Example (0441U)

A 72-year-old-female who has dementia presents to the emergency department with altered mental status. Blood is submitted to determine the risk of sepsis vs alternate diagnoses.

Description of Procedure (0441U)

Insert whole blood into a sample preparation module that isolates white blood cells (WBCs) in suspension. Add the WBC suspension to a microfluidics cartridge and insert the cartridge into the instrument. A qualified laboratory professional reviews the score provided by the instrument and reports the results to the ordering physician.

Clinical Example (0442U)

A 50-year-old patient who has asthma presents to the clinic after developing a new onset runny nose, sore throat, cough, and fever. A finger-stick sample is submitted to differentiate bacterial from nonbacterial etiologies and assess the patient's need for antibiotics.

Description of Procedure (0442U)

Transfer blood from the finger stick by capillary action to a test strip. A button releases the buffer to transfer blood across the test strip. When the test lines are visible, a qualified laboratory professional reads the results and sends them to the ordering provider.

Clinical Example (0443U)

A 31-year-old male is diagnosed with amyotrophic lateral sclerosis. He carries a rare variant in the SOD1 gene suspected to be pathogenic. Serum is submitted to identify neuronal injury.

Description of Procedure (0443U)

Serum, plasma, or cerebrospinal fluid undergo digital immunoassay for the quantitative determination of neurofilament-light. A qualified laboratory professional reviews the data and reports the results to the ordering provider.

Clinical Example (0444U)

A 67-year-old male who has stage IIIB lung cancer underwent a mediastinal biopsy. Formalin-fixed paraffin-embedded tissue is submitted to assess the potential presence of actionable gene fusions.

Description of Procedure (0444U)

Dewax and rehydrate the formalin-fixed paraffin-embedded tumor tissue. Digest crosslinked DNA with restriction enzymes. Biotinylate and ligate spatially proximal DNA and capture the sequence and genome structure. Mechanically shear this DNA, prepare the libraries, and enrich and sequence the biotinylated DNA. Perform a bioinformatic analysis to call and visualize structural variants (eg, gene fusions). Annotate clinically significant variants and report to the ordering provider.

Pathology and Laboratory 80047-89398, 0001U-0520U

Clinical Example (0445U)

A 62-year-old is evaluated by a neurologist for worsening memory complaints, mood changes, and anxiety for the past year. Routine laboratory tests are not informative. Cerebrospinal fluid is submitted to evaluate the cause of cognitive decline.

Description of Procedure (0445U)

Subject cerebrospinal fluid to immunoassay analysis. A qualified laboratory professional reports the ratio to the ordering physician.

Clinical Example (0446U)

A 26-year-old female, who was previously diagnosed with systemic lupus erythematosus, presents to her physician. Plasma is submitted for immunoassay analysis to assess the patient's current disease activity.

Description of Procedure (0446U)

Isolate and subject plasma from a blood sample to immunoassay for BAFF/BLyS, CXCL10/IP-10, IFNα-2, IFN-γ, IL-10, IL-15, IL-4, IL-7, OPN, and TRAIL protein biomarkers. A proprietary algorithm yields a risk-index score corresponding to the current disease activity. A qualified laboratory professional reviews and communicates the results to the ordering physician.

Clinical Example (0447U)

A 26-year-old female, who was previously diagnosed with systemic lupus erythematosus, presents to her physician. Plasma is submitted for immunoassay analysis to assess the patient's likelihood of experiencing a flare within the next 12 weeks.

Description of Procedure (0447U)

Isolate and subject plasma from a blood sample to immunoassay for MCP1/CCL2, IL-5, IL-17A, IL-7, IL-4, TNF-α, MCP3/CCL7, BAFF/BLyS, OPN, TNFR1/TNFRSF1A, and TNFR2/TNFRSF1B protein biomarkers. A proprietary algorithm yields a risk-index score corresponding to the likelihood of the patient developing a lupus flare in the next 12 weeks. A qualified laboratory professional reviews the report and communicates the results to the ordering physician.

Clinical Example (0448U)

A 67-year-old female presents with non-small cell lung cancer. Formalin-fixed paraffin-embedded (FFPE) tumor tissue is submitted for polymerase chain reaction (PCR) analysis to assess for actionable mutations.

Description of Procedure (0448U)

Extract and subject DNA from FFPE tumor tissue to gene-specific PCR and next-generation sequencing for EGFR and KRAS. A qualified laboratory professional prepares a report and communicates the results to the ordering provider.

Clinical Example (0449U)

A 32-year-old primigravida presents to her obstetrician at 10 weeks gestation with no known family history of genetic conditions. A blood sample is submitted for carrier screening.

Description of Procedure (0449U)

Isolate and subject maternal DNA from blood to genomic analysis of CFTR, SMN1, HBA1, HBA2, and HBB to identify carrier status. A qualified laboratory professional examines the mutation calls for each gene, generates a report specifying the patient's carrier status for each condition, and sends the report to the ordering physician.

Clinical Example (0450U)

A 72-year-old female presents with an immunoglobulin G kappa monoclonal myeloma. Serum-based proteomic assay to define baseline specific clonotypic peptides quantification is ordered.

Description of Procedure (0450U)

Enrich, enzymatically digest, and analyze the serum by liquid chromatography-tandem mass spectrometry using two fragmentation methods (HCD and EThcD) to increase the amount of detectable protein fragments. Use up to eight abundantly detected paraprotein-specific (clonotypic) peptides to create a patient-specific panel. A qualified laboratory professional reviews the results and issues a report.

Clinical Example (0451U)

A 72-year-old female presents with a history of multiple myeloma status post-treatment and complete response serum protein electrophoresis. Serum-based proteomic follow-up assay is ordered and compared with previous assay to evaluate for residual disease.

Description of Procedure (0451U)

Enzymatically digest and analyze the serum by liquid chromatography-tandem mass spectrometry using targeted parallel reaction monitoring. Quantify and use up to eight previously detected clonotypic peptides to calculate the monoclonal paraprotein abundance. A qualified laboratory professional reviews the results and issues a report.

★ = Telemedicine   ◀ = Audio-only   ✛ = Add-on code   ✗ = FDA approval pending   # = Resequenced code   ⦸ = Modifier 51 exempt

Clinical Example (0452U)

A 48-year-old male presents with intermittent, painless hematuria that was confirmed on urinalysis. Urine is submitted to further assess the risk of bladder cancer before undergoing an invasive cystoscopy.

Description of Procedure (0452U)

Extract and analyze DNA from urine for methylated PENK by linear target enrichment. The qualified laboratory professional examines the test results, composes a report, and sends it to the ordering provider.

Clinical Example (0453U)

A 55-year-old male, who has a family history of colon cancer, presents with abdominal pain and blood in his stool. A blood sample is submitted for methylation-based quantitative polymerase chain reaction (qPCR) analysis to detect circulating-tumor DNA.

Description of Procedure (0453U)

Isolate and subject cell-free DNA from plasma to bisulfite conversion followed by real-time PCR with fluorescence monitoring for the methylation status of six colon cancer–specific genes regions (Septin9, IKZF1, BCAT1, Septin9-2, VAV3, BCAN). A qualified laboratory professional composes a report for the clinician.

Clinical Example (0454U)

A 3-year-old male, who has a developmental delay/intellectual disability, hypotonia, and multiple congenital anomalies, presents to a geneticist. Optical genome mapping is ordered.

Description of Procedure (0454U)

Extract and subject DNA from whole blood to optical genome mapping. A qualified laboratory professional interprets the results, prepares a report, and communicates the results to the ordering provider.

Clinical Example (0455U)

A 24-year-old female presents to her physician with vaginal discharge with burning sensation while urinating. The physician orders a multiplex amplified probe testing on the vagina swab for Chlamydia trachomatis (CT), Neisseria gonorrhoeae (NG), and Trichomonas vaginalis (TV).

Description of Procedure (0455U)

Isolate high-quality nucleic acid from the vaginal swab. Perform polymerase chain reaction amplification using probes for CT, NG, and TV with a control. A qualified

laboratory professional reviews the results and issues a report to the ordering provider.

Clinical Example (0456U)

A 51-year-old female who has rheumatoid arthritis and is on methotrexate continues to have high-disease activity despite adequate dosing. Blood is submitted to determine the likelihood of an inadequate response to a tumor necrosis factor inhibitor (TNFi).

Description of Procedure (0456U)

Extract and subject RNA from whole blood to next-generation sequencing for NOD2, CFLAR, NOTCH1, TRIM25, BCL2, ALPL, IL1B, ZFP36, LIMK2, JAK3, CDK11A, GOLGA1, IMPDH2, SPON2, SPINT2, ATRAID, COMMD5, KLHDC3, STOML2. Combine the gene-expression data and additional biological features, including anti-CCP (analyzed from serum) and demographic variables (body mass index, patient sex, and patient global assessment), in an algorithm to generate a likelihood of inadequate response to a TNFi score. A qualified laboratory professional reviews the findings and reports the findings to the ordering provider.

Clinical Example (0457U)

A 40-year-old female presents after learning she lives in a region with known perfluoroalkyl substances (PFAS) contamination in the drinking water. Plasma is submitted to determine the presence of PFAS and assess the risk of PFAS-associated health conditions.

Description of Procedure (0457U)

Analyze plasma or serum by liquid chromatography with tandem mass spectrometry for methylperfluorooctane sulfonamidoacetic acid, perfluorohexanesulfonic acid, perfluorooctanoic acid, perfluorooctanoic acid isomers, perfluorodecanoic acid, perfluoroundecanoic acid, perfluorooctane sulfonic acid, perfluoromethylheptane sulfonic acid isomers, and perfluorononanoic acid. A qualified laboratory professional reviews the findings and reports the findings to the ordering provider.

Clinical Example (0458U)

A 45-year-old female presents for evaluation of breast health. A tear sample is submitted for protein analysis to assess the patient's risk level and active breast abnormality.

Description of Procedure (0458U)

Evaluate the tear fluid sample using a standard sandwich enzyme-linked immunosorbent assay for the concentration of S100 A8 and A9 proteins. A qualified laboratory professional reviews the findings and issues a report that shows a high-, medium-, or low-risk for active breast abnormality.

Clinical Example (0459U)

A 62-year-old male presents with worsening memory complaints for the past year. The family also noticed mood changes and anxiety. The neurologist suspects Alzheimer disease and recommends lumbar puncture for cerebrospinal fluid (CSF) biomarkers.

Description of Procedure (0459U)

Subject CSF to analysis by immunoassay for tTau/Abeta42 ratio. A laboratory professional reviews the results and reports the findings to the ordering provider.

Clinical Example (0460U)

A 55-year-old male, who has a new diagnosis of colorectal cancer on a chemotherapy regime, including fluorouracil, presents with a worsening of his major depression. A buccal swab is submitted for a pharmacogenomic analysis.

Description of Procedure (0460U)

Isolate and subject high-quality genomic DNA from the buccal or blood sample to genotyping using real-time polymerase chain reaction for targeted variants in CYP1A2, CYP2B6, CYP2C9, CYP2C19, CYP2C cluster, CYP2D6, CYP3A4, CYP3A5, CYP4F2, COMT, DPYD, F2, F5, GRIK4, HLA-A, HLA-B, HTR2A, NUDT15, OPRM1, SLC6A4, SLCOB1, TPMT, UGT1A1, and VKORC1 genes. Generate report with genotype results and phenotypic interpretation. A qualified laboratory director approves the report, and it is delivered to the ordering provider.

Clinical Example (0461U)

A 55-year-old male who has a history of depression presents with a new diagnosis of colorectal cancer. Upon learning of the diagnosis, his depression worsened and medical therapy is warranted. A buccal swab is submitted for a pharmacogenomic analysis to evaluate the metabolizer status of a selection of genes.

Description of Procedure (0461U)

Isolate and subject high-quality genomic DNA from the buccal or blood sample to genotyping using real-time polymerase chain reaction for targeted variants in CYP1A2, CYP2B6, CYP2C9, CYP2C19, CYP2C cluster, CYP2D6, CYP3A4, CYP3A5, CYP4F2, COMT, DPYD, F2, F5, GRIK4, HLA-A, HLA-B, HTR2A, NUDT15, OPRM1, SLC6A4, SLCOB1, TPMT, UGT1A1, and VKORC1 genes. Generate a report with genotype results, phenotypic interpretation,

and likely effects of the genetic variants on drug metabolism. A qualified laboratory director approves the report, and it is delivered to the ordering provider.

Clinical Example (0462U)

A 40-year-old female presents with a history of chronic sleep disturbances. The physician orders a melatonin-level test.

Description of Procedure (0462U)

Isolate and subject melatonin from saliva to quantitative immunoassay. Chart results for pattern observation of the increase or decrease of melatonin concentrations over time. A qualified laboratory professional prepares a report, which is delivered to the ordering provider.

Clinical Example (0463U)

A 30-year-old female is diagnosed with abnormal results (eg, atypical squamous cells of undetermined significance and/or human papillomavirus [HPV] primary screen positive test results) in routine cervical cancer screening. A cervical epithelial cell sample is sent for HPV messenger RNA gene expression profiling, providing the current risk status of progression to cervical cancer.

Description of Procedure (0463U)

Extract and subject nucleic acid from cervical swab to nucleic acid amplification and simultaneous detection with molecular beacon probes for HPV E6 and E7 and high-risk types 16, 18, 31, 33, 45, 52, 58. A qualified laboratory professional analyzes the results, and a report is sent to the ordering provider.

Clinical Example (0464U)

A 50-year-old female presents to her physician for a yearly wellness evaluation. Given her age, her physician recommends colon cancer screening and orders a multi-target stool DNA test.

Description of Procedure (0464U)

Isolate and subject high-quality DNA from stool samples to bisulfite treatment and quantitative real-time target and signal amplification for detection of specific methylated DNA markers, including LASS4, LRRC4, and PPP2R5C (a reference marker ZDHHC1). Detect fecal hemoglobin using a quantitative enzyme-linked immunosorbent assay. Generate a qualitative positive or negative result using an algorithm that incorporates the results of the DNA methylation and hemoglobin assays. A qualified laboratory professional issues a report to the provider.

Clinical Example (0465U)

A 53-year-old male presents with hematuria and negative results from urinary cytology and fluorescence in situ hybridization tests. A urine sample is sent for methylation quantitative polymerase chain reaction (qPCR) to evaluate for bladder cancer.

Description of Procedure (0465U)

Extract and subject high-quality DNA from urine-exfoliated cells to fluorescence qPCR following bisulfite treatment to detect the reference gene, ACTB, and the methylation of ONECUT2 and VIM. A qualified laboratory professional reviews the results and issues a report to the ordering physician.

Clinical Example (0466U)

A 42-year-old male, who has a family history of coronary artery disease, presents for an annual health evaluation. His atherosclerotic cardiovascular disease risk estimator was 3.7%. The physician orders genome-wide association studies to determine the polygenic risk of acquired heart disease.

Description of Procedure (0466U)

Extract and subject high-quality DNA from the cheek/buccal swab to genotyping using an array. Impute and use the array results to calculate a polygenic risk score. A qualified laboratory professional reviews the results and issues a report to the ordering provider.

Clinical Example (0467U)

A 67-year-old male presents to his urologist for surveillance of previously treated non-muscle, invasive bladder cancer. A urine specimen is sent for evaluation of minimal residual disease.

Description of Procedure (0467U)

Extract and subject high-quality DNA from urine to deep sequencing on exons and noncoding regions of 60 genes and low-pass whole-genome sequencing. A qualified laboratory professional reviews the results and issues a report to the ordering physician.

Clinical Example (0468U)

A 47-year-old female who has diabetes presents following a recent computed tomography scan that showed a fatty liver. Blood is submitted to determine the risk level of nonalcoholic steatohepatitis (NASH) and fibrosis.

Description of Procedure (0468U)

Test samples for HbA1c, YKL40, alpha 2-macroglobulin, and miR-34a-5p using immunoturbidimetry, enzyme-linked immunosorbent assay, and quantitative reverse transcription polymerase chain reaction. Combine the results using an algorithm that reports a single score reflecting both NASH activity and fibrosis.

Clinical Example (0469U)

A 35-year-old pregnant female presents for her 12-week fetal ultrasound that shows an intracardiac echogenic focus. Amniotic fluid is submitted to assess the fetus for constitutional/heritable genetic changes.

Description of Procedure (0469U)

Sequence the genomic DNA from the fetal specimen and establish the backup cell cultures for maternal cell contamination (MCC), if needed. A qualified laboratory professional examines fetal DNA sequence variants, correlates these variants with the fetus's phenotype, and confirms the absence of MCC. Analyze parental samples as comparators or for maternal cell contamination in some cases. Evaluate and report variants best matching the phenotype for pathogenicity based on the American College of Medical Genetics and Genomics guidelines.

Clinical Example (0470U)

A 68-year-old patient, who has a biopsy-confirmed p16-positive squamous cell carcinoma, presents for treatment. Before treatment initiation, a baseline test is performed to identify the human papillomavirus (HPV) subtype and initial copy-number. Following treatment, the cell-free HPV DNA is evaluated to assess treatment efficacy and minimal residual disease.

Description of Procedure (0470U)

Isolate, amplify, and sequence the cell-free DNA from plasma, to identify specific HPV 16 and 18 subtypes. Based on sequencing, report results as "detected or not detected" in copies/mL. Identify the changes in HPV copy-numbers over time based on historical data and compose and provide the report to the ordering provider.

Clinical Example (0471U)

A 65-year-old male, who recently had a colonoscopy-confirmed colon carcinoma, reports blood in his stool. Tissue is submitted for biomarker testing to assess the patient's KRAS and NRAS mutation status.

Description of Procedure (0471U)

Isolate and subject DNA from formalin-fixed paraffin-embedded tissue to real-time polymerase chain reaction to assess the mutation status of exons 2, 3, and 4 of KRAS and NRAS genes. A qualified laboratory professional examines the test results and composes a report that specifies the patient's mutation status.

Clinical Example (0472U)

A 46-year-old female presents to a rheumatologist with a history of dry eyes and has been using saline eye drops for 2 years. Her serum is submitted for semiqualitative detection of early Sjogren's syndrome antibodies.

Description of Procedure (0472U)

Assay serum using an enzyme-linked immunosorbent assay–based semiquantitative assay to detect immunoglobulin G, M, A antibodies against carbonic anhydrase VI (CA VI), parotid specific/secretory protein, and salivary protein. A qualified laboratory professional reviews the findings and compiles a report with specific levels of autoantibodies, and the report is sent to the ordering provider.

Clinical Example (0473U)

A 53-year-old male, who has colorectal carcinoma, undergoes a peripheral blood draw and a tumor biopsy. The matched blood and tissue specimens are submitted for somatic cancer mutation testing.

Description of Procedure (0473U)

Isolate extracted DNA from tumor tissue and blood for cancer mutation testing using next-generation sequencing. Custom software identifies somatic mutations in the tumor and filters out germline variants identified from the patient's normal DNA. Assess and report sequence variants, copy-number variants, rearrangements, microsatellite instability, and tumor mutational burden to a qualified health care professional with information on clinical significance.

Clinical Example (0474U)

A 42-year-old female, who has a recent diagnosis of breast cancer and has a family history of multiple malignancies, is recommended for germline testing by the genetic counselor. Saliva is submitted for testing.

Description of Procedure (0474U)

Isolate and subject DNA from blood or saliva to next-generation sequencing to identify single-nucleotide variants/indels in 88 genes and copy number variants in 20 genes. A bioinformatician compiles a sequencing report with identified germline variants. A qualified laboratory professional reviews the findings and issues a report to the ordering provider.

Clinical Example (0475U)

A 50-year-old male presents with an elevated prostate-specific antigen and a family history of cancer. A prostate biopsy shows a Gleason score of 3+4 prostate cancer. Saliva is submitted for germline testing.

Description of Procedure (0475U)

Isolate and subject DNA from blood or saliva to next-generation sequencing to identify single-nucleotide variants/indels in 23 genes, copy number variants in 15 genes, and 223 single-nucleotide polymorphisms associated with prostate cancer risk. A qualified laboratory professional compiles a sequencing report with the identified germline variants and issues a report to the ordering physician.

Clinical Example (0476U)

A 35-year-old female presents to a clinic with major depressive disorder after having no success with one antidepressant. Medication therapy is needed given clinical findings. A buccal swab is submitted for pharmacogenomic testing to evaluate the metabolizer status.

Description of Procedure (0476U)

Isolate and subject high-quality genomic DNA from a buccal sample to genotyping using real-time polymerase chain reaction for a group of variants in the 14 genes (ie, CYP1A2, CYP2B6, CYP2C19, CYP2D6, CYP3A4, CYP3A5, COMT, DRD2, GRIK4, HLA-A, HLA-B, HTR2A, HTR2C, SLC6A4). A qualified laboratory director prepares a report with genotype results and phenotypic interpretation and delivers it to the ordering provider.

Clinical Example (0477U)

A 35-year-old female presents to a clinic with major depressive disorder after having no success with one antidepressant. A buccal swab is submitted for pharmacogenomic testing to evaluate the metabolizer status.

Description of Procedure (0477U)

Isolate and subject high-quality genomic DNA from a buccal sample to genotyping using real-time polymerase chain reaction for a group of variants in the 14 genes (ie, CYP1A2, CYP2B6, CYP2C19, CYP2D6, CYP3A4, CYP3A5, COMT, DRD2, GRIK4, HLA-A, HLA-B, HTR2A, HTR2C, SLC6A4). A qualified laboratory director prepares a report with genotype results, phenotypic interpretation, and impacted gene-drug interactions and sends the report to the ordering provider.

Clinical Example (0478U)

A 70-year-old male is diagnosed with metastatic non-small cell lung cancer. Formalin-fixed paraffin-embedded (FFPE) tissue is submitted to determine targeted and immunotherapy eligibility.

Description of Procedure (0478U)

Extract and analyze RNA and DNA from FFPE tissue using digital polymerase chain reaction for EGFR, KRAS, BRAF, ALK, ROS1, RET, NTRK 1/2/3, ERBB2, and MET. A qualified laboratory professional examines the results, composes a report that specifies the patient's mutation status, and reports the findings to the ordering provider.

Clinical Example (0479U)

A 70-year-old female, who has a one-year history of forgetfulness and occasional spatial confusion when driving, presents to a neurologist for evaluation. A blood sample is submitted for pTau217 analysis.

Description of Procedure (0479U)

Subject plasma to a digital immunoassay for pTau217. A qualified laboratory professional reviews the results and reports them to the ordering provider.

Clinical Example (0480U)

A 35-year-old male, who was hospitalized with a 10-day history of headache, fever, and malaise, has negative conventional testing for meningitis/encephalitis. Cerebrospinal fluid is submitted for metagenomic analysis.

Description of Procedure (0480U)

Extract and subject DNA and RNA from cerebrospinal fluid to next-generation sequencing and bioinformatic analysis to identify pathogenic bacteria, DNA and RNA viruses, fungi, and parasites. A qualified laboratory professional prepares a report and sends it to the ordering provider.

Clinical Example (0481U)

A 60-year-old male is diagnosed with a lower-grade infiltrating astrocytoma without necrosis or microvascular proliferation (histological diagnostic criteria for glioblastoma). Testing is ordered for IDH1, IDH2, and TERT.

Description of Procedure (0481U)

Extract and subject DNA from formalin-fixed paraffin-embedded tissue to next-generation sequencing for TERT promoter and IDH1 and IDH2. A qualified laboratory professional prepares a report and communicates the results to the ordering provider.

Clinical Example (0482U)

A 32-year-old female, who is at 25 weeks of gestation, presents with clinical signs and symptoms of hypertension that might progress into preeclampsia with severe features within 2 weeks. Testing for the soluble fms-like tyrosine kinase 1 (sFlt-1)/placental growth factor (PlGF) ratio is ordered for risk assessment.

Description of Procedure (0482U)

Measure sFlt-1 and PlGF from the serum. Report the sFlt-1/PlGF ratio and the risk of progression for severe features of preeclampsia.

Clinical Example (0483U)

A 23-year-old female has tested positive for N. gonorrhoeae. The provider submits an oral, rectal, or vaginal swab for gyrA S91F point mutations to determine ciprofloxacin resistance.

Description of Procedure (0483U)

Extract and analyze DNA from an oral, rectal, or vaginal swab using a polymerase chain reaction assay for the presence of N. gonorrhoeae gyrA S91F mutation and associated findings to predict ciprofloxacin resistance. A qualified laboratory professional reviews the result and reports it to the ordering provider.

Clinical Example (0484U)

A 24-year-old male presents to his physician with M. genitalium. His physician orders a test on a rectal swab to predict sensitivity to macrolide antibiotics.

Description of Procedure (0484U)

Extract and analyze DNA from rectal swab for the presence of 23S ribosomal RNA variants of M. genitalium. A qualified health care professional analyzes the results and algorithm, composes a report, and communicates the results to the ordering physician.

Clinical Example (0485U)

A 49-year-old female, who has ovarian serous adenocarcinoma, presents with findings concerning for colonic metastases. Liquid biopsy testing is ordered to determine actionable mutations due to the insufficient availability of tumor biopsy material.

Description of Procedure (0485U)

Isolate and subject high-quality cell-free DNA/cell-free RNA and genomic DNA/RNA from plasma and the buffy coat to whole exome and whole transcriptome sequencing. Generate reports for germline mutations, clonal hematopoiesis of indeterminate potential, tumor-derived single-nucleotide variants, small insertions/deletions, copy-number alterations, fusions, microsatellite instability, and tumor mutational burden.

A qualified laboratory professional analyzes the data and prepares the report for the ordering provider.

Clinical Example (0486U)

A 52-year-old female presents to her oncologist with a history of stage IV non-small cell lung cancer and has started a new line of systemic therapy that is causing side effects. A blood sample is submitted to assess for baseline changes.

Description of Procedure (0486U)

Isolate cell-free tumor DNA from the patient's blood sample. Perform next-generation sequencing analysis of >500 tumor methylation markers. A qualified health care professional analyzes the results, compares to previous results, if applicable, composes a report, and communicates the results to the appropriate caregiver.

Clinical Example (0487U)

A 52-year-old female presents to her oncologist with recurrent stage IV non-small cell lung cancer. A blood test that may inform targeted treatment or immunotherapy treatment options and/or clinical trials is ordered.

Description of Procedure (0487U)

Isolate cell-free tumor DNA from the patient's blood sample. Perform next-generation sequencing of 84 genes to detect therapeutically relevant variants (eg, single-nucleotide variants), indels, and copy-number amplifications, and copy-number losses and fusions. A qualified laboratory professional examines the calls and composes a report with pathogenic variants and quantification. Communicate the report to the ordering provider.

Clinical Example (0488U)

A 32-year-old female who is primigravida Rh-negative and alloimmunized to Kell (K) antigens presents to maternal-fetal medicine at 13 weeks gestation. Her reproductive partner is unknown. A blood sample is submitted to assess the fetal Kell (K) antigen status.

Description of Procedure (0488U)

Isolate and subject cell-free fetal DNA from the alloimmunized pregnant patient's blood sample to multiplex polymerase chain reaction amplification and next-generation sequencing for identification of the ordered blood antigen marker (Rh, C, c, D, E, Duffy (Fya) or Kell [K]). A qualified health care professional analyzes the results, composes a report, and communicates the results to the appropriate caregiver.

Clinical Example (0489U)

A 32-year-old female who is pregnant is identified as a carrier of the F508del pathogenic variant in the CFTR gene. Her physician orders a test to determine if the fetus is at risk of being affected.

Description of Procedure (0489U)

Subject cell-free fetal DNA from maternal plasma to targeted DNA sequence analysis of one gene. A qualified health care professional analyzes the results, composes a report, and communicates the results to the appropriate caregiver.

Clinical Example (0490U)

A 78-year-old male, who has node-positive stage III cutaneous melanoma, is in remission for 12 months post-treatment. His oncologist submits a blood sample to evaluate circulating melanoma cell status to assess whether the patient's cancer may be relapsing and if treatment should be reinitiated.

Description of Procedure (0490U)

Subject blood to fixation, immunomagnetic selection, and immunofluorescence staining for CD146, high-molecular weight melanoma-associated antigen, CD34, and CD45. A qualified health care professional analyzes the results, composes a report, and communicates the results to the ordering oncologist.

Clinical Example (0491U)

A 69-year-old female who has estrogen receptor (ER)-negative metastatic breast cancer on treatment with endocrine therapy shows initial signs of disease progression. Her oncologist submits a blood sample to evaluate circulating tumor cells-ER status to assess whether her prognosis has changed and whether a different treatment approach should be considered.

Description of Procedure (0491U)

Subject blood to fixation, immunomagnetic selection, and immunofluorescence staining for protein biomarkers associated with tumor cells. Identify stained cells, characterize morphologically, enumerate, and score for ER protein biomarker positivity relative to controls via proprietary imaging software. A laboratory scientist reviews images and generates a report with absolute and ER-positive cell count and reference range. A laboratory director reviews the report from the laboratory scientist and issues a report to the ordering oncologist.

★=Telemedicine ◀=Audio-only ➕=Add-on code ⭘=FDA approval pending #=Resequenced code ⊘=Modifier 51 exempt

Clinical Example (0492U)

A 57-year-old male, who has metastatic non-small cell lung cancer on treatment with a PD-1 inhibitor therapy, has an uncertain therapeutic response. His oncologist submits a blood sample to evaluate circulating tumor cells-PD-L1 status to assess whether a different treatment approach should be considered.

Description of Procedure (0492U)

Subject blood to fixation, immunomagnetic selection, and immunofluorescence staining for protein biomarkers associated with tumor cells. Identify stained cells, characterize morphologically, enumerate, and score for PD-L1 protein biomarker positivity relative to controls via proprietary imaging software. A laboratory scientist reviews images and generates a report with absolute and PD-L1 positive cell count and reference range. A laboratory director reviews the report from the laboratory scientist and issues a report to the ordering oncologist.

Clinical Example (0493U)

A 55-year-old male, who had orthotopic heart transplantation 6 months ago, presents to his physician for a routine six-month follow-up visit. A blood test is analyzed for donor-derived cell-free DNA (dd-cfDNA) to assess the patient's risk for rejection and the need for an endomyocardial biopsy.

Description of Procedure (0493U)

Subject cell-free DNA to targeted next-generation sequencing to collect genotypes specific to the patient and donor organ. Quantify the percentage of dd-cfDNA (dd-cfDNA%) in the specimen using an algorithm. A qualified health care professional analyzes the results, composes a report, and communicates the results to the appropriate caregiver.

Clinical Example (0494U)

A 28-year-old female who is pregnant presents for her first obstetrics appointment. The patient is Rh negative, so blood is drawn to screen for the fetus's Rh status.

Description of Procedure (0494U)

Isolate and subject the cell-free DNA sample from the patient's blood to targeted next-generation sequencing of the RHD gene. Use an algorithm to generate and report a positive or negative result. A qualified health care professional analyzes the results, composes a report, and communicates the results to the ordering obstetrician.

Clinical Example (0495U)

A 66-year-old male is referred to a urologist based on elevated prostate-specific antigen. His physician orders a test to determine the risk of clinically significant prostate cancer.

Description of Procedure (0495U)

Subject plasma protein concentrations to sandwich-based immunoassays for tPSA, fPSA, KLK2, PSP94, and GDF15. Perform DNA genotyping for 60 variants. Perform an algorithm using DNA and protein results, as well as an analysis of patient-specific questions. A qualified health care professional analyzes the results, composes a report, and communicates the results to the ordering physician.

Clinical Example (0496U)

A 50-year-old male presents with metastatic colorectal cancer and symptoms of bowel obstruction and weight loss. Blood is submitted to assess the patient's risk for recurrent disease.

Description of Procedure (0496U)

Isolate and test cell-free DNA from blood for mutations (KRAS, APC, CTNNB1, BRAF, TP53, NRAS, PIK3CA, SMAD4) and methylation (C9Orf50, KCNQ5, MYO1G, CLIP4, FLI1, TWIST1, ZNF132), and evaluate plasma by enzyme-linked immunosorbent assay for CA19-9, OPN, CEA, and IL-8. A qualified laboratory professional reviews the findings and composes a report describing the colorectal cancer or advanced adenoma risk and sends it to the ordering provider.

Clinical Example (0497U)

A 63-year-old male presents with an abnormal prostate-specific antigen to his physician. Testing is ordered on the formalin-fixed paraffin-embedded biopsy to evaluate his risk for aggressive prostate cancer.

Description of Procedure (0497U)

Extract and subject RNA tumor tissue to quantitative reverse transcription polymerase chain reaction for FOXM1, MCM3, MTUS1, TTC21B, ALAS1, and PPP2CA. Enter the gene expression data and clinical and pathological information into an algorithm to produce a risk score. A qualified health care professional analyzes the results, composes a report, and communicates the results to the appropriate caregiver.

Clinical Example (0498U)

A 48-year-old male presents with stage III colorectal cancer. The blood and formalin-fixed paraffin-embedded (FFPE) samples are submitted for cell-free DNA (cfDNA) and DNA isolation, respectively, to assess targeted mutation and methylation pattern.

Description of Procedure (0498U)

Isolate cfDNA from blood. Isolate and subject genomic DNA from an FFPE specimen to next-generation sequencing in 43 genes and methylation pattern in 45 genes. Bioinformatics software identifies oncogenic mutations, microsatellite instability status, and aberrantly methylated regions. Use other software to extract variants and methylation levels from genomic data. Analytics classify variants based on their oncogenic level. A qualified laboratory professional reviews the data and prepares a report for the ordering provider to inform treatment decisions.

Clinical Example (0499U)

A 50-year-old male, who has stage III colorectal cancer, presents to his physician with symptoms of bleeding in the rectum, weight loss, and constipation. The physician orders a targeted mutation panel.

Description of Procedure (0499U)

Subject DNA from the formalin-fixed paraffin-embedded sample to targeted next-generation sequencing for NRAS, EGFR, CTNNB1, PIK3CA, APC, BRAF, KRAS, and TP53. A qualified health care professional analyzes the results, composes a report, and communicates the results to the ordering physician.

Clinical Example (0500U)

A 60-year-old male, who has inflammatory arthritis, dermatitis, and relapsing chondritis, presents to his physician with macrocytic anemia and thrombo-cytopenia. Blood is submitted to evaluate the patient for VEXAS syndrome.

Description of Procedure (0500U)

Subject DNA from whole blood to mutation detection for M41T, M41V, M41L, c.118-2A>C, c.118-1G>C, c.118- 9_118-2del, S56F, and S621C. A qualified health care professional analyzes the results, composes a report, and communicates the results to the appropriate caregiver.

Clinical Example (0501U)

A 55-year-old male presents to his physician with fecal immunochemical test–positive result. His physician orders a test to evaluate his risk for colorectal cancer.

Description of Procedure (0501U)

Isolate the plasma from the blood samples and measure cell-free DNA concentration using a luminometer. A qualified health care professional analyzes the results, composes a report, and communicates the results to the ordering physician.

Clinical Example (0502U)

A 33-year-old female presents to her physician with a history of multiple sex partners. Her physician orders HPV testing.

Description of Procedure (0502U)

Collect, lyse, and subject cells from pap smear to branched-chain capture hybridization. A qualified health care professional analyzes the results, composes a report, and communicates the results to the ordering physician.

Clinical Example (0503U)

A 71-year-old female presents to her physician with symptoms of cognitive decline. Her physician orders a blood test to determine the risk of Alzheimer disease.

Description of Procedure (0503U)

Immunoprecipitate and subject whole blood to liquid chromatography-tandem mass spectrometry to detect Aβ40, Aβ42, pTau217, and npTau217. Combine the ratios using an algorithm to calculate an amyloid probability score. A qualified laboratory professional reviews the results and provides a report to the ordering physician.

Clinical Example (0504U)

An 18-year-old female presents with dysuria. Urine is submitted to assess for a urinary tract infection.

Description of Procedure (0504U)

Isolate and subject DNA from urine to real-time polymerase chain reaction to determine the presence or absence of Acinetobacter baumannii, Candida albicans, Citrobacter freundii, Enterobacter aerogenes, Enterobacter cloacae, Enterococcus faecalis, Enterococcus faecium, Escherichia coli, Klebsiella oxytoca, Klebsiella pneumoniae, Morganella morganii, Proteus mirabilis, Proteus vulgaris, Providencia stuarttii, Pseudomonas aeruginosa, Staphylococcus saprophyticus, and Streptococcus agalactiae (group B strep). A qualified laboratory professional reviews the findings, composes a report, and communicates the findings to the ordering provider.

Clinical Example (0505U)

An 18-year-old female presents with dysuria. A vaginal swab is submitted to assess for the presence of a vaginal tract infection.

Description of Procedure (0505U)

Isolate and subject DNA isolated from the vaginal swab to real-time polymerase chain reaction to detect Atopobium vaginae; Bacteroides fragilis; Bacterial Vaginosis-Associated Bacteria (BVABl, BVAB2, and BVAB3); Mycoplasma hominis; Gardnerella vagina/is (trivalent pool); Haemophilus ducreyi; Megasphaera Type 1; Megasphaera Type 2; Mobiluncus spp. (M. curtisii and M. mulieris); Ureaplasma urealyticum; Prevotella bivia; Enterococcus faecalis; Treponema pallidum (Syphilis); Candida albicans; Candida Group (C. dubliniensis, C. lusitaniae, and C. tropicalis); Candida glabrata; Candida krusei; Candida parapsilosis; Mycoplasma genitalium; Chlamydia trachomatis; Trichomonas vaginalis; Herpes Simplex Virus 1; Herpes Simplex Virus 2; Klebsiella pneumoniae; Neisseria gonorrhoeae; Staphylococcus aureus; Streptococcus agalactiae (group B strep); and Escherichia coli, Lactobacillus crispatus, Lactobacillus gasseri, Lactobacillus iners, or Lactobacillus jensenii. A qualified health care professional analyzes the results, composes a report, and communicates the results to the appropriate caregiver.

Clinical Example (0506U)

A 50-year-old male smoker, who has obesity, presents with a five-year history of gastroesophageal reflux disease. His physician ordered testing for the likelihood of Barrett's esophagus.

Description of Procedure (0506U)

Subject DNA from esophageal cell to a methylation next-generation sequencing panel containing 89 targeted genomic regions. Apply an algorithm. A qualified health care professional analyzes the results, composes a report, and communicates the results to the ordering physician.

Clinical Example (0507U)

A 32-year-old female, who has a maternal history of ovarian cancer and a BRCA1 gene, presents to her gynecologist. Blood is submitted to evaluate her for the presence or absence of ovarian cancer.

Description of Procedure (0507U)

Extract and subject cell-free DNA (cfDNA) from the plasma to next-generation sequencing of 5-hydroxymethylation (5hmC)-enriched cfDNA and total cfDNA. Enter data into an algorithm to report the detection or non-detection of an abnormal epigenomic sequence. A qualified laboratory professional reviews the findings and provides a report to the ordering physician.

Clinical Example (0508U)

A 50-year-old male presents to a clinic 60 days post-renal transplant for end-stage renal failure. A test is ordered to determine the risk of transplant failure.

Description of Procedure (0508U)

Extract and subject cell-free DNA from plasma to digital polymerase chain reaction for 40 variants to monitor donor vs recipient. A qualified health care professional analyzes the results, composes a report, and communicates the results to the appropriate caregiver.

Clinical Example (0509U)

A 50-year-old male presents 90 days post-renal transplant with concern for transplant rejection. Plasma is submitted to evaluate the risk for active rejection using a comparison to previously archived data.

Description of Procedure (0509U)

Extract and subject cell-free DNA from plasma to digital polymerase chain reaction for 12 variants to monitor donor vs recipient and compared to the previous profile. A qualified health care professional analyzes the results, composes a report, and communicates the results to the appropriate caregiver.

Clinical Example (0510U)

A 65-year-old female, who has stage IV pancreatic cancer, had previously received whole-transcriptome RNA sequencing. The sequencing data are submitted for augmentative algorithmic analysis to predict tumor molecular subtype, which the patient's provider uses to help inform first-line therapy selection.

Description of Procedure (0510U)

Evaluate normalized gene-expression data from 16 genes (GPR87, REG4, KRT6A, ANXA10, BCAR3, GATA6, PTGES, CLDN18, ITGA3, LGALS4, C16orf74, DDC, S100A2, SLC40A1, KRT5, CLRN3) from previously sequenced whole-transcriptome RNA using a proprietary augmentative algorithm to classify specimens into one of two molecular subtypes (basal-like or classical). A qualified health care professional reviews the report and communicates the results to the ordering provider.

Clinical Example (0511U)

A 54-year-old female, who has chemorefractory ovarian cancer stage IIIC, presents to her oncologist. The physician orders a test to assess the tumor's response to drug therapies to determine potential treatment selection.

Description of Procedure (0511U)

Grow tumor cells isolated from tumor specimens in cell culture to derive tumor organoids in a three-dimensional microenvironment. Expose culture cells to therapeutic agents, and then assess cell viability via luminescence. Algorithms combine the absolute and relative measures of drug response to produce a response score for each drug. A qualified laboratory professional reviews, edits, and prepares the report, and communicates the results to the ordering physician.

Clinical Example (0512U)

A 57-year-old male presents following a biopsy-confirmed diagnosis of prostate cancer. The physician orders a test to predict the patient's risk for microsatellite instability-high (MSI-H) status.

Description of Procedure (0512U)

Analyze digitized hematoxylin and eosin stained slides from prostate cancer formalin-fixed paraffin-embedded tissue using deep neural networks. The algorithm identifies patients whose tumors are likely to be MSI-H. A qualified health care professional analyzes the results, reviews the report, and communicates the results to the ordering physician.

Clinical Example (0513U)

A 57-year-old male presents following a biopsy-confirmed diagnosis of prostate cancer. The physician orders a test to predict the patient's risk for microsatellite instability status and homologous recombination deficiency (HRD) status.

Description of Procedure (0513U)

Analyze digitized hematoxylin and eosin stained slides from prostate cancer formalin-fixed paraffin-embedded tissue using deep neural networks. The algorithm identifies patients whose tumors are likely to be microsatellite instability-high and HRD. A qualified health care professional analyzes the results, reviews the report, and communicates the results to the ordering physician.

Clinical Example (0514U)

A 24-year-old male treated for Crohn's disease with adalimumab presents with recurring symptoms. Serum is submitted to assess adalimumab levels.

Description of Procedure (0514U)

Subject serum to fluorescence resonance energy transfer signal to detect adalimumab presence and quantity. Report results using a numerical value in micrograms per milliliter (µg/mL). A qualified health care professional analyzes the results, composes a report, and communicates the results to the appropriate caregiver.

Clinical Example (0515U)

A 24-year-old male treated for Crohn's disease with infliximab presents with recurring symptoms. Serum is submitted to assess infliximab levels.

Description of Procedure (0515U)

Subject serum to fluorescence resonance energy transfer signal to detect infliximab presence and quantity. Report results using a numerical value in micrograms per milliliter (µg/mL). A qualified health care professional analyzes the results, composes a report, and communicates the results to the appropriate caregiver.

Clinical Example (0516U)

A 54-year-old male presents to a clinic with severe pain after surgery despite taking opioids. A whole-blood sample is sent for pharmacogenomic testing to evaluate the metabolizer status.

Description of Procedure (0516U)

Isolate and subject high-quality genomic DNA from whole blood to genotyping using next-generation sequencing for 40 genes (ie, ABCB1, ABCG2, ADRA2A, ANKK1, APOE, COMT, CYP1A2, CYP2B6, CYP2C19, CYP2C8, CYP2C9, CYP2D6, CYP3A4, CYP3A5, DBH, DPYD, DRD1, DRD4, F2, F5, FLOT1 [HLA-B], GABRA6, GABRP, GRIK4, HCP5 [HLA-B], HLA-A, HTR2A, HTR2C, ITGB3, KIF6, MTHFR, OPRD1, OPRK1, OPRM1, SLCO1B1, TPMT, UGT1A1, UGT2B15, UGT2B7, VKORC1). A qualified laboratory director interprets and prepares a report with genotype results and phenotypic interpretation and reports the results to the ordering provider.

Clinical Example (0517U)

A 58-year-old female presents with a history of anxiety and worsening depression. She reports worsening depression after being on a serotonin and norepinephrine reuptake inhibitor for 2 months. Plasma is submitted to determine drug levels to guide further therapy.

★=Telemedicine   ◀=Audio-only   ✚=Add-on code   ✗=FDA approval pending   #=Resequenced code   ⊘=Modifier 51 exempt

Description of Procedure (0517U)

Subject plasma to liquid chromatography-tandem mass spectrometry. Then follow up with algorithmic analysis to identify and quantify psychoactive drugs and metabolites (antidepressant, anxiolytic, antipsychotic, mood stabilizer, and pain medications) with spectral data analysis for at least 80 analytes, which results in the evaluation of each analyte within its therapeutic range; evaluation of drug-drug interactions; and reconciliation of drugs identified with those reported. A qualified laboratory professional analyzes the results, composes a report, and communicates the results to the ordering provider.

Clinical Example (0518U)

A 62-year-old female presents with a history of L3/L4 spinal fusion, chronic arthritis, and major depressive disorder. She reports worsening back pain despite current medications that include gabapentin, duloxetine, acetaminophen, ibuprofen, and oxycodone. Plasma is submitted to determine drug levels to guide further therapy.

Description of Procedure (0518U)

Subject plasma to liquid chromatography-tandem mass spectrometry. Then follow up with algorithmic analysis to identify and quantify mental health drugs and metabolites with spectral data analysis of at least 90 analytes, which results in the evaluation of each analyte within its detectable range; evaluation of drug-drug interactions; and reconciliation of drugs identified with those reported. A qualified laboratory professional analyzes the results, composes a report, and communicates the results to the ordering provider.

Clinical Example (0519U)

A 55-year-old male, who has a substance use disorder, depression, anxiety, and chronic pain, presents to his physician. His physician orders therapeutic drug monitoring.

Description of Procedure (0519U)

Extract plasma from blood, place on a dried plasma card, and subject to liquid chromatography-tandem mass spectrometry for identification of parent drug compounds and their metabolites. A qualified laboratory scientist examines the spectral data for 110 or more analytes in the specimen, which results in an evaluation of each analyte within its therapeutic range. A qualified health care professional analyzes the results, composes a report, and communicates the results to the ordering physician.

Clinical Example (0520U)

A 50-year-old male presents to his primary care physician with a history of hypertension, depression, anxiety, and hypercholesterolemia. He reports worsening depression and high blood pressure. His physician orders therapeutic drug monitoring.

Description of Procedure (0520U)

Subject plasma to liquid chromatography-tandem mass spectrometry. Then follow up with algorithmic analysis to identify and quantify multiple classes of drugs and metabolites with spectral data analysis of at least 200 analytes, which results in the evaluation of each analyte within its therapeutic range; evaluation of drug-drug interactions; and reconciliation of drugs identified with those reported. A qualified laboratory professional analyzes the results, composes a report, and communicates the results to the ordering physician.

Notes

Medicine

Summary of Additions, Deletions, and Revisions

The summary of changes shows the actual changes that have been made to the code descriptors.

New codes appear with a bullet (●) and are indicated as "Code added." Revised codes are preceded with a triangle (▲). Within revised codes, or if a code symbol has been deleted, the deleted language and code symbol appear with a ~~strikethrough~~, while new text appears underlined.

The ✗ symbol is used to identify codes for vaccines that are pending FDA approval. The # symbol is used to identify codes that have been resequenced. CPT add-on codes are annotated by the ✚ symbol. The ⊘ symbol is used to identify codes that are exempt from the use of modifier 51. The ★ symbol is used to identify codes that may be used for reporting telemedicine services. The ✣ symbol is used to identify a proprietary laboratory analyses (PLA) test that has an identical descriptor as another PLA test. A PLA code that satisfies Category I code criteria and has been accepted by the CPT Editorial Panel is annotated with the ⇅ symbol. The ◀ symbol is used to identify codes that may be used to report audio-only telemedicine services when appended by modifier 93 (see Appendix T).

Code	Description
~~0001A~~	~~Immunization administration by intramuscular injection of severe acute respiratory syndrome coronavirus 2 (SARS-CoV-2) (coronavirus disease [COVID-19]) vaccine, mRNA-LNP, spike protein, preservative free, 30 mcg/0.3 mL dosage, diluent reconstituted; first dose~~
~~0002A~~	~~second dose~~
~~0003A~~	~~third dose~~
~~0004A~~	~~booster dose~~
~~0051A~~	~~Immunization administration by intramuscular injection of severe acute respiratory syndrome coronavirus 2 (SARS-CoV-2) (coronavirus disease [COVID-19]) vaccine, mRNA-LNP, spike protein, preservative free, 30 mcg/0.3 mL dosage, tris-sucrose formulation; first dose~~
~~0052A~~	~~second dose~~
~~0053A~~	~~third dose~~
~~0054A~~	~~booster dose~~
~~0121A~~	~~Immunization administration by intramuscular injection of severe acute respiratory syndrome coronavirus 2 (SARS-CoV-2) (coronavirus disease [COVID-19]) vaccine, mRNA-LNP, bivalent spike protein, preservative free, 30 mcg/0.3 mL dosage, tris-sucrose formulation; single dose~~
~~0124A~~	~~additional dose~~
~~0071A~~	~~Immunization administration by intramuscular injection of severe acute respiratory syndrome coronavirus 2 (SARS-CoV-2) (coronavirus disease [COVID-19]) vaccine, mRNA-LNP, spike protein, preservative free, 10 mcg/0.2 mL dosage, diluent reconstituted, tris-sucrose formulation; first dose~~
~~0072A~~	~~second dose~~
~~0073A~~	~~third dose~~
~~0074A~~	~~booster dose~~

Code	Description
0151A	~~Immunization administration by intramuscular injection of severe acute respiratory syndrome coronavirus 2 (SARS-CoV-2) (coronavirus disease [COVID-19]) vaccine, mRNA-LNP, bivalent spike protein, preservative free, 10 mcg/0.2 mL dosage, diluent reconstituted, tris-sucrose formulation; single dose~~
0154A	~~additional dose~~
0081A	~~Immunization administration by intramuscular injection of severe acute respiratory syndrome coronavirus 2 (SARS-CoV-2) (coronavirus disease [COVID-19]) vaccine, mRNA-LNP, spike protein, preservative free, 3 mcg/0.2 mL dosage, diluent reconstituted, tris-sucrose formulation; first dose~~
0082A	~~second dose~~
0083A	~~third dose~~
0171A	~~Immunization administration by intramuscular injection of severe acute respiratory syndrome coronavirus 2 (SARS-CoV-2) (coronavirus disease [COVID-19]) vaccine, mRNA-LNP, bivalent spike protein, preservative free, 3 mcg/0.2 mL dosage, diluent reconstituted, tris-sucrose formulation; first dose~~
0172A	~~second dose~~
0173A	~~third dose~~
0174A	~~additional dose~~
0011A	~~Immunization administration by intramuscular injection of severe acute respiratory syndrome coronavirus 2 (SARS-CoV-2) (coronavirus disease [COVID-19]) vaccine, mRNA-LNP, spike protein, preservative free, 100 mcg/0.5 mL dosage; first dose~~
0012A	~~second dose~~
0013A	~~third dose~~
0064A	~~Immunization administration by intramuscular injection of severe acute respiratory syndrome coronavirus 2 (SARS-CoV-2) (coronavirus disease [COVID-19]) vaccine, mRNA-LNP, spike protein, preservative free, 50 mcg/0.25 mL dosage, booster dose~~
0134A	~~Immunization administration by intramuscular injection of severe acute respiratory syndrome coronavirus 2 (SARS-CoV-2) (coronavirus disease [COVID-19]) vaccine, mRNA-LNP, spike protein, bivalent, preservative free, 50 mcg/0.5 mL dosage, additional dose~~
0141A	~~Immunization administration by intramuscular injection of severe acute respiratory syndrome coronavirus 2 (SARS-CoV-2) (coronavirus disease [COVID-19]) vaccine, mRNA-LNP, spike protein, bivalent, preservative free, 25 mcg/0.25 mL dosage; first dose~~
0142A	~~second dose~~
0144A	~~additional dose~~
0091A	~~Immunization administration by intramuscular injection of severe acute respiratory syndrome coronavirus 2 (SARS-CoV-2) (coronavirus disease [COVID-19]) vaccine, mRNA-LNP, spike protein, preservative free, 50 mcg/0.5 mL dosage; first dose, when administered to individuals 6 through 11 years~~
0092A	~~second dose, when administered to individuals 6 through 11 years~~
0093A	~~third dose, when administered to individuals 6 through 11 years~~
0094A	~~booster dose, when administered to individuals 18 years and older~~
0021A	~~Immunization administration by intramuscular injection of severe acute respiratory syndrome coronavirus 2 (SARS-CoV-2) (coronavirus disease [COVID-19]) vaccine, DNA, spike protein, chimpanzee adenovirus Oxford 1 (ChAdOx1) vector, preservative free, 5×10^{10} viral particles/0.5 mL dosage; first dose~~

★ =Telemedicine   ◀ =Audio-only   ✚ =Add-on code   ✔ =FDA approval pending   # =Resequenced code   ⊘ =Modifier 51 exempt

Code	Description
0022A	~~second dose~~
0031A	~~Immunization administration by intramuscular injection of severe acute respiratory syndrome coronavirus 2 (SARS-CoV-2) (coronavirus disease [COVID-19]) vaccine, DNA, spike protein, adenovirus type 26 (Ad26) vector, preservative free, 5x10¹⁰ viral particles/0.5 mL dosage; single dose~~
0034A	~~booster dose~~
0041A	~~Immunization administration by intramuscular injection of severe acute respiratory syndrome coronavirus 2 (SARS-CoV-2) (coronavirus disease [COVID-19]) vaccine, recombinant spike protein nanoparticle, saponin-based adjuvant, preservative free, 5 mcg/0.5 mL dosage; first dose~~
0042A	~~second dose~~
0044A	~~booster dose~~
0104A	~~Immunization administration by intramuscular injection of severe acute respiratory syndrome coronavirus 2 (SARS-CoV-2) (coronavirus disease [COVID-19]) vaccine, monovalent, preservative free, 5 mcg/0.5 mL dosage, adjuvant AS03 emulsion, booster dose~~
0111A	~~Immunization administration by intramuscular injection of severe acute respiratory syndrome coronavirus 2 (SARS-CoV-2) (coronavirus disease [COVID-19]) vaccine, mRNA-LNP, spike protein, preservative free, 25 mcg/0.25 mL dosage; first dose~~
0112A	~~second dose~~
0113A	~~third dose~~
0164A	~~Immunization administration by intramuscular injection of severe acute respiratory syndrome coronavirus 2 (SARS-CoV-2) (coronavirus disease [COVID-19]) vaccine, mRNA-LNP, spike protein, bivalent, preservative free, 10 mcg/0.2 mL dosage, additional dose~~
#●90480	Code added
91300	~~Severe acute respiratory syndrome coronavirus 2 (SARS-CoV-2) (coronavirus disease [COVID-19]) vaccine, mRNA-LNP, spike protein, preservative free, 30 mcg/0.3 mL dosage, diluent reconstituted, for intramuscular use~~
91305	~~Severe acute respiratory syndrome coronavirus 2 (SARS-CoV-2) (coronavirus disease [COVID-19]) vaccine, mRNA-LNP, spike protein, preservative free, 30 mcg/0.3 mL dosage, tris-sucrose formulation, for intramuscular use~~
91312	~~Severe acute respiratory syndrome coronavirus 2 (SARS-CoV-2) (coronavirus disease [COVID-19]) vaccine, mRNA-LNP, bivalent spike protein, preservative free, 30 mcg/0.3 mL dosage, tris-sucrose formulation, for intramuscular use~~
91307	~~Severe acute respiratory syndrome coronavirus 2 (SARS-CoV-2) (coronavirus disease [COVID-19]) vaccine, mRNA-LNP, spike protein, preservative free, 10 mcg/0.2 mL dosage, diluent reconstituted, tris-sucrose formulation, for intramuscular use~~
91315	~~Severe acute respiratory syndrome coronavirus 2 (SARS-CoV-2) (coronavirus disease [COVID-19]) vaccine, mRNA-LNP, bivalent spike protein, preservative free, 10 mcg/0.2 mL dosage, diluent reconstituted, tris-sucrose formulation, for intramuscular use~~
91308	~~Severe acute respiratory syndrome coronavirus 2 (SARS-CoV-2) (coronavirus disease [COVID-19]) vaccine, mRNA-LNP, spike protein, preservative free, 3 mcg/0.2 mL dosage, diluent reconstituted, tris-sucrose formulation, for intramuscular use~~
91317	~~Severe acute respiratory syndrome coronavirus 2 (SARS-CoV-2) (coronavirus disease [COVID-19]) vaccine, mRNA-LNP, bivalent spike protein, preservative free, 3 mcg/0.2 mL dosage, diluent reconstituted, tris-sucrose formulation, for intramuscular use~~
91301	~~Severe acute respiratory syndrome coronavirus 2 (SARS-CoV-2) (coronavirus disease [COVID-19]) vaccine, mRNA-LNP, spike protein, preservative free, 100 mcg/0.5 mL dosage, for intramuscular use~~

Code	Description
~~91306~~	~~Severe acute respiratory syndrome coronavirus 2 (SARS-CoV-2) (coronavirus disease [COVID-19]) vaccine, mRNA-LNP, spike protein, preservative free, 50 mcg/0.25 mL dosage, for intramuscular use~~
~~91313~~	~~Severe acute respiratory syndrome coronavirus 2 (SARS-CoV-2) (coronavirus disease [COVID-19]) vaccine, mRNA-LNP, spike protein, bivalent, preservative free, 50 mcg/0.5 mL dosage, for intramuscular use~~
~~91314~~	~~Severe acute respiratory syndrome coronavirus 2 (SARS-CoV-2) (coronavirus disease [COVID-19]) vaccine, mRNA-LNP, spike protein, bivalent, preservative free, 25 mcg/0.25 mL dosage, for intramuscular use~~
~~91311~~	~~Severe acute respiratory syndrome coronavirus 2 (SARS-CoV-2) (coronavirus disease [COVID-19]) vaccine, mRNA-LNP, spike protein, preservative free, 25 mcg/0.25 mL dosage, for intramuscular use~~
~~91316~~	~~Severe acute respiratory syndrome coronavirus 2 (SARS-CoV-2) (coronavirus disease [COVID-19]) vaccine, mRNA-LNP, spike protein, bivalent, preservative free, 10 mcg/0.2 mL dosage, for intramuscular use~~
~~91309~~	~~Severe acute respiratory syndrome coronavirus 2 (SARS-CoV-2) (coronavirus disease [COVID-19]) vaccine, mRNA-LNP, spike protein, preservative free, 50 mcg/0.5 mL dosage, for intramuscular use~~
~~91302~~	~~Severe acute respiratory syndrome coronavirus 2 (SARS-CoV-2) (coronavirus disease [COVID-19]) vaccine, DNA, spike protein, chimpanzee adenovirus Oxford 1 (ChAdOx1) vector, preservative free, $5x10^{10}$ viral particles/0.5 mL dosage, for intramuscular use~~
~~91303~~	~~Severe acute respiratory syndrome coronavirus 2 (SARS-CoV-2) (coronavirus disease [COVID-19]) vaccine, DNA, spike protein, adenovirus type 26 (Ad26) vector, preservative free, $5x10^{10}$ viral particles/0.5 mL dosage, for intramuscular use~~
#▲91304	Severe acute respiratory syndrome coronavirus 2 (SARS-CoV-2) (coronavirus disease [COVID-19]) vaccine, recombinant spike protein nanoparticle, saponin-based adjuvant, ~~preservative free,~~ 5 mcg/0.5 mL dosage, for intramuscular use
~~91310~~	~~Severe acute respiratory syndrome coronavirus 2 (SARS-CoV-2) (coronavirus disease [COVID-19]) vaccine, monovalent, preservative free, 5 mcg/0.5 mL dosage, adjuvant AS03 emulsion, for intramuscular use~~
#●91318	Code added
#●91319	Code added
#●91320	Code added
#●91321	Code added
#●91322	Code added
~~90654~~	~~Influenza virus vaccine, trivalent (IIV3), split virus, preservative-free, for intradermal use~~
~~90630~~	~~Influenza virus vaccine, quadrivalent (IIV4), split virus, preservative free, for intradermal use~~
▲90661	Influenza virus vaccine, trivalent (ccIIV3), derived from cell cultures, subunit, ~~preservative and~~ antibiotic free, 0.5 mL dosage, for intramuscular use
#⚡●90695	Code added
#●90684	Code added
#⚡●90637	Code added
#⚡●90638	Code added
#⚡●90624	Code added
▲92132	~~Scanning c~~Computerized ophthalmic diagnostic imaging (eg, optical coherence tomography [OCT]), anterior segment, with interpretation and report, unilateral or bilateral

★=Telemedicine ◀=Audio-only ✚=Add-on code ⚡=FDA approval pending #=Resequenced code ⊘=Modifier 51 exempt

Code	Description
▲92133	~~Scanning c~~Computerized ophthalmic diagnostic imaging <u>(eg, optical coherence tomography [OCT])</u>, posterior segment, with interpretation and report, unilateral or bilateral; optic nerve
▲92134	retina
#●92137	Code added
▲93656	Comprehensive electrophysiologic evaluation ~~including~~<u>with</u> transseptal catheterizations, insertion and repositioning of multiple electrode catheters<u>, induction or attempted induction of an arrhythmia including left or right atrial pacing/recording,</u> ~~with~~<u>and</u> intracardiac catheter ablation of atrial fibrillation by pulmonary vein isolation, including intracardiac electrophysiologic 3-dimensional mapping, intracardiac echocardiography ~~including~~<u>with</u> imaging supervision and interpretation,~~ induction or attempted induction of an arrhythmia including left or right atrial pacing/recording,~~ right ventricular pacing/recording, and His bundle recording, when performed
93890	~~vasoreactivity study~~
▲93893	~~emboli~~<u>venous-arterial shunt</u> detection with intravenous microbubble injection
#✛●93896	Code added
#✛●93897	Code added
#✛●93898	Code added
96003	~~Dynamic fine wire electromyography, during walking or other functional activities, 1 muscle~~
96040	~~Medical genetics and genetic counseling services, each 30 minutes face-to-face with patient/family~~
★◀●96041	Code added
#●96380	Code added
#●96381	Code added
✛▲97811	without electrical stimulation, each additional 15 minutes of personal one-on-one contact with the patient, with ~~re-~~insertion of needle(s) (List separately in addition to code for primary procedure)
✛▲97814	with electrical stimulation, each additional 15 minutes of personal one-on-one contact with the patient, with ~~re-~~insertion of needle(s) (List separately in addition to code for primary procedure)
★▲98960	Education and training for patient self-management by a <u>nonphysician </u>qualified~~, nonphysician~~ health care professional using a standardized curriculum, face-to-face with the patient (could include caregiver/family) each 30 minutes; individual patient
★▲98961	2-4 patients
★▲98962	5-8 patients
▲98966	Telephone assessment and management service provided by a <u>nonphysician </u>qualified ~~nonphysician ~~health care professional to an established patient, parent, or guardian not originating from a related assessment and management service provided within the previous 7 days nor leading to an assessment and management service or procedure within the next 24 hours or soonest available appointment; 5-10 minutes of medical discussion
▲98967	11-20 minutes of medical discussion
▲98968	21-30 minutes of medical discussion
▲98970	<u>Nonphysician Q</u>qualified ~~nonphysician ~~health care professional online digital assessment and management, for an established patient, for up to 7 days, cumulative time during the 7 days; 5-10 minutes
▲98971	11-20 minutes

Code	Description
▲98972	21 or more minutes
▲98975	Remote therapeutic monitoring (eg, therapy adherence, therapy response, digital therapeutic intervention); initial set-up and patient education on use of equipment
▲98976	device(s) supply for data access or data transmissions to support monitoring of ~~with scheduled (eg, daily) recording(s) and/or programmed alert(s) transmission to monitor~~ respiratory system, each 30 days
▲98977	device(s) supply for data access or data transmissions to support monitoring of ~~with scheduled (eg, daily) recording(s) and/or programmed alert(s) transmission to monitor~~ musculoskeletal system, each 30 days
▲98978	device(s) supply for data access or data transmissions to support monitoring of ~~with scheduled (eg, daily) recording(s) and/or programmed alert(s) transmission to monitor~~ cognitive behavioral therapy, each 30 days

★ = Telemedicine   ◀ = Audio-only   ✚ = Add-on code   ✗ = FDA approval pending   # = Resequenced code   ⊘ = Modifier 51 exempt

Medicine

Immune Globulins, Serum or Recombinant Products

90380   Respiratory syncytial virus, monoclonal antibody, seasonal dose; 0.5 mL dosage, for intramuscular use

90381   1 mL dosage, for intramuscular use

▶(Do not report 90380, 90381 in conjunction with 96372)◀

▶(For administration of respiratory syncytial virus, monoclonal antibody, seasonal dose, see 96380, 96381)◀

Rationale

Parenthetical notes have been added following codes 90380 and 90381. The first parenthetical note restricts reporting codes 90380 and 90381 in conjunction with the therapeutic, prophylactic, or diagnostic injection code because there are specific codes for reporting the administration of the respiratory syncytial virus (RSV) vaccine. The second parenthetical note directs users to the appropriate codes for the administration of an RSV, monoclonal antibody, and seasonal dose (90380, 90381).

Refer to the codebook and the Rationale for codes 96380 and 96381 for a full discussion of these changes.

90384   Rho(D) immune globulin (RhIg), human, full-dose, for intramuscular use

Immunization Administration for Vaccines/Toxoids

▶Report vaccine immunization administration codes (90460, 90461, 90471-90474, 90480) in addition to the vaccine and toxoid code(s) (90476-90759, 91304, 91318, 91319, 91320, 91321, 91322).◀

Report codes 90460 and 90461 only when the physician or other qualified health care professional provides face-to-face counseling of the patient/family during the administration of a vaccine other than when performed for severe acute respiratory syndrome coronavirus 2 (SARS-CoV-2) (coronavirus disease [COVID-19]) vaccines. For immunization administration of any vaccine, other than SARS-CoV-2 (coronavirus disease [COVID-19]) vaccines, that is not accompanied by face-to-face physician or other qualified health care professional counseling to the patient/family/guardian or for administration of vaccines to patients over 18 years of age, report codes 90471-90474. (See also **Instructions for Use of the CPT Codebook** for definition of reporting qualifications.)

▶Report 90480 for immunization administration of SARS-CoV-2 (coronavirus disease [COVID-19]) vaccines only. This code is used for administration and counseling that involves the use of COVID-19 vaccines for immunization against contracting disease. This includes administration of COVID-19 vaccine for all age populations.◀

Rationale

The guidelines for the Immunization Administration for Vaccines/Toxoids subsection have been revised to: (1) reference new COVID-19 vaccine administration code 90480; (2) delete codes and instructions that were previously used to report the administration of coronavirus disease 2019 (COVID-19) vaccines; and (3) add instructional language about the appropriate use of code 90480.

Refer to the codebook and the Rationale for code 90480 for a full discussion of these changes.

If a significant separately identifiable evaluation and management service (eg, new or established patient office or other outpatient services [99202-99215], office or other outpatient consultations [99242, 99243, 99244, 99245], emergency department services [99281-99285], preventive medicine services [99381-99429]) is performed, the appropriate E/M service code should be reported in addition to the vaccine and toxoid administration codes.

A component refers to all antigens in a vaccine that prevent disease(s) caused by one organism (90460 and 90461). Multi-valent antigens or multiple serotypes of antigens against a single organism are considered a single component of vaccines. Combination vaccines are those vaccines that contain multiple vaccine components. Conjugates or adjuvants contained in vaccines are not considered to be component parts of the vaccine as defined above.

▶For immune globulins and monoclonal antibodies immunizations, see 90281-90399. For administration of immune globulins and monoclonal antibodies immunizations, see 96365, 96366, 96367, 96368, 96369, 96370, 96371, 96372, 96374, 96375, 96380, 96381.◀

(For allergy testing, see 95004 et seq)

(For skin testing of bacterial, viral, fungal extracts, see 86485-86580)

(For therapeutic or diagnostic injections, see 96372-96379)

Rationale

New guidelines have been added to provide instructions for reporting immune globulin products and their administration for immunizations, including for RSV.

Refer to the codebook and the Rationale for codes 96380 and 96381 for a full discussion of these changes.

90460 Immunization administration through 18 years of age via any route of administration, with counseling by physician or other qualified health care professional; first or only component of each vaccine or toxoid administered

+ 90461 each additional vaccine or toxoid component administered (List separately in addition to code for primary procedure)

(Use 90460 for each vaccine administered. For vaccines with multiple components [combination vaccines], report 90460 in conjunction with 90461 for each additional component in a given vaccine)

▶(Do not report 90460, 90461 in conjunction with 91304, 91318, 91319, 91320, 91321, 91322, unless both a severe acute respiratory syndrome coronavirus 2 [SARS-CoV-2] [coronavirus disease {COVID-19}] vaccine/toxoid product and at least one vaccine/toxoid product from 90476-90759 are administered at the same encounter)◀

90471 Immunization administration (includes percutaneous, intradermal, subcutaneous, or intramuscular injections); 1 vaccine (single or combination vaccine/toxoid)

(Do not report 90471 in conjunction with 90473)

+ 90472 each additional vaccine (single or combination vaccine/toxoid) (List separately in addition to code for primary procedure)

(Use 90472 in conjunction with 90460, 90471, 90473)

▶(Do not report 90471, 90472 in conjunction with 91304, 91318, 91319, 91320, 91321, 91322, unless both a severe acute respiratory syndrome coronavirus 2 [SARS-CoV-2] [coronavirus disease {COVID-19}] vaccine/toxoid product and at least one vaccine/toxoid product from 90476-90759 are administered at the same encounter)◀

(For intravesical administration of BCG vaccine, see 51720, 90586)

Rationale

Parenthetical notes in the Immunization Administration for Vaccines/Toxoids subsection have been revised to reflect the replacement of deleted COVID-19 vaccine codes with five new COVID-19 vaccine product codes (91318-91322) and the retention of existing code 91304, whose emergency use authorization (EUA) is still valid.

Refer to the codebook and the Rationale for code 90480 for a full discussion of these changes.

90473 Immunization administration by intranasal or oral route; 1 vaccine (single or combination vaccine/toxoid)

(Do not report 90473 in conjunction with 90471)

+ 90474 each additional vaccine (single or combination vaccine/toxoid) (List separately in addition to code for primary procedure)

(Use 90474 in conjunction with 90460, 90471, 90473)

▶(Do not report 90473, 90474 in conjunction with 91304, 91318, 91319, 91320, 91321, 91322, unless both a severe acute respiratory syndrome coronavirus 2 [SARS-CoV-2] [coronavirus disease {COVID-19}] vaccine/toxoid product and at least one vaccine/toxoid product from 90476-90759 are administered at the same encounter)◀

▶(0001A, 0002A, 0003A, 0004A have been deleted. To report administration of COVID-19 vaccine, use 90480)◀

▶(0051A, 0052A, 0053A, 0054A have been deleted. To report administration of COVID-19 vaccine, use 90480)◀

▶(0121A, 0124A have been deleted. To report administration of COVID-19 vaccine, use 90480)◀

▶(0071A, 0072A, 0073A, 0074A have been deleted. To report administration of COVID-19 vaccine, use 90480)◀

▶(0151A, 0154A have been deleted. To report administration of COVID-19 vaccine, use 90480)◀

▶(0081A, 0082A, 0083A have been deleted. To report administration of COVID-19 vaccine, use 90480)◀

▶(0171A, 0172A, 0173A, 0174A have been deleted. To report administration of COVID-19 vaccine, use 90480)◀

▶(0011A, 0012A, 0013A have been deleted. To report administration of COVID-19 vaccine, use 90480)◀

▶(0064A has been deleted. To report administration of COVID-19 vaccine, use 90480)◀

▶(0134A has been deleted. To report administration of COVID-19 vaccine, use 90480)◀

▶(0141A, 0142A, 0144A have been deleted. To report administration of COVID-19 vaccine, use 90480)◀

▶(0091A, 0092A, 0093A, 0094A have been deleted. To report administration of COVID-19 vaccine, use 90480)◀

▶(0021A, 0022A have been deleted. To report administration of COVID-19 vaccine, use 90480)◀

▶(0031A, 0034A have been deleted. To report administration of COVID-19 vaccine, use 90480)◀

▶(0041A, 0042A, 0044A have been deleted. To report administration of COVID-19 vaccine, use 90480)◀

▶(0104A has been deleted. To report administration of COVID-19 vaccine, use 90480)◀

★ = Telemedicine   ◀ = Audio-only   ✛ = Add-on code   ✗ = FDA approval pending   # = Resequenced code   ⊘ = Modifier 51 exempt

▶(0111A, 0112A, 0113A have been deleted. To report administration of COVID-19 vaccine, use 90480)◀

▶(0164A has been deleted. To report administration of COVID-19 vaccine, use 90480)◀

Rationale

Parenthetical notes in the Immunization Administration for Vaccines/Toxoids subsection have been deleted and new parenthetical notes have been added to reflect the replacement of deleted COVID-19 vaccine administration codes with new code 90480.

Refer to the codebook and the Rationale for code 90480 for a full discussion of these changes.

#● **90480** Immunization administration by intramuscular injection of severe acute respiratory syndrome coronavirus 2 (SARS-CoV-2) (coronavirus disease [COVID-19]) vaccine, single dose

▶(Report 90480 for the administration of vaccine 91304, 91318, 91319, 91320, 91321, 91322)◀

▶(Do not report 90480 in conjunction with 90476-90759)◀

Rationale

Code 90480 has been established to report the administration of any COVID-19 vaccine. In addition, instructional and exclusionary parenthetical notes have been added to direct users to the appropriate vaccine product codes that may be reported in conjunction with code 90480 and to restrict its reporting for non-COVID-19 vaccine products.

Refer to the codebook and the Rationale for codes 91318-91322 for a full discussion of these changes.

Clinical Example (90480)

A parent or guardian of a 1-year-old child seeks immunization against severe acute respiratory syndrome coronavirus 2 (SARS-CoV-2) to decrease the risk of contracting this disease, consistent with evidence-supported guidelines. The parent or guardian is offered and agrees to an intramuscular injection of SARS-CoV-2 vaccine for the child for this purpose.

Description of Procedure (90480)

The physician or other qualified health care professional reviews the patient's chart to confirm that vaccination to decrease the risk of COVID-19 is indicated. Counsel the parent or guardian on the benefits and risks of vaccination to decrease the risk of COVID-19 and obtain consent. Administer the dose of the COVID-19 vaccine by intramuscular injection. Monitor the patient for any adverse reaction. Update the patient's immunization record (and registry when applicable) to reflect the vaccine administered.

Vaccines, Toxoids

To assist users to report the most recent new or revised vaccine product codes, the American Medical Association (AMA) currently uses the CPT website (ama-assn.org/cpt-cat-i-immunization-codes), which features updates of CPT Editorial Panel actions regarding these products. See the Introduction section of the CPT code set for a complete list of the dates of release and implementation.

The CPT Editorial Panel, in recognition of the public health interest in vaccine products, has chosen to publish new vaccine product codes prior to approval by the US Food and Drug Administration (FDA). These codes are indicated with the ✗ symbol and will be tracked by the AMA to monitor FDA approval status. Once the FDA status changes to approval, the ✗ symbol will be removed. CPT users should refer to the AMA CPT website (ama-assn.org/cpt-cat-i-immunization-codes) for the most up-to-date information on codes with the ✗ symbol.

▶Codes 90476-90759, 91304, 91318, 91319, 91320, 91321, 91322 identify the vaccine product **only**. To report the administration of a vaccine/toxoid other than SARS-CoV-2 (coronavirus disease [COVID-19]), the vaccine/toxoid product codes (90476-90759) must be used in addition to an immunization administration code(s) (90460, 90461, 90471, 90472, 90473, 90474). To report the administration of a SARS-CoV-2 (coronavirus disease [COVID-19]) vaccine, the vaccine/toxoid product codes 91304, 91318, 91319, 91320, 91321, 91322 should be reported with the corresponding immunization administration code (90480).

Do not report 90476-90759 in conjunction with the SARS-CoV-2 (coronavirus disease [COVID-19]) immunization administration code 90480, unless both a SARS-CoV-2 (coronavirus disease [COVID-19]) vaccine/toxoid product and at least one vaccine/toxoid product from 90476-90759 are administered at the same encounter.

Modifier 51 should not be reported with vaccine/toxoid codes 90476-90759, 91304, 91318, 91319, 91320, 91321, 91322, when reported in conjunction with administration codes 90460, 90461, 90471, 90472, 90473, 90474, 90480.◀

Medicine 90281-99607

If a significantly separately identifiable Evaluation and Management (E/M) service (eg, office or other outpatient services, preventive medicine services) is performed, the appropriate E/M service code should be reported in addition to the vaccine and toxoid administration codes.

To meet the reporting requirements of immunization registries, vaccine distribution programs, and reporting systems (eg, Vaccine Adverse Event Reporting System) the exact vaccine product administered needs to be reported. Multiple codes for a particular vaccine are provided in the CPT codebook when the schedule (number of doses or timing) differs for two or more products of the same vaccine type (eg, hepatitis A, Hib) or the vaccine product is available in more than one chemical formulation, dosage, or route of administration.

The "when administered to" age descriptions included in CPT vaccine codes are not intended to identify a product's licensed age indication. The term "preservative free" includes use for vaccines that contain no preservative and vaccines that contain trace amounts of preservative agents that are not present in a sufficient concentration for the purpose of preserving the final vaccine formulation. The absence of a designation regarding a preservative does not necessarily indicate the presence or absence of preservative in the vaccine. Refer to the product's prescribing information (PI) for the licensed age indication before administering vaccine to a patient.

Separate codes are available for combination vaccines (eg, Hib-HepB, DTap-IPV/Hib). It is inappropriate to code each component of a combination vaccine separately. If a specific vaccine code is not available, the unlisted procedure code should be reported, until a new code becomes available.

▶The immunization/vaccine/toxoid abbreviations listed in codes 90380, 90381, 90476-90759, 91304, 91318, 91319, 91320, 91321, 91322 reflect the most recent US vaccine abbreviation references used in the Advisory Committee on Immunization Practices (ACIP) recommendations at the time of CPT code set publication. Interim updates to vaccine code descriptors will be made following abbreviation approval by the ACIP on a timely basis via the AMA CPT website (ama-assn.org/cpt-cat-i-immunization-codes). The accuracy of the ACIP vaccine abbreviation designations in the CPT code set does not affect the validity of the vaccine code and its reporting function.◀

Rationale

Guidelines for the Vaccines/Toxoids subsection have been deleted and revised to reflect the replacement of deleted COVID-19 vaccine administration and product codes. In addition, a single COVID-19 vaccine administration code (90480) and five COVID-19 product codes (91318-91322) have been added to report COVID-19 vaccination services.

Furthermore, codes 90380 and 90381 and the term "immunization" have been added to reflect their intended use for immunizations and the RSV vaccine products.

Refer to the codebook and the Rationale for codes 90380, 90381, 90480, and 91318-91322 for a full discussion of these changes.

▶(For immune globulins and monoclonal antibodies immunizations, see 90281-90399)◀

▶(For administration of immune globulins and monoclonal antibodies immunizations, with the exception of respiratory syncytial virus, monoclonal antibody, seasonal product, see 96365-96375)◀

▶(For administration of respiratory syncytial virus, monoclonal antibody, seasonal product, see 96380, 96381)◀

Rationale

Two existing parenthetical notes in the Vaccines/Toxoids subsection have been revised to: (1) reflect the use of immune globulin product codes (90281-90399) for immune globulins and monoclonal antibodies; and (2) note the codes that may be used for the administration of non-RSV immune globulin products (96365-96375). In addition, a new parenthetical note has been added to provide separate instructions for reporting the administration of RSV immunizations (96380, 96381).

Refer to the codebook and the Rationale for codes 96380 and 96381 for a full discussion of these changes.

▶(91300 has been deleted. To report severe acute respiratory syndrome coronavirus 2 [SARS-CoV-2] [coronavirus disease {COVID-19}] vaccine product immunization, see 91318, 91319, 91320, 91321, 91322)◀

▶(91305 has been deleted. To report severe acute respiratory syndrome coronavirus 2 [SARS-CoV-2] [coronavirus disease {COVID-19}] vaccine product immunization, see 91318, 91319, 91320, 91321, 91322)◀

▶(91312 has been deleted. To report severe acute respiratory syndrome coronavirus 2 [SARS-CoV-2] [coronavirus disease {COVID-19}] vaccine product immunization, see 91318, 91319, 91320, 91321, 91322)◀

▶(91307 has been deleted. To report severe acute respiratory syndrome coronavirus 2 [SARS-CoV-2] [coronavirus disease {COVID-19}] vaccine product immunization, see 91318, 91319, 91320, 91321, 91322)◀

▶(91315 has been deleted. To report severe acute respiratory syndrome coronavirus 2 [SARS-CoV-2] [coronavirus disease {COVID-19}] vaccine product immunization, see 91318, 91319, 91320, 91321, 91322)◀

★=Telemedicine   ◀=Audio-only   ✚=Add-on code   ✗=FDA approval pending   #=Resequenced code   ⦸=Modifier 51 exempt

►(91308 has been deleted. To report severe acute respiratory syndrome coronavirus 2 [SARS-CoV-2] [coronavirus disease {COVID-19}] vaccine product immunization, see 91318, 91319, 91320, 91321, 91322)◄

►(91317 has been deleted. To report severe acute respiratory syndrome coronavirus 2 [SARS-CoV-2] [coronavirus disease {COVID-19}] vaccine product immunization, see 91318, 91319, 91320, 91321, 91322)◄

►(91301 has been deleted. To report severe acute respiratory syndrome coronavirus 2 [SARS-CoV-2] [coronavirus disease {COVID-19}] vaccine product immunization, see 91318, 91319, 91320, 91321, 91322)◄

►(91306 has been deleted. To report severe acute respiratory syndrome coronavirus 2 [SARS-CoV-2] [coronavirus disease {COVID-19}] vaccine product immunization, see 91318, 91319, 91320, 91321, 91322)◄

►(91313 has been deleted. To report severe acute respiratory syndrome coronavirus 2 [SARS-CoV-2] [coronavirus disease {COVID-19}] vaccine product immunization, see 91318, 91319, 91320, 91321, 91322)◄

►(91314 has been deleted. To report severe acute respiratory syndrome coronavirus 2 [SARS-CoV-2] [coronavirus disease {COVID-19}] vaccine product immunization, see 91318, 91319, 91320, 91321, 91322)◄

►(91311 has been deleted. To report severe acute respiratory syndrome coronavirus 2 [SARS-CoV-2] [coronavirus disease {COVID-19}] vaccine product immunization, see 91318, 91319, 91320, 91321, 91322)◄

►(91316 has been deleted. To report severe acute respiratory syndrome coronavirus 2 [SARS-CoV-2] [coronavirus disease {COVID-19}] vaccine product immunization, see 91318, 91319, 91320, 91321, 91322)◄

►(91309 has been deleted. To report severe acute respiratory syndrome coronavirus 2 [SARS-CoV-2] [coronavirus disease {COVID-19}] vaccine product immunization, see 91318, 91319, 91320, 91321, 91322)◄

►(91302 has been deleted. To report severe acute respiratory syndrome coronavirus 2 [SARS-CoV-2] [coronavirus disease {COVID-19}] vaccine product immunization, see 91318, 91319, 91320, 91321, 91322)◄

►(91303 has been deleted. To report severe acute respiratory syndrome coronavirus 2 [SARS-CoV-2] [coronavirus disease {COVID-19}] vaccine product immunization, see 91318, 91319, 91320, 91321, 91322)◄

Rationale

To accommodate the replacement of the previously created COVID-19 vaccine product codes, a number of COVID-19 codes and their associated parenthetical notes have been deleted.

Refer to the codebook and the Rationale for codes 91318-91322 for a full discussion of these changes.

\#▲ **91304** Severe acute respiratory syndrome coronavirus 2 (SARS-CoV-2) (coronavirus disease [COVID-19]) vaccine, recombinant spike protein nanoparticle, saponin-based adjuvant, 5 mcg/0.5 mL dosage, for intramuscular use

►(Report 91304 with administration code 90480)◄

Rationale

Code 91304 has been revised by removing the term "preservative free" as part of the effort to remove obsolete language from vaccine descriptors.

Code 91304 has been retained because the EUA for this specific COVID-19 vaccine product is still valid. The parenthetical note following code 91304 has been revised to direct users to report code 90480 for the administration of this specific vaccine product.

Refer to the codebook and the Rationale for code 91322 for a full discussion of these changes.

►(91310 has been deleted. To report severe acute respiratory syndrome coronavirus 2 [SARS-CoV-2] [coronavirus disease {COVID-19}] vaccine product immunization, see 91318, 91319, 91320, 91321, 91322)◄

\#● **91318** Severe acute respiratory syndrome coronavirus 2 (SARS-CoV-2) (coronavirus disease [COVID-19]) vaccine, mRNA-LNP, spike protein, 3 mcg/0.3 mL dosage, tris-sucrose formulation, for intramuscular use

►(Report 91318 with administration code 90480)◄

\#● **91319** Severe acute respiratory syndrome coronavirus 2 (SARS-CoV-2) (coronavirus disease [COVID-19]) vaccine, mRNA-LNP, spike protein, 10 mcg/0.3 mL dosage, tris-sucrose formulation, for intramuscular use

►(Report 91319 with administration code 90480)◄

\#● **91320** Severe acute respiratory syndrome coronavirus 2 (SARS-CoV-2) (coronavirus disease [COVID-19]) vaccine, mRNA-LNP, spike protein, 30 mcg/0.3 mL dosage, tris-sucrose formulation, for intramuscular use

►(Report 91320 with administration code 90480)◄

\#● **91321** Severe acute respiratory syndrome coronavirus 2 (SARS-CoV-2) (coronavirus disease [COVID-19]) vaccine, mRNA-LNP, spike protein, 25 mcg/0.25 mL dosage, for intramuscular use

►(Report 91321 with administration code 90480)◄

\#● **91322** Severe acute respiratory syndrome coronavirus 2 (SARS-CoV-2) (coronavirus disease [COVID-19]) vaccine, mRNA-LNP, 50 mcg/0.5 mL dosage, for intramuscular use

►(Report 91322 with administration code 90480)◄

▲ = Revised code   ● = New code   ► ◄ = Contains new or revised text   ✖ = Duplicate PLA test   ⇅ = Category I PLA   American Medical Association   **125**

Medicine 90281-99607

Medicine 90281-99607

Rationale

To address the urgent health care crisis and curtail the rapid spread of COVID-19 throughout the United States, an EUA was provided by the Food and Drug Administration (FDA). The EUA allowed the rapid development of COVID-19 vaccines from multiple manufacturers and made COVID-19 vaccine products available earlier for code development.

As a result, multiple codes were included in the Vaccine/Toxoids subsection to enable the reporting of: (1) separate COVID-19 vaccine product codes according to the manufacturer of the product and (2) specific administration codes that were unique to the various COVID-19 vaccine products that had obtained EUA. This was exemplified by the inclusion of multiple vaccine administration and COVID-specific product codes that were reported based on the COVID-19 vaccine product administered.

With the end of the pandemic, the accommodations to address the then-urgent health needs have been removed. As a result, the reporting of COVID-19 vaccine products and administration procedures has been simplified in the CPT code set.

The simplification is achieved with: (1) the removal of all COVID-19 vaccine product and administration codes that no longer have EUA for protection against contracting COVID-19; (2) the removal of the Appendix Q table and its information that crosswalked nonconventional information (eg, vaccine manufacturer, national drug code numbers) with CPT COVID-19 codes; (3) the removal and revision of guidelines and parenthetical notes that referenced and explained the intention of various COVID-19 vaccine product and administration codes previously included in the code set; and (4) the addition of one new COVID-19 administration (90480) and five new COVID-19 vaccine product codes (91318-91322) to enable reporting COVID-19 vaccines that have received FDA approval. In addition, because the EUA status of the COVID-19 vaccine product it represents is still valid, code 91304 has been retained, and the administration of this vaccine product should be reported with code 90480. Because of the simplification, code 90480 is the only administration code that should be reported for the administration of any COVID-19 vaccine product.

Parenthetical notes and guidelines have been revised to provide users with instructions on the separate reporting of COVID-19 vaccine products according to its formulation and dosage. Instructions have been included in the Evaluation and Management and Medicine sections to indicate that COVID-19 administration code 90480 should be used only with COVID-19 vaccine products, ie, non-COVID-19 administration codes should not be used with any COVID-19 vaccine product codes. Guidelines and parenthetical notes have been revised to provide instructions regarding when non-COVID-19 vaccine administration codes may be additionally reported (ie, when a COVID-19 vaccine product is also administered in addition to a non-COVID-19 vaccine product).

Clinical Example (91318)

A parent or guardian of a 1-year-old child seeks immunization against severe acute respiratory syndrome coronavirus 2 (SARS-CoV-2) to decrease the risk of contracting this disease, consistent with evidence-supported guidelines. The parent or guardian is offered and agrees to an intramuscular injection of SARS-CoV-2 vaccine for the child for this purpose.

Description of Procedure (91318)

The physician or other qualified health care professional determines that the SARS-CoV-2 vaccine is appropriate for this patient and dispenses the vaccine according to the dose scheduled in the administration code for the SARS-CoV-2 vaccine.

Clinical Example (91319)

A parent or guardian of a 7-year-old child seeks immunization against severe acute respiratory syndrome coronavirus 2 (SARS-CoV-2) to decrease the risk of contracting this disease, consistent with evidence-supported guidelines. The individual is offered and accepts an intramuscular injection of SARS-CoV-2 vaccine for this purpose.

Description of Procedure (91319)

The physician or other qualified health care professional determines that the SARS-CoV-2 vaccine is appropriate for this patient and dispenses the vaccine according to the dose scheduled in the administration code for the SARS-CoV-2 vaccine.

Clinical Example (91320)

A 33-year-old individual seeks immunization against severe acute respiratory syndrome coronavirus 2 (SARS-CoV-2) to decrease the risk of contracting this disease, consistent with evidence-supported guidelines. The individual is offered and accepts an intramuscular injection of SARS-CoV-2 vaccine for this purpose.

Description of Procedure (91320)

The physician or other qualified health care professional determines that the SARS-CoV-2 vaccine is appropriate for this patient and dispenses the vaccine according to the dose scheduled in the administration code for the SARS-CoV-2 vaccine.

★=Telemedicine ◀=Audio-only +=Add-on code ✚=FDA approval pending #=Resequenced code ⊘=Modifier 51 exempt

Clinical Example (91321)

A parent or guardian of a 1-year-old child seeks immunization against severe acute respiratory syndrome coronavirus 2 (SARS-CoV-2) to decrease the risk of contracting this disease, consistent with evidence-supported guidelines. The parent or guardian is offered and agrees to an intramuscular injection of SARS-CoV-2 vaccine for the child for this purpose.

Description of Procedure (91321)

The physician or other qualified health care professional determines that the SARS-CoV-2 vaccine is appropriate for this patient and dispenses the vaccine according to the dose scheduled in the administration code for the SARS-CoV-2 vaccine.

Clinical Example (91322)

A 33-year-old individual seeks immunization against severe acute respiratory syndrome coronavirus 2 (SARS-CoV-2) to decrease the risk of contracting this disease, consistent with evidence-supported guidelines. The individual is offered and accepts an intramuscular injection of SARS-CoV-2 vaccine for this purpose.

Description of Procedure (91322)

The physician or other qualified health care professional determines that the SARS-CoV-2 vaccine is appropriate for this patient and dispenses the vaccine according to the dose scheduled in the administration code for the SARS-CoV-2 vaccine.

90476	Adenovirus vaccine, type 4, live, for oral use
90480	Code is out of numerical sequence. See 90473-90477
# **90589**	Chikungunya virus vaccine, live attenuated, for intramuscular use
90624	Code is out of numerical sequence. See 90717-90739
90636	Hepatitis A and hepatitis B vaccine (HepA-HepB), adult dosage, for intramuscular use
90637	Code is out of numerical sequence. See 90689-90691
90638	Code is out of numerical sequence. See 90689-90691
90644	Code is out of numerical sequence. See 90717-90739
90647	Haemophilus influenzae type b vaccine (Hib), PRP-OMP conjugate, 3 dose schedule, for intramuscular use

▶(90654 has been deleted. To report influenza vaccine, see 90653, 90655, 90656, 90657, 90658, 90660, 90661, 90662, 90664, 90666, 90667, 90668, 90672, 90673, 90674, 90682, 90685, 90686, 90687, 90688, 90689, 90694, 90756)◀

▶(90630 has been deleted. To report influenza vaccine, see 90653, 90655, 90656, 90657, 90658, 90660, 90661, 90662, 90664, 90666, 90667, 90668, 90672, 90673, 90674, 90682, 90685, 90686, 90687, 90688, 90689, 90694, 90756)◀

Rationale

Codes 90654 and 90630 have been deleted from the code set because the vaccine products described in those codes are no longer used. Therefore, the deletion of these two codes is congruent with efforts to streamline immunization reporting. Parenthetical notes have been included to indicate the obsolete vaccine-product codes' deletion and direct users to the appropriate product codes for influenza immunizations.

▲ **90661** Influenza virus vaccine, trivalent (ccIIV3), derived from cell cultures, subunit, antibiotic free, 0.5 mL dosage, for intramuscular use

Rationale

Code 90661 has been revised by removing "preservative" from its descriptor. This enables the reporting of code 90661 for identical formulations of the trivalent (ccIIV3) influenza virus vaccine derived from cell cultures that are antibiotic-free as 0.5 mL dosages, regardless of whether the dosages are obtained from a multi- or single-dose vial.

✗ **90668** Influenza virus vaccine (IIV), pandemic formulation, split virus, for intramuscular use

#✗● **90695** Influenza virus vaccine, H5N8, derived from cell cultures, adjuvanted, for intramuscular use

Rationale

A new code (90695) has been created in the Vaccines, Toxoids subsection to report the H5N8 vaccine product in the CPT 2025 code set. In order to help physicians or other qualified health care professionals (QHPs) offer the H5N8 vaccine if the FDA authorizes or approves it, code 90695's creation was expedited.

The H5N8 is an influenza virus vaccine that is derived from cell cultures and adjuvanted for intramuscular use. The administration of the H5N8 vaccine is reported separately using immunization administration for vaccines/toxoids codes 90460-90472.

Note that code 90695 carries the FDA-approval pending symbol (✗); therefore, interim updates on its status can be found at www.ama-assn.org/system/files/vaccine-long-descriptors.pdf, under the CPT Category I Vaccine Codes. The Centers for Disease Control and Prevention (CDC) Advisory Committee on Immunization Practices (AICP) has not assigned a US vaccine abbreviation for this vaccine. Visit the AMA CPT website for updates on the US vaccine abbreviation status for this vaccine.

Clinical Example (90695)

The H5 avian influenza was detected on a farm, and individuals who were potentially exposed are recommended to obtain the H5N8 immunization due to their increased risk. The patient agrees to receive the H5N8 immunization.

Description of Procedure (90695)

A physician or other qualified health care professional determines that the pre-pandemic influenza vaccine is appropriate for the patient. A vaccine information sheet that reviews the risks and benefits of vaccination and potential side effects is provided to the patient. After receiving the patient's consent, inject the vaccine intramuscularly. Report the administration of the immunization separately from the vaccine.

 # 90677 Pneumococcal conjugate vaccine, 20 valent (PCV20), for intramuscular use

#● 90684 Pneumococcal conjugate vaccine, 21 valent (PCV21), for intramuscular use

Rationale

New vaccine product code 90684 has been established in the Vaccines/Toxoids subsection to report the pneumococcal 21 valent conjugate vaccine (PCV21) for immunization against pneumococcal pneumonia caused by Streptococcus pneumoniae serotypes 3, 6A/C, 7F, 8, 9N, 10A, 11A, 12F, 15A, 15B/C, 16F, 17F, 19A, 20, 22F, 23A, 23B, 24F, 31, 33F, and 35B. The administration of PCV21 is reported separately using codes 90460-90472 (immunization administration for vaccines or toxoids). Note that code 90684 carries the FDA approval pending symbol (〃); therefore, interim updates on the status of this code can be found at www.ama-assn.org/system/files/vaccine-long-descriptors.pdf. The CDC ACIP has not assigned a US vaccine abbreviation for this vaccine. Visit the AMA CPT website for updates on the US vaccine abbreviation status for this vaccine.

Clinical Example (90684)

A 67-year-old male presents for an annual physical. The physician or other qualified health care professional reviews the patient's medical history and immunization record and determines that the patient should receive the pneumococcal 21-valent conjugate vaccine.

Description of Procedure (90684)

Administer the pneumococcal 21-valent conjugate vaccine by intramuscular injection.

 # 90683 Respiratory syncytial virus vaccine, mRNA lipid nanoparticles, for intramuscular use

►(For seasonal respiratory syncytial virus [RSV] monoclonal antibodies immunization codes, see 90380, 90381. For administration of seasonal RSV monoclonal antibodies immunizations, see 96380, 96381)◄

Rationale

In the parenthetical note following code 90683, code 96372 has been replaced with new codes 96380 and 96381 to report the immunization administration of seasonal RSV monoclonal antibodies.

Refer to the codebook and the Rationale for codes 96380 and 96381 for a full description of these changes.

90680 Rotavirus vaccine, pentavalent (RV5), 3 dose schedule, live, for oral use

90684 Code is out of numerical sequence. See 90670-90676

90689 Influenza virus vaccine, quadrivalent (IIV4), inactivated, adjuvanted, preservative free, 0.25 mL dosage, for intramuscular use

 # 90694 Influenza virus vaccine, quadrivalent (aIIV4), inactivated, adjuvanted, preservative free, 0.5 mL dosage, for intramuscular use

#〃● 90637 Influenza virus vaccine, quadrivalent (qIRV), mRNA; 30 mcg/0.5 mL dosage, for intramuscular use

#〃● 90638 60 mcg/0.5 mL dosage, for intramuscular use

Rationale

New vaccine product codes 90637 and 90638 have been established in the Vaccines/Toxoids subsection to report quadrivalent influenza virus vaccine products for immunization against influenza. Code 90637 identifies a "half" dose of product (30 mcg/0.5 mL); and code 90638 identifies a "full" dose of product (60 mcg/0.5 mL). The administration of the influenza vaccine is reported separately using codes 90460-90472. Note that codes 90637 and 90638 carry the FDA approval pending symbol (✗); therefore, interim updates on the FDA status of this code can be found at www.ama-assn.org/system/files/vaccine-long-descriptors.pdf. The CDC ACIP has not assigned a US vaccine abbreviation for this vaccine. Visit the AMA CPT website for updates on the US vaccine abbreviation status for this vaccine.

Clinical Example (90637)

A 40-year-old female seeks an annual influenza immunization against infection to decrease the risk of contracting the disease. The physician or other qualified health care professional determines that the patient is an appropriate candidate for the quadrivalent messenger RNA (mRNA) influenza vaccine and orders its administration.

Description of Procedure (90637)

A physician or other qualified health care professional determines that the quadrivalent mRNA influenza vaccine is appropriate for this patient. After counseling and obtaining consent, administer the immunization intramuscularly. Report the administration of the immunization separately from the vaccine.

Clinical Example (90638)

A 66-year-old male seeks an annual influenza immunization against infection to decrease the risk of contracting the disease. The physician or other qualified health care professional determines that the patient is an appropriate candidate for quadrivalent messenger RNA (mRNA) influenza vaccine and orders its administration.

Description of Procedure (90638)

A physician or other qualified health care professional determines that the quadrivalent high-dose mRNA influenza vaccine is appropriate for this patient. After counseling and obtaining consent, administer the immunization intramuscularly. Report the administration of the immunization separately from the vaccine.

90690	Typhoid vaccine, live, oral
90691	Typhoid vaccine, Vi capsular polysaccharide (ViCPs), for intramuscular use
90694	Code is out of numerical sequence. See 90688-90691
90695	Code is out of numerical sequence. See 90667-90671
# **90623**	Meningococcal pentavalent vaccine, conjugated Men A, C, W, Y- tetanus toxoid carrier, and Men B-FHbp, for intramuscular use
#✗● **90624**	Meningococcal pentavalent vaccine, Men B-4C recombinant proteins and outer membrane vesicle and conjugated Men A, C, W, Y-diphtheria toxoid carrier, for intramuscular use

Rationale

New vaccine product code 90624 has been established in the Vaccines/Toxoids subsection to report Meningococcal pentavalent vaccine product for immunization against meningococcal infection for Men B-4C recombinant proteins and conjugated Men A, C, W, and Y. The administration of the Meningococcal pentavalent vaccine is reported separately using codes 90460-90472. Note that code 90624 carries the FDA approval pending symbol (✗); therefore, interim updates on the FDA status of this code can be found at www.ama-assn.org/system/files/vaccine-long-descriptors.pdf. The CDC ACIP has not assigned a US vaccine abbreviation for this vaccine. Visit the AMA CPT website for updates on the US vaccine abbreviation status for this vaccine.

Clinical Example (90624)

A 16-year-old male seeks immunization against meningococcal infection to decrease the risk of contracting the disease. A physician or other qualified health care professional (QHP) determines that the patient is an appropriate candidate for the pentavalent meningococcal vaccine and orders its administration.

Description of Procedure (90624)

A physician or other QHP determines that the pentavalent meningococcal vaccine is appropriate for this patient. After counseling and obtaining informed consent, administer the immunization intramuscularly. Report the vaccination administration separately from the vaccine product.

Psychiatry

Psychiatric Diagnostic Procedures

★◀ **90792**   Psychiatric diagnostic evaluation with medical services

▶(Do not report 90791 or 90792 in conjunction with 99202-99316, 99341-99350, 99366-99368, 99401, 99402, 99403, 99404, 99406, 99407, 99408, 99409, 99411, 99412, 97151, 97152, 97153, 97154, 97155, 97156, 97157, 97158, 0362T, 0373T)◀

(Use 90785 in conjunction with 90791, 90792 when the diagnostic evaluation includes interactive complexity services)

Rationale

In accordance with the deletion of codes 99441-99443 and the establishment of codes 98008-98016, the exclusionary parenthetical note following code 90792 has been revised to reflect these changes.

Refer to the codebook and the Rationale for codes 99441-99443 and 98008-98016 for a full discussion of these changes.

Other Psychiatric Services or Procedures

90867   Therapeutic repetitive transcranial magnetic stimulation (TMS) treatment; initial, including cortical mapping, motor threshold determination, delivery and management

(Report only once per course of treatment)

▶(Do not report 90867 in conjunction with 90868, 90869, 95860, 95870, 95928, 95929, 95939, 0889T, 0890T, 0891T, 0892T)◀

(For peripheral nerve transcutaneous magnetic stimulation, see 0766T, 0767T)

Rationale

In accordance with the establishment of Category III codes 0889T-0892T, an exclusionary parenthetical note has been revised to restrict reporting these new codes with therapeutic repetitive transcranial magnetic stimulation treatment code 90867.

Refer to the codebook and the Rationale for changes to codes 0889T-0892T for a full discussion of these changes.

90868   subsequent delivery and management, per session

▶(Do not report 90868 in conjunction with 0889T, 0890T, 0891T, 0892T)◀

Rationale

In accordance with the establishment of Category III codes 0889T-0892T, a new exclusionary parenthetical note has been added following code 90868 to restrict reporting code 90868 with these new codes.

Refer to the codebook and the Rationale for changes to codes 0889T-0892T for a full discussion of these changes.

90869   subsequent motor threshold re-determination with delivery and management

▶(Do not report 90869 in conjunction with 90867, 90868, 95860-95870, 95928, 95929, 95939, 0889T, 0890T, 0891T, 0892T)◀

(If a significant, separately identifiable evaluation and management, medication management, or psychotherapy service is performed, the appropriate E/M or psychotherapy code may be reported in addition to 90867-90869. Evaluation and management activities directly related to cortical mapping, motor threshold determination, delivery and management of TMS are not separately reported)

Rationale

In accordance with the establishment of Category III codes 0889T-0892T, an existing exclusionary parenthetical note has been revised to restrict reporting these new codes with therapeutic repetitive transcranial magnetic stimulation treatment code 90869.

Refer to the codebook and the Rationale for changes to codes 0889T-0892T for a full discussion of these changes.

Dialysis

Hemodialysis

Codes 90935, 90937 are reported to describe the hemodialysis procedure with all evaluation and management services related to the patient's renal disease on the day of the hemodialysis procedure. These codes are used for inpatient end-stage renal disease (ESRD) and non-ESRD procedures or for outpatient non-ESRD dialysis services. Code 90935 is reported if only one evaluation of the patient is required related to that hemodialysis procedure. Code 90937 is reported when patient re-evaluation(s) is required during a hemodialysis procedure. Use modifier 25 with evaluation and management codes, including new or established patient office or other outpatient services (99202-99215), office or other outpatient consultations (99242, 99243, 99244,

99245), hospital inpatient or observation care including admission and discharge (99234, 99235, 99236), initial and subsequent hospital inpatient or observation care (99221, 99222, 99223, 99231, 99232, 99233), hospital inpatient or observation discharge services (99238, 99239), new or established patient emergency department services (99281-99285), critical care services (99291, 99292), inpatient neonatal intensive care services and pediatric and neonatal critical care services (99466-99480), nursing facility services (99304, 99305, 99306, 99307, 99308, 99309, 99310, 99315, 99316), and home or residence services (99341-99350), for separately identifiable services unrelated to the dialysis procedure or renal failure that cannot be rendered during the dialysis session.

▶(For home visit hemodialysis services performed by a nonphysician qualified health care professional, use 99512)◀

(For cannula declotting, see 36831, 36833, 36860, 36861)

(For declotting of implanted vascular access device or catheter by thrombolytic agent, use 36593)

(For collection of blood specimen from a partially or completely implantable venous access device, use 36591)

(For prolonged attendance by a physician or other qualified health care professional, use 99360)

90935   Hemodialysis procedure with single evaluation by a physician or other qualified health care professional

Rationale

In accordance with efforts to standardize references to nonphysician QHPs throughout the CPT 2025 code set, the parenthetical note preceding code 90935 has been revised.

Refer to the codebook and the Rationale for the Medical Team Conferences guidelines in the Evaluation and Management section for a full discussion of these changes.

Gastroenterology

Gastric Physiology

91132   Electrogastrography, diagnostic, transcutaneous;

91133   with provocative testing

▶(Do not report 91132, 91133 in conjunction with 0779T, 0868T)◀

Rationale

In accordance with the establishment of code 0868T, an exclusionary parenthetical note has been added following code 91133 to restrict reporting codes 91132 and 91133 in conjunction with codes 0779T and 0868T.

Refer to the codebook and the Rationale for code 0868T for a full discussion of these changes.

Other Procedures

91299   Unlisted diagnostic gastroenterology procedure

91318   Code is out of numerical sequence. See 90473-90477

91319   Code is out of numerical sequence. See 90473-90477

91320   Code is out of numerical sequence. See 90473-90477

91321   Code is out of numerical sequence. See 90473-90477

91322   Code is out of numerical sequence. See 90473-90477

Ophthalmology

Special Ophthalmological Services

▲ **92132**   Computerized ophthalmic diagnostic imaging (eg, optical coherence tomography [OCT]), anterior segment, with interpretation and report, unilateral or bilateral

(Do not report 92132 in conjunction with 0730T)

▶(For computerized ophthalmic diagnostic imaging of the optic nerve and retina, see 92133, 92134, 92137)◀

(For specular microscopy and endothelial cell analysis, use 92286)

(For tear film imaging, use 0330T)

▲ **92133**   Computerized ophthalmic diagnostic imaging (eg, optical coherence tomography [OCT]), posterior segment, with interpretation and report, unilateral or bilateral; optic nerve

▲ **92134**   retina

#● **92137**   retina, including OCT angiography

▶(Do not report 92133, 92134, 92137 at the same patient encounter)◀

▶(Report 92137 separately when performed at same encounter as 92235, 92240, 92242)◀

Rationale

As a result of changes and modernization in clinical practice and terminology, codes 92133 and 92134 have been revised, code 92137 has been added, and parenthetical notes have been added and revised throughout the CPT 2025 code set to report computerized ophthalmic diagnostic imaging of the posterior segment of the eye, which includes optical coherence tomography (OCT). In addition, code 92132 has been revised by adding OCT to the descriptor.

These changes were implemented because the AMA/Specialty Society Relative Value Scale (RVS) Update Committee (RUC) Relativity Assessment Workgroup (RAW) screen showed a substantial increase in the utilization of code 92134, which was attributed to the growth in active medical treatment of age-related macular degeneration and diabetic retinopathy, especially macular edema, and the introduction of OCT of the retina into routine clinical practice that includes noninjection, fluorescein-free angiography.

Besides the creation of code 92137 to report computerized ophthalmic diagnostic imaging of the retina, including OCT angiography, the other change is the removal of the term "scanning" from codes 92132-92134 because it is no longer used to describe these tests, and adding the updated example in parenthesis, ie, "(eg, optical coherence tomography [OCT])" in their descriptors. In addition, the parenthetical note following code 76513 has been revised by deleting "scanning" and including code 92137.

These updated, newer tests involve computerized diagnostic imaging that scans multiple layers of the retina and nerve fiber layer. OCT retinal angiography is performed by the same technician in addition to retinal OCT imaging of the structures at the same sitting using an upgraded imaging instrument, with the physician providing additional interpretation of the vasculature and blood flow through multiple layers.

The addition of code 92137 has generated other corresponding changes in the Diagnostic Ultrasound subsection of the Radiology section and the Ophthalmoscopy subsection of the Medicine section. These corresponding changes include the addition of parenthetical notes that direct users to codes for other procedures, the deletion of parenthetical notes that no longer apply because of the language revision in the existing codes, the addition of a conditional parenthetical note that provides instruction regarding reporting services provided during the same encounter, and when code 92137 may be separately reported. In addition, instructions have been added to direct users to code 92137 in other subsections of the code set.

Clinical Example (92132)

A 45-year-old male complains of an inability to read small print. The patient has temporal narrowing of the anterior chamber angle in the left eye. Imaging is ordered to evaluate the risk of angle closure.

Description of Procedure (92132)

Evaluate the quality of the study. Analyze the images and numerical values and cross-reference them to normative data. Review prior studies if available and compare for an evaluation of interval change. Enter the interpretation into the electronic health record.

Clinical Example (92133)

A 65-year-old female presents with elevated levels of intraocular pressure in both eyes. Visual field examinations reveal no evidence of visual-field loss attributable to glaucoma. Examination of the nerve fiber layer by optical coherence tomography in both eyes to look for evidence of retinal nerve fiber layer damage consistent with glaucoma is indicated.

Description of Procedure (92133)

Evaluate the quality of the study. Analyze the images and numerical values and cross-reference them to normative data. Review and compare prior studies for an evaluation of interval change. Enter the interpretation into the electronic health record.

Clinical Example (92134)

A 75-year-old male, who has a recent history of intravitreal drug injection, presents with exudative age-related macular degeneration. Optical coherence tomography is indicated to evaluate the subretinal fluid thickness and intraretinal edema in one eye.

Description of Procedure (92134)

Evaluate the quality of the study. Analyze the images and numerical values and cross-reference them to normative data. Review and compare prior studies for an evaluation of interval change. Enter the interpretation into the electronic health record.

Clinical Example (92137)

A 67-year-old male, who has a history of non-insulin-dependent diabetes mellitus, notes blurred vision and is found to have diabetic macular edema. Optical coherence tomography (OCT) and OCT angiography are ordered to examine the retinal structure in depth and determine the cause of the edema and identify any associated foveal ischemia with non-dye angiography.

Description of Procedure (92137)

Evaluate the quality of the study. Analyze and cross-reference the OCT images and numerical values to normative data. Reformat the images for angiography. Analyze the OCT angiography images for artifacts in comparison to the non-angiographic OCT images. Evaluate the OCT angiography images of the vasculature of the posterior segment at multiple levels of the retina and choriod for evidence of ischemia, microaneurysms, and neovascularization. If available, review prior studies and make a comparison for the assessment of interval change. Enter the interpretation into the electronic health record.

92136	Ophthalmic biometry by partial coherence interferometry with intraocular lens power calculation
92137	Code is out of numerical sequence. See 92133-92145
92145	Corneal hysteresis determination, by air impulse stimulation, unilateral or bilateral, with interpretation and report

Ophthalmoscopy

92235 Fluorescein angiography (includes multiframe imaging) with interpretation and report, unilateral or bilateral

▶(For optical coherence tomography [OCT] retinal angiography, use 92137)◀

(When fluorescein and indocyanine-green angiography are performed at the same patient encounter, use 92242)

92240 Indocyanine-green angiography (includes multiframe imaging) with interpretation and report, unilateral or bilateral

▶(For optical coherence tomography [OCT] retinal angiography, use 92137)◀

(When indocyanine-green and fluorescein angiography are performed at the same patient encounter, use 92242)

92242 Fluorescein angiography and indocyanine-green angiography (includes multiframe imaging) performed at the same patient encounter with interpretation and report, unilateral or bilateral

▶(For optical coherence tomography [OCT] retinal angiography, use 92137)◀

(To report fluorescein angiography and indocyanine-green angiography not performed at the same patient encounter, see 92235, 92240)

Rationale

In support of the establishment of code 92137, new cross-reference parenthetical notes directing users to report this code for OCT have been added following codes 92235, 92240, and 92242.

Refer to the codebook and the Rationale for code 92137 for a full discussion of these changes.

Cardiovascular

Therapeutic Services and Procedures

Coronary Therapeutic Services and Procedures

(To report transcatheter placement of radiation delivery device for coronary intravascular brachytherapy, use 92974)

(For intravascular radioelement application, see 77770, 77771, 77772)

(For nonsurgical septal reduction therapy [eg, alcohol ablation], use 93799)

▶(For percutaneous transcatheter therapeutic drug delivery by intracoronary drug-delivery balloon, see 0913T, 0914T)◀

 # 92920 Percutaneous transluminal coronary angioplasty; single major coronary artery or branch

▶(Do not report 92920 in conjunction with 0913T)◀

#+ 92921 each additional branch of a major coronary artery (List separately in addition to code for primary procedure)

(Use 92921 in conjunction with 92920, 92924, 92928, 92933, 92937, 92941, 92943)

▶(For percutaneous transcatheter therapeutic drug delivery by intracoronary drug-delivery balloon, see 0913T, 0914T)◀

 # 92924 Percutaneous transluminal coronary atherectomy, with coronary angioplasty when performed; single major coronary artery or branch

▶(Do not report 92924 in conjunction with 0913T)◀

#+ 92925 each additional branch of a major coronary artery (List separately in addition to code for primary procedure)

(Use 92925 in conjunction with 92924, 92928, 92933, 92937, 92941, 92943)

▶(For percutaneous transcatheter therapeutic drug delivery by intracoronary drug-delivery balloon, see 0913T, 0914T)◀

92928 Percutaneous transcatheter placement of intracoronary stent(s), with coronary angioplasty when performed; single major coronary artery or branch

▶(Do not report 92928 in conjunction with 0913T)◀

#✚ 92929   each additional branch of a major coronary artery (List separately in addition to code for primary procedure)

(Use 92929 in conjunction with 92928, 92933, 92937, 92941, 92943)

▶(For percutaneous transcatheter therapeutic drug delivery by intracoronary drug-delivery balloon, see 0913T, 0914T)◀

92933 Percutaneous transluminal coronary atherectomy, with intracoronary stent, with coronary angioplasty when performed; single major coronary artery or branch

▶(Do not report 92933 in conjunction with 0913T)◀

#✚ 92934   each additional branch of a major coronary artery (List separately in addition to code for primary procedure)

(Use 92934 in conjunction with 92933, 92937, 92941, 92943)

▶(For percutaneous transcatheter therapeutic drug delivery by intracoronary drug-delivery balloon, see 0913T, 0914T)◀

92937 Percutaneous transluminal revascularization of or through coronary artery bypass graft (internal mammary, free arterial, venous), any combination of intracoronary stent, atherectomy and angioplasty, including distal protection when performed; single vessel

▶(Do not report 92937 in conjunction with 0913T)◀

#✚ 92938   each additional branch subtended by the bypass graft (List separately in addition to code for primary procedure)

(Use 92938 in conjunction with 92937)

▶(For percutaneous transcatheter therapeutic drug delivery by intracoronary drug-delivery balloon, see 0913T, 0914T)◀

92941 Percutaneous transluminal revascularization of acute total/subtotal occlusion during acute myocardial infarction, coronary artery or coronary artery bypass graft, any combination of intracoronary stent, atherectomy and angioplasty, including aspiration thrombectomy when performed, single vessel

▶(Do not report 92941 in conjunction with 0913T for intervention in the same major coronary artery or in the same bypass graft)◀

▶(For additional vessels treated, see 92920-92938, 92943, 92944, 0913T, 0914T)◀

(For transcatheter intra-arterial hyperoxemic reperfusion/supersaturated oxygen therapy [SSO2], use 0659T)

92943 Percutaneous transluminal revascularization of chronic total occlusion, coronary artery, coronary artery branch, or coronary artery bypass graft, any combination of intracoronary stent, atherectomy and angioplasty; single vessel

▶(Do not report 92943 in conjunction with 0913T)◀

#✚ 92944   each additional coronary artery, coronary artery branch, or bypass graft (List separately in addition to code for primary procedure)

(Use 92944 in conjunction with 92924, 92928, 92933, 92937, 92941, 92943)

(For intravascular radioelement application, see 77770, 77771, 77772)

(To report transcatheter placement of radiation delivery device for coronary intravascular brachytherapy, use 92974)

▶(For percutaneous transcatheter therapeutic drug delivery by intracoronary drug-delivery balloon, see 0913T, 0914T)◀

#✚ 92972 Percutaneous transluminal coronary lithotripsy (List separately in addition to code for primary procedure)

(Use 92972 in conjunction with 92920, 92924, 92928, 92933, 92937, 92941, 92943, 92975)

#✚ 92973 Percutaneous transluminal coronary thrombectomy mechanical (List separately in addition to code for primary procedure)

(Use 92973 in conjunction with 92920, 92924, 92928, 92933, 92937, 92941, 92943, 92975, 93454-93461, 93563, 93564)

▶(Do not report 92973 in conjunction with 0913T for intervention in the same major coronary artery or in the same bypass graft)◀

(Do not report 92973 for aspiration thrombectomy)

#✚ 92974 Transcatheter placement of radiation delivery device for subsequent coronary intravascular brachytherapy (List separately in addition to code for primary procedure)

(Use 92974 in conjunction with 92920, 92924, 92928, 92933, 92937, 92941, 92943, 93454-93461)

(For intravascular radioelement application, see 77770, 77771, 77772)

92975 Thrombolysis, coronary; by intracoronary infusion, including selective coronary angiography

92977   by intravenous infusion

(For thrombolysis of vessels other than coronary, see 37211-37214)

(For cerebral thrombolysis, use 37195)

#✚ 92978 Endoluminal imaging of coronary vessel or graft using intravascular ultrasound (IVUS) or optical coherence tomography (OCT) during diagnostic evaluation and/or therapeutic intervention including imaging supervision, interpretation and report; initial vessel (List separately in addition to code for primary procedure)

(Use 92978 in conjunction with 92975, 92920, 92924, 92928, 92933, 92937, 92941, 92943, 93454-93461, 93563, 93564)

(Report 92978 once per session)

▶(Do not report 92978 in conjunction with 0913T, 0914T for intervention in the same major coronary artery or in the same bypass graft)◀

#+ 92979   each additional vessel (List separately in addition to code for primary procedure)

(Report 92979 once per additional vessel)

(Use 92979 in conjunction with 92978)

(Intravascular ultrasound and optical coherence tomography services include all transducer manipulations and repositioning within the specific vessel being examined, both before and after therapeutic intervention [eg, stent placement])

Rationale

In accordance with the establishment of Category III codes 0913T and 0914T to report percutaneous transcatheter therapeutic drug delivery by intracoronary drug-delivery balloon, parenthetical notes following codes 92920-92944, 92973, and 92978 have been revised and added to accommodate the inclusion of codes 0913T and 0914T.

Refer to the codebook and the Rationale for codes 0913T and 0914T for a full discussion of these changes.

Cardiovascular Monitoring Services

93224   External electrocardiographic recording up to 48 hours by continuous rhythm recording and storage; includes recording, scanning analysis with report, review and interpretation by a physician or other qualified health care professional

93225   recording (includes connection, recording, and disconnection)

93226   scanning analysis with report

93227   review and interpretation by a physician or other qualified health care professional

(For less than 12 hours of continuous recording, use modifier 52)

▶(For greater than 48 hours of monitoring, see 93241, 93242, 93243, 93244, 93245, 93246, 93247, 93248, 0937T, 0938T, 0939T, 0940T)◀

93241   External electrocardiographic recording for more than 48 hours up to 7 days by continuous rhythm recording and storage; includes recording, scanning analysis with report, review and interpretation

93242   recording (includes connection and initial recording)

93243   scanning analysis with report

93244   review and interpretation

▶(Do not report 93241, 93242, 93243, 93244 in conjunction with 93224, 93225, 93226, 93227, 93228, 93229, 93245, 93246, 93247, 93248, 93268, 93270, 93271, 93272, 99091, 99453, 99454, 0937T, 0938T, 0939T, 0940T, for the same monitoring period)◀

93245   External electrocardiographic recording for more than 7 days up to 15 days by continuous rhythm recording and storage; includes recording, scanning analysis with report, review and interpretation

93246   recording (includes connection and initial recording)

93247   scanning analysis with report

93248   review and interpretation

▶(Do not report 93245, 93246, 93247, 93248 in conjunction with 93224, 93225, 93226, 93227, 93228, 93229, 93241, 93242, 93243, 93244, 93268, 93270, 93271, 93272, 99091, 99453, 99454, 0937T, 0938T, 0939T, 0940T, for the same monitoring period)◀

Rationale

Parenthetical notes following codes 93227, 93244, and 93248 have been updated to include new Category III codes for external electrocardiogram (ECG) recording (0937T-0940T).

Refer to the codebook and the Rationale for codes 0937T-0940T for a full discussion of these changes.

Implantable, Insertable, and Wearable Cardiac Device Evaluations

93264   Remote monitoring of a wireless pulmonary artery pressure sensor for up to 30 days, including at least weekly downloads of pulmonary artery pressure recordings, interpretation(s), trend analysis, and report(s) by a physician or other qualified health care professional

(Report 93264 only once per 30 days)

(Do not report 93264 if download[s], interpretation[s], trend analysis, and report[s] do not occur at least weekly during the 30-day time period)

(Do not report 93264 if review does not occur at least weekly during the 30-day time period)

(Do not report 93264 if monitoring period is less than 30 days)

▶(For remote monitoring of an implantable wireless left atrial pressure sensor, use 0934T)◀

Rationale

In accordance with the addition of Category III code 0934T, a cross-reference parenthetical note has been added following code 93264.

Refer to the codebook and the Rationale for codes 0933T and 0934T for a full discussion of these changes.

93286 Peri-procedural device evaluation (in person) and programming of device system parameters before or after a surgery, procedure, or test with analysis, review and report by a physician or other qualified health care professional; single, dual, or multiple lead pacemaker system, or leadless pacemaker system

(Report 93286 once before and once after surgery, procedure, or test, when device evaluation and programming is performed before and after surgery, procedure, or test)

▶(Do not report 93286 in conjunction with 93279, 93280, 93281, 93288, 0408T, 0409T, 0410T, 0411T, 0414T, 0415T, 0915T-0925T)◀

Rationale

An existing exclusionary parenthetical note following code 93286 has been revised to include code 93280 to report programming device evaluation and new Category III codes 0915T-0925T to report the insertion, removal, relocation, and repositioning of a cardiac contractility modulation-defibrillation system.

Refer to the codebook and the Rationale for codes 0915T-0931T for a full discussion of these changes.

93287 single, dual, or multiple lead implantable defibrillator system

(Use 93286, 93287 in conjunction with 0696T when body surface–activation mapping to optimize electrical synchrony is also performed)

(Report 93287 once before and once after surgery, procedure, or test, when device evaluation and programming is performed before and after surgery, procedure, or test)

▶(Do not report 93287 in conjunction with 93260, 93261, 93282, 93283, 93284, 93289, 0408T, 0409T, 0410T, 0411T, 0414T, 0415T, 0915T-0925T)◀

Rationale

An existing exclusionary parenthetical note following code 93287 has been revised to include new Category III codes 0915T-0925T to report the insertion, removal, relocation, and repositioning of a cardiac contractility modulation-defibrillation system.

Refer to the codebook and the Rationale for codes 0915T-0931T for a full discussion of these changes.

Cardiac Catheterization

✚ 93571 Intravascular Doppler velocity and/or pressure derived coronary flow reserve measurement (coronary vessel or graft) during coronary angiography including pharmacologically induced stress; initial vessel (List separately in addition to code for primary procedure)

▶(Use 93571 in conjunction with 92920, 92924, 92928, 92933, 92937, 92941, 92943, 92975, 93454-93461, 93563, 93564, 93593, 93594, 93595, 93596, 93597, 0913T)◀

(Do not report 93571 in conjunction with 0523T)

✚ 93572 each additional vessel (List separately in addition to code for primary procedure)

(Use 93572 in conjunction with 93571)

(Do not report 93572 in conjunction with 0523T)

(Intravascular distal coronary blood flow velocity measurements include all Doppler transducer manipulations and repositioning within the specific vessel being examined, during coronary angiography or therapeutic intervention [eg, angioplasty])

(For unlisted cardiac catheterization procedure, use 93799)

Rationale

In accordance with the establishment of Category III codes 0913T and 0914T to report percutaneous transcatheter therapeutic drug delivery by intracoronary drug-delivery balloon, the parenthetical note following code 93571 has been revised by adding code 0913T.

Refer to the codebook and the Rationale for codes 0913T and 0914T for a full discussion of these changes.

★ =Telemedicine   ◀ =Audio-only   ✚ =Add-on code   ✗ =FDA approval pending   # =Resequenced code   ⊘ =Modifier 51 exempt

Medicine 90281-99607

Intracardiac Electrophysiological Procedures/Studies

Intracardiac electrophysiologic studies (EPS) are invasive diagnostic medical procedures which include the insertion and repositioning of electrode catheters, recording of electrograms before and during pacing, programmed stimulation of multiple locations in the heart, analysis of recorded information, and report of the procedure. In many circumstances, patients with arrhythmias are evaluated and treated at the same encounter. In this situation, a diagnostic *electrophysiologic study* is performed, induced tachycardia(s) are *mapped*, and on the basis of the diagnostic and mapping information, the tissue is *ablated*.

Definitions

Mapping is a distinct procedure performed in addition to a diagnostic electrophysiologic study or ablation procedure and may be separately reported using 93609 or 93613. Do not report standard mapping (93609) in addition to 3-dimensional mapping (93613).

▶*Ablation:* Once the part of the heart involved in the tachycardia is localized, the tachycardia may be treated by ablation to the area to selectively destroy cardiac tissue. Ablation procedures (93653-93657) are performed at the same session as electrophysiology studies and therefore represent a combined code descriptor. When reporting ablation therapy codes (93653-93657), the single site electrophysiology studies (93600-93603, 93610, 93612, 93618) and the comprehensive electrophysiology studies (93619, 93620) may not be reported separately. Code 93622 may be reported separately with 93653 and 93656. Code 93623 may be reported separately with 93653, 93654, and 93656. However, 93621 for left atrial pacing and recording from coronary sinus or left atrium should not be reported in conjunction with 93656, as this procedure is a component of 93656. Codes 93653 and 93654 include right ventricular pacing and recording and His bundle recording when clinically indicated. When performance of one or more components is not possible or indicated, document the reason for not performing. Code 93656 includes each of left atrial pacing/recording, right ventricular pacing/recording, and His bundle recording when clinically indicated. When performance of one or more components is not possible or indicated, document the reason for not performing.◀

The differences in the techniques involved for ablation of supraventricular arrhythmias, ventricular arrhythmias, and atrial fibrillation are reflected within the descriptions for 93653-93657. Code 93653 is a primary code for catheter ablation for treatment of supraventricular tachycardia caused by dual atrioventricular nodal pathways, accessory atrioventricular connections, or other atrial foci. Code 93654 describes catheter ablation for treatment of ventricular tachycardia or focus of ventricular ectopy. Code 93656 is a primary code for reporting treatment of atrial fibrillation by ablation to achieve complete pulmonary vein electrical isolation. Codes 93653, 93654, and 93656 are distinct primary procedure codes and may not be reported together.

▲ **93656**   Comprehensive electrophysiologic evaluation with transseptal catheterizations, insertion and repositioning of multiple electrode catheters, induction or attempted induction of an arrhythmia including left or right atrial pacing/recording, and intracardiac catheter ablation of atrial fibrillation by pulmonary vein isolation, including intracardiac electrophysiologic 3-dimensional mapping, intracardiac echocardiography with imaging supervision and interpretation, right ventricular pacing/recording, and His bundle recording, when performed

(Do not report 93656 in conjunction with 93279, 93280, 93281, 93282, 93283, 93284, 93286, 93287, 93288, 93289, 93462, 93600, 93602, 93603, 93610, 93612, 93613, 93618, 93619, 93620, 93621, 93653, 93654, 93662)

Rationale

For the CPT 2025 code set, the Intracardiac Electrophysiological Procedures/Studies guidelines have been editorially revised to clarify the current ablation methods for treating atrial fibrillation. Code 93656 has also been editorially revised.

Deleting specific methods from the guidelines (ie, radiofrequency and cryo-energy) enable the inclusion and use of new emerging technologies, such as laser and pulsed-field ablation. In addition, code 93656 has been editorially revised to clarify that the catheter placement in the atrium is necessary and not optional for the catheter ablation of atrial fibrillation. The term "including" has been deleted in the code descriptor to avoid confusion.

Home and Outpatient International Normalized Ratio (INR) Monitoring Services

Home and outpatient international normalized ratio (INR) monitoring services describe the management of warfarin therapy, including ordering, review, and interpretation of new INR test result(s), patient instructions, and dosage adjustments as needed.

If a significantly, separately identifiable evaluation and management (E/M) service is performed on the same day as 93792, the appropriate E/M service may be reported using modifier 25.

Do not report 93793 on the same day as an E/M service.

▶Do not report 93792, 93793 in conjunction with 98012, 98013, 98014, 98015, 98016, 98966, 98967, 98968, 98970, 98971, 98972, 99421, 99422, 99423, when telephone or online digital evaluation and management services address home and outpatient INR monitoring.◀

Do not count time spent in 93792, 93793 in the time of 99439, 99487, 99489, 99490, 99491, when reported in the same calendar month.

93792   Patient/caregiver training for initiation of home international normalized ratio (INR) monitoring under the direction of a physician or other qualified health care professional, face-to-face, including use and care of the INR monitor, obtaining blood sample, instructions for reporting home INR test results, and documentation of patient's/caregiver's ability to perform testing and report results

(For provision of test materials and equipment for home INR monitoring, see 99070 or the appropriate supply code)

Rationale

In accordance with the deletion of codes 99441-99443 and the establishment of codes 98012-98016, the Home and Outpatient International Normalized Ratio (INR) Monitoring Services subsection guidelines have been revised to reflect these changes.

Refer to the codebook and the Rationale for codes 98012-98016 for a full discussion of these changes.

Noninvasive Vascular Diagnostic Studies

Cerebrovascular Arterial Studies

A complete transcranial Doppler (TCD) study (93886) includes ultrasound evaluation of the right and left anterior circulation territories and the posterior circulation territory (to include vertebral arteries and basilar artery). In a limited TCD study (93888) there is ultrasound evaluation of two or fewer of these territories. For TCD, ultrasound evaluation is a reasonable and concerted attempt to identify arterial signals through an acoustic window.

▶Use TCD study codes (93886, 93888, 93892, 93893) when a single study is performed. Use 93896, 93897, 93898, when a vasoreactivity study, emboli detection without intravenous microbubble injection, or venous-arterial shunt detection with intravenous microbubble

injection is performed in conjunction with a complete TCD on the same day.◀

Code 93895 includes the acquisition and storage of images of the common carotid arteries, carotid bulbs, and internal carotid arteries bilaterally with quantification of intima media thickness (common carotid artery mean and maximal values) and determination of presence of atherosclerotic plaque.

93880   Duplex scan of extracranial arteries; complete bilateral study

(Do not report 93880 in conjunction with 93895)

93882   unilateral or limited study

(Do not report 93882 in conjunction with 93895)

93886   Transcranial Doppler study of the intracranial arteries; complete study

93888   limited study

▶(Do not report 93888 in conjunction with 93886, 93892, 93893, 93896, 93897, 93898)◀

▶(93890 has been deleted. To report vasoreactivity study, use 93896)◀

93892   emboli detection without intravenous microbubble injection

▲ **93893**   venous-arterial shunt detection with intravenous microbubble injection

▶(Do not report 93892, 93893 in conjunction with 93886, 93888)◀

#+● **93896**   Vasoreactivity study performed with transcranial Doppler study of intracranial arteries, complete (List separately in addition to code for primary procedure)

▶(Use 93896 in conjunction with 93886)◀

▶(Do not report 93896 in conjunction with 93888)◀

#+● **93897**   Emboli detection without intravenous microbubble injection performed with transcranial Doppler study of intracranial arteries, complete (List separately in addition to code for primary procedure)

▶(Use 93897 in conjunction with 93886)◀

▶(Do not report 93897 in conjunction with 93888)◀

#+● **93898**   Venous-arterial shunt detection with intravenous microbubble injection performed with transcranial Doppler study of intracranial arteries, complete (List separately in addition to code for primary procedure)

▶(Use 93898 in conjunction with 93886)◀

▶(Do not report 93898 in conjunction with 93888)◀

93895   Quantitative carotid intima media thickness and carotid atheroma evaluation, bilateral

(Do not report 93895 in conjunction with 93880, 93882)

★ =Telemedicine   ◀ =Audio-only   ✚ =Add-on code   ✔ =FDA approval pending   # =Resequenced code   ⊘ =Modifier 51 exempt

93896   Code is out of numerical sequence. See 93892-93922

93897   Code is out of numerical sequence. See 93892-93922

93898   Code is out of numerical sequence. See 93892-93922

Rationale

Changes have been made regarding the reporting of transcranial Doppler (TCD) procedures of intracranial arteries. Specifically, code 93890 has been deleted, code 93893 revised, and three add-on codes (93896-93898) have been established. The Cerebrovascular Arterial Studies guidelines have also been revised.

Changes to the reporting of TCD procedures were initiated following the identification of Doppler procedures described by codes 93886, 93890, and 93892 in a RUC RAW screen for codes inherently performed together. It was determined that a coding solution was necessary to eliminate duplicate reporting of pre- and postservice work when a complete TCD study of intracranial arteries is performed with a vasoreactivity study, with emboli detection but without intravenous microbubble injection, or with venous-arterial shunt detection with intravenous microbubble injection. To remedy this issue, three add-on codes have been established to report when the following are performed with a complete TCD study of intracranial arteries (93886): vasoreactivity study (93896), emboli detection without intravenous microbubble injection (93897), or venous-arterial shunt detection with intravenous microbubble injection (93898). Code 93890, which previously described a TCD study with a vasoreactivity study, has been deleted. Code 93893, which previously described emboli detection with intravenous microbubble injection, has been revised to describe venous-arterial shunt detection with an intravenous microbubble technique.

The Cerebrovascular Arterial Studies guidelines have been revised to clarify that a single TCD study is reported with codes 93886, 93888, 93892, or 93893, as appropriate, and to provide instructions on the appropriate use of codes 93896-93898. Inclusionary and exclusionary parenthetical notes have been added to clarify which codes may and may not be reported together.

Clinical Example (93893)

A 50-year-old male has had an episode of stroke-like symptoms. A transcranial Doppler with agitated saline injection is ordered to assess for a right-to-left intracardiac shunt or pulmonary AV fistula.

Description of Procedure (93893)

Supervise the vascular technologist with patient preparation and performance of the test as needed. Review acquired Doppler spectral waveforms, flow direction, mean systolic and diastolic flow velocity, depth of sampling, and pulsatility index values, including waveforms obtained before, during, and after the agitated saline injection(s). Identify and review any high-intensity transient signal events and classify them as embolic or artifact. Count the total number of post-injection embolic signals and note any "shower" or "curtain" appearance of embolic signals and the vessel segment(s) in which they were identified. Record the relationship to the time after intravenous injection and to the Valsalva maneuver. Document the procedure results. Integrate the findings with clinical presentations to formulate and document an examination interpretation. Dictate, review, and approve the report.

Clinical Example (93896)

A 65-year-old female is referred to the transcranial Doppler (TCD) laboratory after a carotid duplex ultrasound examination identified a 90% left internal carotid artery stenosis. During the complete TCD, vasoreactivity testing is ordered to assess cerebrovascular reserve adequacy of collateral flow. [**Note:** This is an add-on code. Only consider the additional work related to vasoreactivity testing.]

Description of Procedure (93896)

Supervise the vascular technologist with patient preparation and performance of the TCD test as needed. Review clinical history in relation to the safety of administering carbon dioxide (CO_2) or acetazolamide. Review the recorded data, including demographics, vital signs, and blood gases. Scan the right and left anterior circulation territories and the posterior circulation territory to include vertebral arteries and basilar arteries. Compare with findings from prior examinations. Assist technologist with the identification of vessels to insonate. Review acquired Doppler spectral waveforms, flow direction, mean systolic and diastolic flow velocities, depth of sampling, pulsatility index values, and capnometer values throughout the duration of the CO_2 administration in the resting values for the arterial segments studied. Document procedure results. Integrate findings with clinical presentation to formulate and document examination interpretation.

Clinical Example (93897)

A 65-year-old female is referred to the transcranial Doppler (TCD) laboratory after presenting with a right hemisphere infarct. During the complete TCD study, embolus detection is ordered to assess for evidence of a

Medicine 90281-99607

proximal embolic source. [**Note:** This is an add-on code. Only consider the additional work related to emboli detection.]

Description of Procedure (93897)

Supervise the vascular technologist with patient preparation and performance of the TCD test as needed. Review the recorded data, including demographics, vital signs, and blood gases. Scan the right and left anterior circulation territories and the posterior circulation territory to include vertebral arteries and basilar arteries. Compare with findings from prior examinations. Emboli detection is performed in the cerebral arteries to monitor high-intensity transients consistent with thromboembolic phenomena. Document procedure results. Integrate findings with clinical presentation to formulate and document examination interpretation.

Clinical Example (93898)

A 50-year-old male is referred to the transcranial Doppler (TCD) laboratory following an episode of aphasia and right hemiparesis. During the complete TCD study, an agitated saline injection is ordered to assess for right-to-left intracardiac shunt or pulmonary AV fistula. [**Note:** This is an add-on code. Only consider the additional work related to shunt detection.]

Description of Procedure (93898)

Supervise the vascular technologist with patient preparation and performance of the TCD test as needed. Review acquired Doppler spectral waveforms, flow direction, mean systolic and diastolic flow velocity, depth of sampling, and pulsatility index values, including waveforms obtained before, during, and after the agitated saline injection(s). Identify and review any high-intensity, transient signal events, and classify them as embolic or artifact. Count the total number of postinjection embolic signals and note any "shower" or "curtain" appearance of embolic signals and the vessel segment(s) in which they were identified. Record the relationship to the time after the intravenous injection and to the Valsalva maneuver. Document procedure results. Integrate findings with clinical presentations to formulate and document exam interpretation.

Extremity Arterial-Venous Studies

93990 Duplex scan of hemodialysis access (including arterial inflow, body of access and venous outflow)

(For measurement of hemodialysis access flow using indicator dilution methods, use 90940)

▶(For limited study of body of hemodialysis fistula using computer-aided ultrasound system, use 0876T)◀

Rationale

In accordance with the establishment of Category III code 0876T, a cross-reference parenthetical note has been added following code 93990 to direct users to code 0876T for a limited study of the body of a hemodialysis fistula using a computer-aided ultrasound system.

Refer to the codebook and the Rationale for code 0876T for a full discussion of these changes.

Pulmonary

Ventilator Management

94002 Ventilation assist and management, initiation of pressure or volume preset ventilators for assisted or controlled breathing; hospital inpatient/observation, initial day

94003 hospital inpatient/observation, each subsequent day

94004 nursing facility, per day

▶(Do not report 94002-94004 in conjunction with evaluation and management services 98000-98016, 99202-99499)◀

Rationale

In accordance with the establishment of codes 98000-98016, the exclusionary parenthetical note following code 94004 has been revised to reflect these changes.

Refer to the codebook and the Rationale for codes 98000-98016 for a full discussion of these changes.

Neurology and Neuromuscular Procedures

Electromyography

95860 Needle electromyography; 1 extremity with or without related paraspinal areas

95861 2 extremities with or without related paraspinal areas

▶(For dynamic electromyography performed during motion analysis studies, use 96002)◀

95863 3 extremities with or without related paraspinal areas

Rationale

In accordance with the deletion of code 96003, the cross-reference parenthetical note following code 95861 has been revised to reflect this change.

Refer to the codebook and the Rationale for code 96003 for a full discussion of this change.

Motion Analysis

▶Codes 96000-96004 describe services performed as part of a major therapeutic or diagnostic decision making process. Motion analysis is performed in a dedicated motion analysis laboratory (ie, a facility capable of performing videotaping from the front, back and both sides, computerized 3D kinematics, 3D kinetics, and dynamic electromyography). Code 96000 may include 3D kinetics and stride characteristics. Code 96002 describes dynamic electromyography.◀

Code 96004 should only be reported once regardless of the number of study(ies) reviewed/interpreted.

(For performance of needle electromyography procedures, see 95860-95870, 95872, 95885-95887)

(For gait training, use 97116)

96000   Comprehensive computer-based motion analysis by video-taping and 3D kinematics;

96001   with dynamic plantar pressure measurements during walking

96002   Dynamic surface electromyography, during walking or other functional activities, 1-12 muscles

▶(Do not report 96002 in conjunction with 95860-95866, 95869-95872, 95885-95887)◀

▶(96003 has been deleted)◀

Rationale

To ensure the CPT 2025 code set reflects current clinical practice, add-on code 96003, *Dynamic fine wire electromyography, during walking or other functional activities, 1 muscle*, has been deleted due to low utilization. A parenthetical note has been added to indicate this deletion. In accordance with this deletion, the Motion Analysis guidelines have been revised to reflect this change.

Medical Genetics and Genetic Counseling Services

▶These services are provided by trained genetic counselors and may include obtaining a structured family genetic history, pedigree construction, analysis for genetic risk assessment, and counseling of the patient and family.◀

▶Total Time of Medical Genetics and Genetic Counseling Services on the Date of the Encounter	Code(s)
Less than 16 minutes	Not reported separately
16-45 minutes	96041 X 1
46-75 minutes	96041 X 2
76-105 minutes	96041 X 3
106-135 minutes	96041 X 4◀

▶(96040 has been deleted. To report medical genetics and genetic counseling services, use 96041)◀

★◀● 96041   Medical genetics and genetic counseling services, each 30 minutes of total time provided by the genetic counselor on the date of the encounter

▶(Do not report 96041 for less than 16 minutes of genetic counselor time)◀

▶(For education regarding genetic risks by a nonphysician to a group, see 98961, 98962)◀

▶(For genetic counseling and education to a group by a physician or other qualified health care professional, use 99078)◀

▶(For genetic counseling and/or risk factor reduction intervention provided to patient[s] without symptoms or established disease, by a physician or other qualified health care professional who may report evaluation and management services, see 99401-99412)◀

▶(For genetic counseling and education provided to an individual by a physician or other qualified health care professional who may report evaluation and management services, see the appropriate evaluation and management codes)◀

Rationale

A new Category I code (96041) has been established to report medical genetics and genetic counseling services. The Medical Genetics and Genetic Counseling Services guidelines and parenthetical notes have been revised and added to reflect this new code. A new table has been added to assist users in reporting the total time of medical genetics and genetic counseling services on the date of the encounter. Code 96040 and all related references have been deleted.

Code 96041 describes the specific and intensive efforts necessary to provide genetic counseling services to patients who may request or require this special type of service. Genetic counseling is a communication process that deals with the human problems associated with the occurrence, or risk thereof, of a genetic disorder in a patient or their family.

Unlike other services represented in the CPT 2025 code set, including the fact that many evaluation and management (E/M) services are performed for patients who clearly present with medical conditions or needs, genetic counseling services are different because patients who may need genetic counseling may be asymptomatic of any birth defect or illness.

Code 96041 describes genetic counseling services for each 30 minutes of the total time provided by the genetic counselor on the date of the encounter, which includes the total time spent with the patient and/or their family.

Code 96041 should not be reported for physician services related to genetics counseling because it is intended to be used by genetic counselors. Therefore, parenthetical notes have been added to identify the appropriate codes for physicians or other QHPs to report when they provide these services. The cross-reference parenthetical note directs users to the E/M codes for genetic counseling services provided by a physician or other QHP. The guidelines have been revised by removing all references to code 96040.

The guidelines for medical genetics and genetic counseling services have also been updated to clarify the current clinical practice and reporting intent, as well as to ensure language synchronicity between the guidelines and the descriptors. As part of the guidelines, a table has been created to delineate the time ranges for time spent on these services on the date of the encounter and how to report these time thresholds using code 96041, including the minimum time that may be reported separately.

Clinical Example (96041)

A 31-year-old female presents with a strong family history of both colon and breast cancer. She is interested in discussing genetic testing and the best ways to assess her future cancer risks and inform her personal medical decision making. She also has questions regarding inheritance and genetic information privacy. Individual genetic counseling services are provided.

Description of Procedure (96041)

N/A

Behavior Management Services

Behavior modification is defined as the process of altering human-behavior patterns over a long-term period using various motivational techniques, namely, consequences and rewards. More simply, behavior modification is the method of changing the way a person reacts either physically or mentally to a given stimulus.

Behavior modification treatment is based on the principles of operant conditioning. The intended clinical outcome for this treatment approach is to replace unwanted or problematic behaviors with more positive, desirable behaviors through the use of evidence-based techniques and methods.

The purpose of the group-based behavioral management/modification training services is to teach the parent(s)/guardian(s)/caregiver(s) interventions that they can independently use to effectively manage the identified patient's illness(es) or disease(s). Codes 96202, 96203 are used to report the total duration of face-to-face time spent by the physician or other qualified health care professional providing group-based parent(s)/guardian(s)/caregiver(s) behavioral management/modification training services. This service involves behavioral treatment training provided to a multiple-family group of parent(s)/guardian(s)/caregiver(s), without the patient present. These services emphasize active engagement and involvement of the parent(s)/guardian(s)/caregiver(s) in the treatment of a patient with a mental or physical health diagnosis. These services do not represent preventive medicine counseling and risk factor reduction interventions.

During these sessions, the parent(s)/guardian(s)/caregiver(s) are trained, using verbal instruction, video and live demonstrations, and feedback from physician or other qualified health care professional or other parent(s)/guardian(s)/caregiver(s) in group sessions, to use skills and strategies to address behaviors impacting the patient's mental or physical health diagnosis. These skills and strategies help to support compliance with the identified patient's treatment and the clinical plan of care.

For counseling and education provided by a physician or other qualified health care professional to a patient and/or family, see the appropriate evaluation and management codes, including office or other outpatient services (99202, 99203, 99204, 99205, 99211, 99212, 99213, 99214, 99215), hospital inpatient and observation care services (99221, 99222, 99223, 99231, 99232, 99233, 99234, 99235, 99236), new or established patient office or other outpatient consultations (99242, 99243, 99244, 99245), inpatient or observation consultations (99252, 99253, 99254, 99255), emergency department services (99281, 99282, 99283, 99284, 99285), nursing facility services (99304, 99305, 99306, 99307, 99308, 99309,

99310, 99315, 99316), home or residence services (99341, 99342, 99344, 99345, 99347, 99348, 99349, 99350), and counseling risk factor reduction and behavior change intervention (99401-99429). See also **Instructions for Use of the CPT Codebook** for definition of reporting qualifications.

Counseling risk factor reduction and behavior change intervention codes (99401, 99402, 99403, 99404, 99406, 99407, 99408, 99409, 99411, 99412) are included and may not be separately reported on the same day as parent(s)/guardian(s)/caregiver(s) training services codes 96202, 96203 by the same provider.

Medical nutrition therapy (97802, 97803, 97804) provided to the identified patient may be reported on the same date of service as parent(s)/guardian(s)/caregiver(s) training service.

> (For health behavior assessment and intervention that is not part of a standardized curriculum, see 96156, 96158, 96159, 96164, 96165, 96167, 96168, 96170, 96171)

> (For educational services that use a standardized curriculum provided to patients with an established illness/disease, see 98960, 98961, 98962)

> ▶(For education provided as genetic counseling services, use 96041. For education to a group regarding genetic risks, see 98961, 98962)◀

96202 Multiple-family group behavior management/ modification training for parent(s)/guardian(s)/ caregiver(s) of patients with a mental or physical health diagnosis, administered by physician or other qualified health care professional (without the patient present), face-to-face with multiple sets of parent(s)/guardian(s)/ caregiver(s); initial 60 minutes

> (Do not report 96202 for behavior management services to the patient and the parent[s]/guardian[s]/caregiver[s] during the same session)

> (Do not report 96202 for less than 31 minutes of service)

Rationale

In accordance with the deletion of code 96040 and the establishment of code 96041, the instructional parenthetical note in the Behavior Management Services subsection has been revised.

Refer to the codebook and the Rationale for codes 96040 and 96041 for a full discussion of these changes.

Hydration, Therapeutic, Prophylactic, Diagnostic Injections and Infusions, and Chemotherapy and Other Highly Complex Drug or Highly Complex Biologic Agent Administration

Therapeutic, Prophylactic, and Diagnostic Injections and Infusions (Excludes Chemotherapy and Other Highly Complex Drug or Highly Complex Biologic Agent Administration)

A therapeutic, prophylactic, or diagnostic IV infusion or injection (other than hydration) is for the administration of substances/drugs. When fluids are used to administer the drug(s), the administration of the fluid is considered incidental hydration and is not separately reportable. These services typically require direct supervision for any or all purposes of patient assessment, provision of consent, safety oversight, and intra-service supervision of staff. Typically, such infusions require special consideration to prepare, dose or dispose of, require practice training and competency for staff who administer the infusions, and require periodic patient assessment with vital sign monitoring during the infusion. These codes are not intended to be reported by the physician or other qualified health care professional in the facility setting.

▶Passive immunizations, such as an immune globulin or monoclonal antibody, provide long-term passive immunization to the patient.◀

Rationale

A new sentence in the guidelines that describes the long-term benefit of passive immunizations using immune globulins and monoclonal antibodies has been added to the Therapeutic, Prophylactic, and Diagnostic Injections and Infusions (Excludes Chemotherapy and Other Highly Complex Drug or Highly Complex Biologic Agent Administration) subsection.

Refer to the codebook and the Rationales for codes 96380, 96381, 90480, and 91318-91322 for a full discussion of these changes.

See codes 96401-96549 for the administration of chemotherapy or other highly complex drug or highly complex biologic agent services. These highly complex services require advanced practice training and competency for staff who provide these services; special considerations for preparation, dosage or disposal; and commonly, these services entail significant patient risk and frequent monitoring. Examples are frequent changes in the infusion rate, prolonged presence of nurse administering the solution for patient monitoring and infusion adjustments, and frequent conferring with the physician or other qualified health care professional about these issues.

(Do not report 96365-96379 with codes for which IV push or infusion is an inherent part of the procedure [eg, administration of contrast material for a diagnostic imaging study])

(For mechanical scalp cooling, see 0662T, 0663T)

96372   Therapeutic, prophylactic, or diagnostic injection (specify substance or drug); subcutaneous or intramuscular

▶(For administration of vaccines/toxoids, see 90460, 90461, 90471, 90472, 90473, 90474, 90480)◀

(Report 96372 for non-antineoplastic hormonal therapy injections)

(Report 96401 for anti-neoplastic nonhormonal injection therapy)

(Report 96402 for anti-neoplastic hormonal injection therapy)

(For intradermal cancer immunotherapy injection, see 0708T, 0709T)

(Do not report 96372 for injections given without direct physician or other qualified health care professional supervision. To report, use 99211. Hospitals may report 96372 when the physician or other qualified health care professional is not present)

(96372 does not include injections for allergen immunotherapy. For allergen immunotherapy injections, see 95115-95117)

Rationale

To accommodate the replacement of COVID-19 vaccine administration codes with a single COVID-19 vaccine administration code (90480) and to complete the parenthetical note by including all non-COVID vaccine administration codes, codes 90473, 90474, and 90480 have been added and all previous COVID-19 vaccine administration codes have been deleted.

Refer to the codebook and the Rationales for codes 96380, 96381, 90480, and 91318-91322 for a full discussion of these changes.

96377   Application of on-body injector (includes cannula insertion) for timed subcutaneous injection

#● **96380**   Administration of respiratory syncytial virus, monoclonal antibody, seasonal dose by intramuscular injection, with counseling by physician or other qualified health care professional

▶(Report 96380 for administration of respiratory syncytial virus, monoclonal antibody, seasonal dose [90380, 90381])◀

#● **96381**   Administration of respiratory syncytial virus, monoclonal antibody, seasonal dose by intramuscular injection

▶(Report 96381 for administration of respiratory syncytial virus, monoclonal antibody, seasonal dose [90380, 90381])◀

96379   Unlisted therapeutic, prophylactic, or diagnostic intravenous or intra-arterial injection or infusion

96380   Code is out of numerical sequence. See 96376-96401

96381   Code is out of numerical sequence. See 96376-96401

Rationale

Codes 96380 and 96381 have been established in the Therapeutic, Prophylactic, and Diagnostic Injections and Infusions (Excludes Chemotherapy and Other Highly Complex Drug or Highly Complex Biologic Agent Administration) subsection to report the administration of seasonal doses of RSV monoclonal antibodies with (96380) and without (96381) physician or other QHP counseling. In addition, several additional and existing guidelines and parenthetical notes have been updated to accommodate the addition of the new codes.

Codes 96380 and 96381 have been added to enable a distinct reporting mechanism for administrations of seasonal RSV monoclonal antibodies. These codes represent intramuscular injections that include counseled (96380) and non-counseled (96381) administration. Other monoclonal antibody administration codes are not specific to RSV and do not include physician or other QHP counseling services.

Parenthetical notes throughout the CPT 2025 code set have been revised with the term "immunization" to reflect the use of immune globulins for immunity. In addition, codes for RSV products (90380, 90381) have been added in guidelines wherever appropriate. Administration codes for RSV immune globulins that have been added to existing and new instructions throughout the CPT 2025 code set exemplify this intention. These changes also include the addition and revision of parenthetical notes that restrict the reporting of RSV product codes 90380 and 90381 in conjunction with the nonspecific therapeutic, prophylactic, or diagnostic injection code 96372. Other instructions direct users to report codes 96380 and 96381 for the administration of seasonal doses of RSV.

Chemotherapy and Other Highly Complex Drug or Highly Complex Biologic Agent Administration

Other Injection and Infusion Services

+ **96547** Intraoperative hyperthermic intraperitoneal chemotherapy (HIPEC) procedure, including separate incision(s) and closure, when performed; first 60 minutes (List separately in addition to code for primary procedure)

+ **96548** each additional 30 minutes (List separately in addition to code for primary procedure)

▶(Use 96547, 96548 in conjunction with 38100, 38101, 38102, 38120, 43611, 43620, 43621, 43622, 43631, 43632, 43633, 43634, 44010, 44015, 44110, 44111, 44120, 44121, 44125, 44130, 44139, 44140, 44141, 44143, 44144, 44145, 44146, 44147, 44150, 44151, 44155, 44156, 44157, 44158, 44160, 44202, 44203, 44204, 44207, 44213, 44227, 47001, 47100, 48140, 48145, 48152, 48155, 49000, 49010, 49320, 58200, 58210, 58575, 58940, 58943, 58950, 58951, 58952, 58953, 58954, 58956, 58958, 58960)◀

Rationale

To accommodate the addition of codes 49186-49190, the parenthetical note following code 96548 has been revised by removing deleted codes 49203-49205 and 58957.

Refer to the codebook and the Rationale for codes 49186-49190 for a full discussion of these changes.

Physical Medicine and Rehabilitation

Therapeutic Procedures

★ **97110** Therapeutic procedure, 1 or more areas, each 15 minutes; therapeutic exercises to develop strength and endurance, range of motion and flexibility

★ **97112** neuromuscular reeducation of movement, balance, coordination, kinesthetic sense, posture, and/or proprioception for sitting and/or standing activities

97113 aquatic therapy with therapeutic exercises

★ **97116** gait training (includes stair climbing)

▶(Use 96000, 96001, 96002 to report comprehensive gait and motion analysis procedures)◀

(For motor-cognitive, semi-immersive virtual reality–facilitated gait training, use 97116 in conjunction with 0791T)

Rationale

In accordance with the deletion of code 96003, the cross-reference parenthetical note following code 97116 has been revised to reflect this change.

Refer to the codebook and the Rationale for code 96003 for a full discussion of this change.

Acupuncture

97810 Acupuncture, 1 or more needles; without electrical stimulation, initial 15 minutes of personal one-on-one contact with the patient

(Do not report 97810 in conjunction with 97813)

+▲ **97811** without electrical stimulation, each additional 15 minutes of personal one-on-one contact with the patient, with insertion of needle(s) (List separately in addition to code for primary procedure)

(Use 97811 in conjunction with 97810, 97813)

97813 with electrical stimulation, initial 15 minutes of personal one-on-one contact with the patient

(Do not report 97813 in conjunction with 97810)

+▲ **97814** with electrical stimulation, each additional 15 minutes of personal one-on-one contact with the patient, with insertion of needle(s) (List separately in addition to code for primary procedure)

(Use 97814 in conjunction with 97810, 97813)

(Do not report 97810, 97811, 97813, 97814 in conjunction with 20560, 20561. When both time-based acupuncture services and needle insertion[s] without injection[s] are performed, report only the time-based acupuncture codes)

Rationale

Codes 97811 and 97814 have been revised by removing "re" from the term "re-insertion" to clarify that any insertion intended for the procedure applies.

Clinical Example (97811)

A 47-year-old patient, who has a diagnosis of lower back pain and left anterior thigh pain, presents for a return office visit. The patient is currently symptomatic, presenting with numbness and tingling in the left anterior and lateral thigh. The pain has been worse for the past 2 days. (**Note:** This is an add-on code. Only consider the additional work related to the additional physician or other qualified health care professional time beyond the initial 15 minutes reported with code 97810.)

Description of Procedure (97811)

Following the removal of the needles from the initial acupuncture service provided, the practitioner adjusts the positioning of the patient. Select new points to complete the treatment. After palpating to locate these new points, mark and prepare the treatment sites with 70% isopropyl alcohol. Select, insert, and manipulate 10 needles to obtain the desired effect. Instruct the patient to rest for 15 minutes and retain the needles. Periodically, the practitioner restimulates the needles.

Clinical Example (97814)

A 58-year-old patient was referred for acupuncture to relieve both neck and shoulder pain. The patient also complains of acute vertex headaches that radiate into the frontal sinus region. (**Note:** This is an add-on code. Only consider the additional work related to the additional physician or other qualified health care professional time beyond the initial 15 minutes reported with code 97813.)

Description of Procedure (97814)

Following the removal of the needles from the initial acupuncture service provided, the practitioner adjusts the positioning of the patient. Select new points to complete the treatment. After palpating to locate these new points, mark and prepare the treatment sites with 70% isopropyl alcohol. Select, insert, and manipulate 10 needles to obtain the desired effect. Attach electrodes to the shafts of the needles and select an appropriate frequency (Hz) and waveform. The practitioner then slowly increases the amplitude of the signal until the patient's tolerance is reached. Instruct the patient to rest for 15 minutes. The practitioner continues to stimulate the needles during this phase of the treatment by adjusting the electrical stimulation until the pain and dysfunction are improved to an acceptable level.

98000	Code is out of numerical sequence. See E/M codes 99214-99222
98001	Code is out of numerical sequence. See E/M codes 99214-99222
98002	Code is out of numerical sequence. See E/M codes 99214-99222
98003	Code is out of numerical sequence. See E/M codes 99214-99222
98004	Code is out of numerical sequence. See E/M codes 99214-99222
98005	Code is out of numerical sequence. See E/M codes 99214-99222
98006	Code is out of numerical sequence. See E/M codes 99214-99222
98007	Code is out of numerical sequence. See E/M codes 99214-99222
98008	Code is out of numerical sequence. See E/M codes 99214-99222
98009	Code is out of numerical sequence. See E/M codes 99214-99222
98010	Code is out of numerical sequence. See E/M codes 99214-99222
98011	Code is out of numerical sequence. See E/M codes 99214-99222
98012	Code is out of numerical sequence. See E/M codes 99214-99222
98013	Code is out of numerical sequence. See E/M codes 99214-99222
98014	Code is out of numerical sequence. See E/M codes 99214-99222
98015	Code is out of numerical sequence. See E/M codes 99214-99222
98016	Code is out of numerical sequence. See E/M codes 99214-99222

Education and Training for Patient Self-Management

▶The following codes are used to report educational and training services prescribed by a physician or other qualified health care professional and provided by a nonphysician qualified health care professional using a standardized curriculum to an individual or a group of patients for the treatment of established illness(s)/disease(s) or to delay comorbidity(s). Education and training for patient self-management may be reported with these codes only when using a standardized curriculum as described below. This curriculum may be modified as necessary for the clinical needs, cultural norms, and health literacy of the individual patient(s).◀

The purpose of the educational and training services is to teach the patient (may include caregiver[s]) how to effectively self-manage the patient's illness(s)/disease(s) or delay disease comorbidity(s) in conjunction with the patient's professional healthcare team. Education and

★ = Telemedicine   ◀ = Audio-only   ✚ = Add-on code   𝒩 = FDA approval pending   # = Resequenced code   ⊘ = Modifier 51 exempt

training related to subsequent reinforcement or due to changes in the patient's condition or treatment plan are reported in the same manner as the original education and training. The type of education and training provided for the patient's clinical condition will be identified by the appropriate diagnosis code(s) reported.

▶The qualifications of the nonphysician qualified health care professionals and the content of the educational and training program must be consistent with guidelines or standards established or recognized by a physician society, nonphysician health care professional society/association, or other appropriate source.◀

(For counseling and education provided by a physician to an individual, see the appropriate evaluation and management codes, including office or other outpatient services [99202-99215], initial and subsequent hospital inpatient or observation care [99221-99223, 99231-99233, 99234, 99235, 99236], new or established patient office or other outpatient consultations [99242, 99243, 99244, 99245], inpatient or observation consultations [99252, 99253, 99254, 99255], emergency department services [99281-99285], nursing facility services [99304-99316], home or residence services [99341-99350], and counseling risk factor reduction and behavior change intervention [99401-99429]. See also **Instructions for Use of the CPT Codebook** for definition of reporting qualifications)

(For counseling and education provided by a physician to a group, use 99078)

(For counseling and/or risk factor reduction intervention provided by a physician to patient[s] without symptoms or established disease, see 99401-99412)

(For medical nutrition therapy, see 97802-97804)

(For health behavior assessment and intervention that is not part of a standardized curriculum, see 96156, 96158, 96159, 96164, 96165, 96167, 96168, 96170, 96171)

▶(For education provided as genetic counseling services, use 96041. For education to a group regarding genetic risks, see 98961, 98962)◀

Rationale

In accordance with the deletion of code 96040 and the establishment of code 96041, the instructional parenthetical note in the Education and Training for Patient Self-Management subsection has been revised.

Refer to the codebook and the Rationale for codes 96040 and 96041 for a full discussion of these changes.

★▲ **98960**   Education and training for patient self-management by a nonphysician qualified health care professional using a standardized curriculum, face-to-face with the patient (could include caregiver/family) each 30 minutes; individual patient

★▲ **98961**   2-4 patients

★▲ **98962**   5-8 patients

Rationale

In accordance with efforts to standardize references to nonphysician QHPs throughout the CPT 2025 code set, the Education and Training for Patient Self-Management subsection guidelines and codes 98960-98962 have been revised.

Refer to the codebook and the Rationale for Medical Team Conferences subsection guidelines in the Evaluation and Management section for a full discussion of these changes.

▶Non-Face-to-Face Nonphysician Qualified Health Care Professional Services◀

Telephone Services

▶Telephone services are non-face-to-face assessment and management services provided by a nonphysician qualified health care professional to a patient using the telephone. These codes are used to report episodes of care by the qualified health care professional initiated by an established patient or guardian of an established patient. If the telephone service ends with a decision to see the patient within 24 hours or the next available urgent visit appointment, the code is not reported; rather the encounter is considered part of the preservice work of the subsequent assessment and management service, procedure, and visit. Likewise, if the telephone call refers to a service performed and reported by the qualified health care professional within the previous seven days (either qualified health care professional requested or unsolicited patient follow-up) or within the postoperative period of the previously completed procedure, then the service(s) are considered part of that previous service or procedure. (Do not report 98966-98968 if reporting 98966-98968 performed in the previous seven days.)◀

▶(For telephone services provided by a physician, see 98012, 98013, 98014, 98015, 98016)◀

▲ **98966**   Telephone assessment and management service provided by a nonphysician qualified health care professional to an established patient, parent, or guardian not originating from a related assessment and management service provided within the previous 7 days nor leading to an assessment and management service or procedure within the next 24 hours or soonest available appointment; 5-10 minutes of medical discussion

▲ 98967   11-20 minutes of medical discussion

▲ 98968   21-30 minutes of medical discussion

(Do not report 98966-98968 during the same month with 99426, 99427, 99439, 99487, 99489, 99490, 99491)

(Do not report 98966, 98967, 98968 in conjunction with 93792, 93793)

Rationale

In accordance with the establishment of codes 98012-98016 and the deletion of codes 99441-99443, the cross-reference parenthetical note preceding code 98966 has been revised to reflect these changes. Refer to the codebook and the Rationale for codes 98012-98016 for a full discussion of these changes.

In addition, in accordance with efforts to standardize references to nonphysician QHPs throughout the CPT 2025 code set, the heading for Non-Face-to-Face Nonphysician Qualified Health Care Professional Services subsection, the Telephone Services subsection guidelines, and codes 98966-98968 have been revised.

Refer to the codebook and the Rationale for the Medical Team Conferences subsection guidelines in the Evaluation and Management section for a full discussion of these changes.

▶Nonphysician Qualified Health Care Professional Online Digital Assessment and Management Service◀

▶Nonphysician qualified health care professional online digital assessment and management services are patient-initiated digital services that require patient evaluation and decision making to generate an assessment and subsequent management of the patient. These services are not for the nonevaluative electronic communication of test results, scheduling of appointments, or other communication that does not include assessment and management. While the patient's problem may be new, the patient is an established patient. Patients initiate these services through Health Insurance Portability and Accountability Act (HIPAA)-compliant, secure platforms, such as through the electronic health record (EHR) portal, email, or other digital applications, which allow digital communication.

Nonphysician qualified health care professional online digital assessments are reported once for the nonphysician qualified health care professional's cumulative time devoted to the service during a seven-day period. The seven-day period begins with the personal review of the patient-generated inquiry. The cumulative service time includes review of the initial inquiry, review of patient records or data pertinent to assessment of the patient's problem, personal interaction with clinical staff focused on the patient's problem, development of management plans, including the generation of prescriptions or ordering of tests, and subsequent communication with the patient through online, telephone, email, or other digitally supported communication. All nonphysician qualified health care professionals in the same group practice who are involved in an online digital assessment contribute to the cumulative service time devoted to the patient's online digital assessment. The online digital assessments require visit documentation and permanent storage (electronic or hard copy) of the encounter.

If the patient generates the initial online digital inquiry within seven days of a previous treatment or assessment and management service and both services relate to the same problem, or the online digital inquiry occurs within the postoperative period of a previously completed procedure, then the online digital assessment may not be reported separately. If the patient generates an initial online digital inquiry for a new problem within seven days of a previous service that addressed a different problem, then the online digital assessment is reported separately. If a separately reported evaluation service occurs within seven days of the initial review of the online digital assessment, codes 98970, 98971, 98972 may not be reported. If the patient presents a new, unrelated problem during the seven-day period of an online digital assessment, then the time spent assessing the additional problem is added to the cumulative service time of the online digital assessment for that seven-day period.◀

▶(Do not report an assessment and management service within 7 days of reporting an online digital assessment and management treatment and/or service)◀

(For an online digital E/M service provided by a physician or other qualified health care professional, see 99421, 99422, 99423)

▲ 98970   Nonphysician qualified health care professional online digital assessment and management, for an established patient, for up to 7 days, cumulative time during the 7 days; 5-10 minutes

▲ 98971   11-20 minutes

▲ 98972   21 or more minutes

(Report 98970, 98971, 98972 once per 7-day period)

▶(Do not report online digital assessment and management services for cumulative visit time less than 5 minutes)◀

(Do not count 98970, 98971, 98972 time otherwise reported with other services)

(Do not report 98970, 98971, 98972 for home and outpatient INR monitoring when reporting 93792, 93793)

(Do not report 98970, 98971, 98972 when using 99091, 99374, 99375, 99377, 99378, 99379, 99380, 99426, 99427, 99437, 99439, 99487, 99489, 99490, 99491, for the same communication[s])

Rationale

In accordance with efforts to standardize references to nonphysician QHPs throughout the CPT 2025 code set, the heading for the Nonphysician Qualified Health Care Professional Online Digital Assessment and Management Service subsection guidelines and codes 98970-98972 have been revised. In addition, an exclusionary parenthetical note has been added to address reporting assessment and management services within 7 days. Furthermore, an exclusionary parenthetical note has been updated by replacing "E/M" with the phrase "assessment and management."

Refer to the codebook and the Rationale for the Medical Team Conferences guidelines in the Evaluation and Management section for a full discussion of these changes.

Remote Therapeutic Monitoring Services

Remote therapeutic monitoring services (eg, musculoskeletal system status, respiratory system status, cognitive behavioral therapy, therapy adherence, therapy response) represent the review and monitoring of data related to signs, symptoms, and functions of a therapeutic response. These data may represent objective device-generated integrated data or subjective inputs reported by a patient. These data are reflective of therapeutic responses that provide a functionally integrative representation of patient status.

▶Codes 98976, 98977, 98978 are used to report remote therapeutic monitoring services during a 30-day period. To report 98975, 98976, 98977, 98978, the service(s) must be ordered by a physician or other qualified health care professional. Code 98975 may be used to report the set-up and patient education on the use of any device(s) utilized for therapeutic data collection generated through digital monitoring or digital therapy. Codes 98976, 98977, 98978 may be used to report supply of the device for data access or data transmissions to support monitoring. To report 98975, 98976, 98977, 98978, the device used must be a medical device as defined by the FDA. In addition to its monitoring functionality, the device may also provide a therapeutic intervention. Codes 98975, 98976, 98977, 98978 are not reported if cumulative monitoring is less than 16 days. Do not report 98975, 98976, 98977, 98978 with other physiologic monitoring services (eg, 95250 for

continuous glucose monitoring requiring a minimum of 72 hours of monitoring or 99453, 99454 for remote monitoring of physiologic parameter[s]).◀

Code 98975 is reported for each episode of care. For reporting remote therapeutic monitoring parameters, an episode of care is defined as beginning when the remote therapeutic monitoring service is initiated and ends with attainment of targeted treatment goals.

▲ **98975** Remote therapeutic monitoring (eg, therapy adherence, therapy response, digital therapeutic intervention); initial set-up and patient education on use of equipment

(Do not report 98975 more than once per episode of care)

▶(Do not report 98975 for less than 16 days of cumulative monitoring during the 30-day period)◀

▲ **98976** device(s) supply for data access or data transmissions to support monitoring of respiratory system, each 30 days

▲ **98977** device(s) supply for data access or data transmissions to support monitoring of musculoskeletal system, each 30 days

▲ **98978** device(s) supply for data access or data transmissions to support monitoring of cognitive behavioral therapy, each 30 days

(Do not report 98975, 98976, 98977, 98978 in conjunction with codes for more specific physiologic parameters [93296, 94760, 99453, 99454])

▶(Do not report 98976, 98977, 98978 for cumulative monitoring of less than 16 days)◀

(For therapeutic monitoring treatment management services, use 98980)

(For remote physiologic monitoring, see 99453, 99454)

(For physiologic monitoring treatment management services, use 99457)

(For self-measured blood pressure monitoring, see 99473, 99474)

Rationale

Codes 98975-98977 have been editorially revised and the Remote Therapeutic Monitoring Services subsection guidelines have been revised. These revisions do not modify the minimum cumulative 16-day monitoring requirement, as noted by the addition of the term "cumulative" to the guidelines' language.

The remote therapeutic monitoring services guidelines have been revised to specify that code 98975 may be reported for the setup and patient education on the use of any device(s) utilized for therapeutic data collection generated through digital monitoring or digital therapy. Clarification has also been given noting that codes

98976-98978 may be reported for supplying the device for data access or data transmissions to support monitoring. Lastly, the guidelines have been revised to indicate that, in addition to its monitoring functionality, the device may also provide therapeutic intervention.

Codes 98975-98978 have been revised to include digital therapeutic intervention as an example of remote therapeutic monitoring. An exclusionary parenthetical note has been added to specify that code 98975 may not be reported for services with less than 16 days of cumulative monitoring during the 30-day period.

Codes 98976-98978 have been revised to include devices supplied for data access or data transmissions to support monitoring. Specifically, "with scheduled (eg, daily) recording(s) and/or programmed alert(s) transmission to monitor" has been removed from their code descriptors. An exclusionary parenthetical note has been added to specify that device supply codes 98976-98978 may not be reported for services less than 16 days.

Remote Therapeutic Monitoring Treatment Management Services

▶Remote therapeutic monitoring treatment management services are provided when a physician or other qualified health care professional uses the results of remote therapeutic monitoring to manage a patient under a specific treatment plan. To report remote therapeutic monitoring, the service must be ordered by a physician or other qualified health care professional. To report 98980, 98981, any device used must be a medical device as defined by the FDA. Do not use 98980, 98981 for time that can be reported using codes for more specific monitoring services. Codes 98980, 98981 may be reported during the same service period as chronic care management services (99439, 99487, 99489, 99490, 99491), transitional care management services (99495, 99496), principal care management services (99424, 99425, 99426, 99427), behavioral health integration services (99484), psychotherapy services (90832-90853), health behavior assessment and intervention services (96156, 96158, 96159, 96160, 96161, 96164, 96165, 96167, 96168, 96170, 96171), and psychiatric collaborative care services (99492, 99493, 99494). However, time spent performing these services should remain separate and no time should be counted toward the required time for both services in a single month. Codes 98980, 98981 require at least one interactive communication with the patient or caregiver. The interactive communication contributes to the total time, but it does not need to represent the entire cumulative reported time of the treatment management service. For the first completed 20 minutes of physician or other qualified health care professional time in a calendar

month, report 98980, and report 98981 for each additional completed 20 minutes. Do not report 98980, 98981 for services of less than 20 minutes. Report 98980 once, regardless of the number of therapeutic monitoring modalities performed in a given calendar month.◀

Do not count any time on a day when the physician or other qualified health care professional reports an E/M service (office or other outpatient services [99202, 99203, 99204, 99205, 99211, 99212, 99213, 99214, 99215], home or residence services [99341, 99342, 99344, 99345, 99347, 99348, 99349, 99350], inpatient or observation care services [99221, 99222, 99223, 99231, 99232, 99233, 99234, 99235, 99236], inpatient consultations [99252, 99253, 99254, 99255]).

▶Do not count any time directly related to other reported services (eg, psychotherapy services [90832, 90833, 90834, 90836, 90837, 90838], interrogation device evaluation services [93290], anticoagulant management services [93793], respiratory monitoring services [94774, 94775, 94776, 94777], health behavior assessment and intervention services [96156, 96158, 96159, 96160, 96161, 96164, 96165, 96167, 96168, 96170, 96171], therapeutic interventions that focus on cognitive function services [97129, 97130], adaptive behavior treatment services [97153, 97154, 97155, 97156, 97157, 97158], therapeutic procedures [97110, 97112, 97116, 97530, 97535], tests and measurements [97750, 97755], physical therapy evaluation services [97161, 97162, 97163, 97164], occupational therapy evaluations [97165, 97166, 97167, 97168], orthotic management and training and prosthetic training services [97760, 97761, 97763], medical nutrition therapy services [97802, 97803, 97804], medication therapy management services [99605, 99606, 99607], critical care services [99291, 99292], principal care management services [99424, 99425, 99426, 99427]) in the cumulative time of the remote therapeutic monitoring treatment management service during the calendar month of reporting. ◀

Rationale

The remote therapeutic monitoring treatment management services guidelines have been revised to include psychotherapy services and health behavior assessment and intervention services as services that may be reported during the same service period as codes 98980 and 98981. In addition, the revised guidelines clarify that any time directly related to other reported services may not be counted. Examples have been identified in the guidelines.

★=Telemedicine ◀=Audio-only ✚=Add-on code ✗=FDA approval pending #=Resequenced code ⊘=Modifier 51 exempt

Home Health Procedures/Services

▶These codes are used by nonphysician qualified health care professionals. Physicians should utilize the home or residence services codes 99341-99350 and utilize CPT codes other than 99500-99600 for any additional procedure/service provided to a patient living in a home or residence.◀

The following codes are used to report services provided in a patient's home or residence (including assisted living facility, group home, custodial care facility, nontraditional private homes, or schools).

Health care professionals who are authorized to use Evaluation and Management (E/M) Home Visit codes (99341-99350) may report 99500-99600 in addition to 99341-99350 if both services are performed. E/M services may be reported separately, using modifier 25, if the patient's condition requires a significant separately identifiable E/M service, above and beyond the home health service(s)/procedure(s) codes 99500-99600.

99500   Home visit for prenatal monitoring and assessment to include fetal heart rate, non-stress test, uterine monitoring, and gestational diabetes monitoring

Rationale

In accordance with efforts to standardize references to nonphysician QHPs throughout the CPT 2025 code set, the Home Health Procedures/Services guidelines have been revised.

Refer to the codebook and the Rationale for the Medical Team Conferences subsection guidelines in the Evaluation and Management section for a full discussion of these changes.

Notes

Category III Codes

Summary of Additions, Deletions, and Revisions

The summary of changes shows the actual changes that have been made to the code descriptors.

New codes appear with a bullet (●) and are indicated as "Code added." Revised codes are preceded with a triangle (▲). Within revised codes, or if a code symbol has been deleted, the deleted language and code symbol appear with a ~~strikethrough~~, while new text appears <u>underlined</u>.

The ⚡ symbol is used to identify codes for vaccines that are pending FDA approval. The # symbol is used to identify codes that have been resequenced. CPT add-on codes are annotated by the ✚ symbol. The ⊘ symbol is used to identify codes that are exempt from the use of modifier 51. The ★ symbol is used to identify codes that may be used for reporting telemedicine services. The ⋇ symbol is used to identify a proprietary laboratory analyses (PLA) test that has an identical descriptor as another PLA test. A PLA code that satisfies Category I code criteria and has been accepted by the CPT Editorial Panel is annotated with the ⇅ symbol. The ◀ symbol is used to identify codes that may be used to report audio-only telemedicine services when appended by modifier 93 (**see Appendix T**).

Code	Description
#●0901T	Code added
0398T	~~Magnetic resonance image guided high intensity focused ultrasound (MRgFUS), stereotactic ablation lesion, intracranial for movement disorder including stereotactic navigation and frame placement when performed~~
#▲0714T	Transperineal laser ablation of benign prostatic hyperplasia, including imaging guidance; <u>prostate volume less than 50 mL</u>
#●0867T	Code added
0500T	~~Infectious agent detection by nucleic acid (DNA or RNA), Human Papillomavirus (HPV) for five or more separately reported high-risk HPV types (eg, 16, 18, 31, 33, 35, 39, 45, 51, 52, 56, 58, 59, 68) (ie, genotyping)~~
0537T	~~Chimeric antigen receptor T-cell (CAR-T) therapy; harvesting of blood-derived T lymphocytes for development of genetically modified autologous CAR-T cells, per day~~
0538T	~~preparation of blood-derived T lymphocytes for transportation (eg, cryopreservation, storage)~~
0539T	~~receipt and preparation of CAR-T cells for administration~~
0540T	~~CAR-T cell administration, autologous~~
0553T	~~Percutaneous transcatheter placement of iliac arteriovenous anastomosis implant, inclusive of all radiological supervision and interpretation, intraprocedural roadmapping, and imaging guidance necessary to complete the intervention~~
0564T	~~Oncology, chemotherapeutic drug cytotoxicity assay of cancer stem cells (CSCs), from cultured CSCs and primary tumor cells, categorical drug response reported based on percent of cytotoxicity observed, a minimum of 14 drugs or drug combinations~~
0567T	~~Permanent fallopian tube occlusion with degradable biopolymer implant, transcervical approach, including transvaginal ultrasound~~
0568T	~~Introduction of mixture of saline and air for sonosalpingography to confirm occlusion of fallopian tubes, transcervical approach, including transvaginal ultrasound and pelvic ultrasound~~

Code	Description
▲0615T	Automated~~Eye-movement~~ analysis <u>of binocular eye movements</u> without spatial calibration, <u>including disconjugacy, saccades, and pupillary dynamics for the assessment of concussion,</u> with interpretation and report
~~0616T~~	~~Insertion of iris prosthesis, including suture fixation and repair or removal of iris, when performed; without removal of crystalline lens or intraocular lens, without insertion of intraocular lens~~
~~0617T~~	~~with removal of crystalline lens and insertion of intraocular lens~~
~~0618T~~	~~with secondary intraocular lens placement or intraocular lens exchange~~
●0868T	Code added
●0869T	Code added
●0870T	Code added
●0871T	Code added
●0872T	Code added
●0873T	Code added
●0874T	Code added
●0875T	Code added
●0876T	Code added
●0877T	Code added
●0878T	Code added
●0879T	Code added
●0880T	Code added
●0881T	Code added
＋●0882T	Code added
＋●0883T	Code added
●0884T	Code added
●0885T	Code added
●0886T	Code added
＋●0887T	Code added
●0888T	Code added
●0889T	Code added
●0890T	Code added
●0891T	Code added
●0892T	Code added
●0893T	Code added
●0894T	Code added
●0895T	Code added

★ = Telemedicine ◀ = Add-on code ＋ = Add-on code ✔ = FDA approval pending # = Resequenced code ⊘ = Modifier 51 exempt

Category III 0042T-0713T

Code	Description
+•0896T	Code added
•0897T	Code added
•0898T	Code added
+•0899T	Code added
+•0900T	Code added
•0902T	Code added
•0903T	Code added
•0904T	Code added
•0905T	Code added
•0906T	Code added
+•0907T	Code added
•0908T	Code added
•0909T	Code added
•0910T	Code added
•0911T	Code added
•0912T	Code added
•0913T	Code added
+•0914T	Code added
•0915T	Code added
•0916T	Code added
•0917T	Code added
•0918T	Code added
•0919T	Code added
•0920T	Code added
•0921T	Code added
•0922T	Code added
•0923T	Code added
•0924T	Code added
•0925T	Code added
•0926T	Code added
•0927T	Code added
•0928T	Code added
•0929T	Code added

▲ = Revised code   ● = New code   ▶ ◀ = Contains new or revised text   ✕ = Duplicate PLA test   ↑↓ = Category I PLA   American Medical Association   **155**

Category III 0042T–0713T

Code	Description
●0930T	Code added
●0931T	Code added
●0932T	Code added
●0933T	Code added
●0934T	Code added
●0935T	Code added
●0936T	Code added
●0937T	Code added
●0938T	Code added
●0939T	Code added
●0940T	Code added
●0941T	Code added
●0942T	Code added
●0943T	Code added
●0944T	Code added
✚●0945T	Code added
●0946T	Code added
●0947T	Code added

★ = Telemedicine   ◀ = Add-on code   ✚ = Add-on code   ✔ = FDA approval pending   # = Resequenced code   ⊘ = Modifier 51 exempt

Category III Codes

0232T Injection(s), platelet rich plasma, any site, including image guidance, harvesting and preparation when performed

(Do not report 0232T in conjunction with 15769, 15771, 15772, 15773, 15774, 20550, 20551, 20600, 20604, 20605, 20606, 20610, 20611, 36415, 36592, 76942, 77002, 77012, 77021, 86965, 0481T)

(Do not report 38220-38230 for bone marrow aspiration for platelet rich stem cell injection. For bone marrow aspiration for platelet rich stem cell injection, use 0232T)

#● 0901T Placement of bone marrow sampling port, including imaging guidance when performed

►(Do not report 0901T in conjunction with 77002, 77012)◄

Rationale

Category III code 0901T has been established to report the placement of a port for bone marrow sampling with imaging guidance. An exclusionary parenthetical note has been added following code 0901T, restricting its use with codes 77002 and 77012.

Patients with leukemia, multiple myeloma, and other bone marrow disorders need frequent bone marrow sampling to monitor the effectiveness of treatment. This procedure involves inserting a bone marrow sampling port to reduce the need for additional access.

Note that existing codes 38220-38222 describe obtaining samples for bone marrow aspiration and/or biopsy but do not include the placement of a permanent device for repeated future sampling.

Clinical Example (0901T)

A 66-year-old female, who is newly diagnosed with leukemia, presents for insertion of a bone marrow sampling port.

Description of Procedure (0901T)

Place the patient in the supine position. Administer intravenous sedation (separately reported). Perform imaging (eg, computed tomography, fluoroscopy) to identify the appropriate portal site. Prepare and drape the site. Infiltrate the surgical site with local anesthetic and make an incision approximately 2-cm in length. Dissect the subcutaneous tissues. Load the port on the screwdriver and drive it into the bone under image guidance. Close the wound in layers and apply a dressing.

0278T Transcutaneous electrical modulation pain reprocessing (eg, scrambler therapy), each treatment session (includes placement of electrodes)

(For peripheral nerve transcutaneous magnetic stimulation, see 0766T, 0767T)

(For implantation of trial or permanent electrode arrays or pulse generators for peripheral subcutaneous field stimulation, use 64999)

(For delivery of thermal energy to the muscle of the anal canal, use 46999)

(For corneal incisions in the recipient cornea created using a laser in preparation for penetrating or lamellar keratoplasty, use 66999)

►(For greater than 48 hours of monitoring of external electrocardiographic recording, see 93241, 93242, 93243, 93244, 93245, 93246, 93247, 93248, 0937T, 0938T, 0939T, 0940T)◄

(For focused microwave thermotherapy of the breast, use 19499)

Rationale

To accommodate the addition of codes 0937T-0940T for reporting external electrocardiogram (ECG) recording services that last more than 15 days and up to 30 days continuously, the parenthetical note following code 0278T has been revised to direct users to the new codes.

Refer to the codebook and the Rationale for codes 0937T-0940T for a full discussion of these changes.

►(0398T has been deleted)◄

►(For magnetic resonance image guided high intensity focused ultrasound [MRgFUS], stereotactic ablation lesion, intracranial, use 61715)◄

Rationale

In accordance with the conversion of Category III code 0398T to Category I code 61715, a deletion parenthetical note and cross-reference parenthetical note for magnetic resonance image-guided high-intensity focused ultrasound [MRgFUS] have been added to the Category III section.

Refer to the codebook and the Rationale for code 61715 for a full discussion of these changes.

0419T Destruction of neurofibroma, extensive (cutaneous, dermal extending into subcutaneous); face, head and neck, greater than 50 neurofibromas

(For excision of neurofibroma, use 64792)

(Report 0419T once per session regardless of the number of lesions treated)

0420T trunk and extremities, extensive, greater than 100 neurofibromas

(For excision of neurofibroma, use 64792)

(Report 0420T once per session regardless of the number of lesions treated)

#▲ **0714T** Transperineal laser ablation of benign prostatic hyperplasia, including imaging guidance; prostate volume less than 50 mL

#● **0867T** prostate volume greater or equal to 50 mL

▶(Do not report 0714T, 0867T in conjunction with 76940, 76942, 77002, 77012, 77021)◀

Rationale

Code 0714T has been revised, and code 0867T has been added to enable separate reporting for transperineal laser ablation of benign prostatic hyperplasia performed for a prostate volume of less than 50 mL (0714T) and greater than or equal to 50 mL (0867T). In addition, a parenthetical note provides additional instruction regarding intended reporting.

Code 0714T describes an image-guided transperineal laser ablation of the prostate, which is a minimally invasive treatment for benign prostatic hypertrophy. Other than changing the language that specifies the volume for which the procedure is used, all other aspects of the code remain the same.

Add-on code 0867T has been established to accommodate more specific reporting for these procedures (ie, a prostate volume greater than or equal to 50 mL). In addition, a new exclusionary parenthetical note has been added following code 0867T to restrict reporting it in conjunction with codes 76940, 76942, 77002, 77012, and 77021, because imaging is included as part of the service.

Clinical Example (0714T)

A 68-year-old male presents with a two-year history of progressive voiding symptoms caused by benign prostatic hypertrophy. A digital rectal examination and an imaging study reveal a benign, enlarged prostate with a volume of 35 mL involving both prostatic lobes. The patient elects to undergo ultrasound-guided transperineal laser ablation of the prostate.

Description of Procedure (0714T)

Position the patient in the lithotomy position, and administer local anesthesia or conscious sedation (separately reported), if required, and antibiotics. Insert the Foley catheter. Monitor vital signs. Using ultrasound imaging, place one introducer needle in each prostatic lobe in the deeper portion of the target lesion, guided by real-time ultrasound imaging. Insert an optical fiber into each introducer needle. Deliver laser energy simultaneously to the target lesion via the two inserted optical fibers. Continuously evaluate the progress of the ablation of the target lesion using ultrasound imaging. Remove the optical fibers and withdraw the introducer needles. Verify that the target lesion is completely ablated. Remove the Foley catheter 12 to 48 hours after the procedure. Perform a postoperative clinic visit within 10 days of the procedure.

Clinical Example (0867T)

A 68-year-old male presents with a two-year history of progressive voiding symptoms caused by benign prostatic hypertrophy. A digital rectal examination and an imaging study reveal a benign, enlarged prostate with a volume of 60 mL involving both prostatic lobes. The patient elects to undergo ultrasound-guided transperineal laser ablation of the prostate.

Description of Procedure (0867T)

Position the patient in the lithotomy position, and administer local anesthesia or conscious sedation (separately reported), if required, and antibiotics. Insert the Foley catheter. Monitor vital signs. Using ultrasound imaging, place two introducer needles in each prostatic lobe, in the deeper portion of the target lesion, guided by real-time ultrasound imaging. Insert an optical fiber into each introducer needle. Deliver laser energy simultaneously to the target lesion via the four inserted optical fibers. Continuously evaluate the progress of the ablation of the target lesion using ultrasound imaging. Remove the optical fibers and withdraw the introducer needles. Verify that the target lesion is completely ablated. Remove the Foley catheter 12 to 48 hours after the procedure. Perform a postoperative clinic visit within 10 days of the procedure.

▶(0500T has been deleted)◀

▶(For singular pooled result of high-risk human papillomavirus [HPV] types [eg, 16, 18, 31, 33, 35, 39, 45, 51, 52, 58, 59, 68], use 87624)◀

▶(For separately reported high-risk human papillomavirus [HPV] types 16 and 18 only, including type 45, if performed, use 87625)◀

★=Telemedicine ◀=Add-on code ✛=Add-on code ⚡=FDA approval pending #=Resequenced code ⊘=Modifier 51 exempt

▶For high-risk human papillomavirus [HPV] types [eg, 16, 18, 31, 45, 51, 52] individually and high-risk pooled result[s] in a single test, use 87626)◀

Rationale

Code 0500T has been deleted from the Category III section and cross-reference parenthetical notes have been added to direct users to codes 87624-87626.

Refer to the codebook and the Rationale for codes 87624 and 87626 for a full discussion of these changes.

Cellular and Gene Therapy

▶(0537T, 0538T, 0539T, 0540T have been deleted)◀

▶(For chimeric antigen receptor T-cell [CAR-T] therapy, see 38225, 38226, 38227, 38228)◀

Rationale

Codes 0537T-0540T and all associated guidelines and parenthetical notes for reporting chimeric antigen receptor T-cell therapy (CAR-T) services have been deleted from the Category III section because they have been converted to Category I codes 38225-38228. Parenthetical notes indicating the deletion and directing users to the new Category I CAR-T therapy codes have been added.

Refer to the codebook and the Rationale for codes 38225-38228 for a full discussion of these changes.

▶(0553T has been deleted)◀

▶(For percutaneous transcatheter placement of iliac arteriovenous anastomosis implant, use 37799)◀

Rationale

In accordance with Current Procedural Terminology (CPT) guidelines for archiving Category III codes, code 0553T has been deleted, and instructions added to report code 37799, *Unlisted procedure, vascular surgery*, for the percutaneous transcatheter placement of an iliac arteriovenous anastomosis implant in a cross-reference parenthetical note.

▶(0564T has been deleted)◀

▶(For chemotherapeutic drug cytotoxicity assay of cancer stem cells, use 89240)◀

Rationale

In accordance with CPT guidelines for archiving Category III codes, code 0564T has been deleted, and instructions added to report code 89240, *Unlisted miscellaneous pathology test*, for the chemotherapeutic drug cytotoxicity assay of cancer stem cells in a cross-reference parenthetical note.

▶(0567T has been deleted)◀

▶(For permanent fallopian tube occlusion with degradable biopolymer implant, transcervical approach, including transvaginal ultrasound, use 58999)◀

Rationale

In accordance with CPT guidelines for archiving Category III codes, code 0567T has been deleted, and instructions added to report code 58999, *Unlisted procedure, female genital system (nonobstetrical)*, for a permanent fallopian tube occlusion with degradable biopolymer implant using a transcervical approach, including transvaginal ultrasound, in a cross-reference parenthetical note.

▶(0568T has been deleted)◀

▶(For introduction of mixture of saline and air for sonosalpingography to confirm occlusion of fallopian tubes, transcervical approach, use 58999)◀

Rationale

In accordance with CPT guidelines for archiving Category III codes, code 0568T has been deleted, and instructions added to report code 58999, *Unlisted procedure, female genital system (nonobstetrical)*, for the introduction of a mixture of saline and air for a sonosalpingography to confirm an occlusion of fallopian tubes using a transcervical approach in a cross-reference parenthetical note.

▲ 0615T   Automated analysis of binocular eye movements without spatial calibration, including disconjugacy, saccades, and pupillary dynamics for the assessment of concussion, with interpretation and report

▶(For recording of saccades with electrooculography, see 92499, 92700)◀

Rationale

Category III code 0615T has been revised, and a cross-reference parenthetical note has been added following code 0615T to direct users to codes 92499 and 92700 for recording saccades with electrooculography. The sunset date for code 0615T has been extended from January 1, 2026, to January 1, 2029.

Prior to its revision, code 0615T described eye-movement analysis without spatial calibration with interpretation and report. The procedure described by code 0615T involves different work than vestibular function codes (92540-92542, 92544-92547); therefore, the descriptor for code 0615T has been modified to clarify that it is for automated analysis of binocular eye movements, including disconjugacy, saccades, and pupillary dynamics for the assessment of a concussion. In addition, the procedure is performed without spatial calibration but does include interpretation and report. Furthermore, code 0615T may be used with codes 92540-92542 or 92544-92547, which is why the exclusionary parenthetical note has been deleted. A cross-reference parenthetical note that directs users to codes 92499 and 92700 for recording saccades with electrooculography has been added as well.

Clinical Example (0615T)

A 16-year-old female, who has suffered a closed head injury, undergoes automated binocular eye movement analysis without spatial calibration to assess for concussion.

Description of Procedure (0615T)

Position the patient's head on the chin rest attached to the eye-movement examination device. Program and activate the device. The device performs an automated analysis of bilateral eye movement without special calibration through pupil tracking, and a report with graphs and data is generated. The physician or other qualified health care professional interprets the results and generates a report.

▶(0616T, 0617T, 0618T have been deleted)◀

▶(For implantation of iris prosthesis, including suture fixation and repair or removal of iris, when performed, use 66683)◀

Rationale

Category III codes 0616T-0618T and their associated parenthetical notes have been deleted, and new Category I code 66683 has been added to report implantation of an iris prosthesis. Cross-reference parenthetical notes have

been added to instruct users regarding the appropriate reporting for this procedure.

Refer to the guidelines and the Rationale for code 66683 for a full discussion of these changes.

0648T Quantitative magnetic resonance for analysis of tissue composition (eg, fat, iron, water content), including multiparametric data acquisition, data preparation and transmission, interpretation and report, obtained without diagnostic MRI examination of the same anatomy (eg, organ, gland, tissue, target structure) during the same session; single organ

(Do not report 0648T in conjunction with 0649T, 0697T, 0698T, when also evaluating same organ, gland, tissue, or target structure)

 # 0697T multiple organs

▶(Do not report 0648T, 0697T in conjunction with 70540, 70542, 70543, 70551, 70552, 70553, 71550, 71551, 71552, 72141, 72142, 72146, 72147, 72148, 72149, 72156, 72157, 72158, 72195, 72196, 72197, 73218, 73219, 73220, 73221, 73222, 73223, 73718, 73719, 73720, 73721, 73722, 73723, 74181, 74182, 74183, 75557, 75559, 75561, 75563, 76390, 76498, 77046, 77047, 77048, 77049, when also evaluating same organ, gland, tissue, or target structure)◀

(Do not report 0697T in conjunction with 0648T, 0649T, 0698T, when also evaluating same organ, gland, tissue, or target structure)

+ 0649T Quantitative magnetic resonance for analysis of tissue composition (eg, fat, iron, water content), including multiparametric data acquisition, data preparation and transmission, interpretation and report, obtained with diagnostic MRI examination of the same anatomy (eg, organ, gland, tissue, target structure); single organ (List separately in addition to code for primary procedure)

(Do not report 0649T in conjunction with 0648T, 0697T, 0698T, when also evaluating same organ, gland, tissue, or target structure)

#+ 0698T multiple organs (List separately in addition to code for primary procedure)

▶(Use 0649T, 0698T in conjunction with 70540, 70542, 70543, 70551, 70552, 70553, 71550, 71551, 71552, 72141, 72142, 72146, 72147, 72148, 72149, 72156, 72157, 72158, 72195, 72196, 72197, 73218, 73219, 73220, 73221, 73222, 73223, 73718, 73719, 73720, 73721, 73722, 73723, 74181, 74182, 74183, 75557, 75559, 75561, 75563, 76390, 76498, 77046, 77047, 77048, 77049, when also evaluating same organ, gland, tissue, or target structure)◀

(Do not report 0698T in conjunction with 0648T, 0649T, 0697T, when also evaluating same organ, gland, tissue, or target structure)

★ = Telemedicine　◀ = Add-on code　✦ = Add-on code　✗ = FDA approval pending　# = Resequenced code　⊘ = Modifier 51 exempt

Rationale

In accordance with the deletion of Category III code 0398T and the establishment of code 61715, the existing cross-reference parenthetical notes following codes 0697T and 0698T have been revised.

Refer to the codebook and the Rationale for code 61715 for a full discussion of these changes.

0779T Gastrointestinal myoelectrical activity study, stomach through colon, with interpretation and report

▶(Do not report 0779T in conjunction with 91020, 91022, 91112, 91117, 91122, 91132, 91133, 0868T)◀

0867T Code is out of numerical sequence. See 0419T-0422T

● **0868T** High-resolution gastric electrophysiology mapping with simultaneous patient-symptom profiling, with interpretation and report

▶(Do not report 0868T in conjunction with 91132, 91133, 0779T)◀

Rationale

Category III code 0868T has been established to report high-resolution gastric electrophysiology mapping with simultaneous patient-symptom profiling, including an interpretation and report. This procedure is useful for identifying conditions such as chronic nausea and vomiting syndrome, gastroparesis, and functional dyspepsia.

In addition, the exclusionary parenthetical note following code 0779T has been revised to include code 0868T and to restrict reporting of these mutually exclusive services.

Clinical Example (0868T)

A 56-year-old female presents with a six-month history of idiopathic nausea, vomiting, and abdominal pain that occur most days per week and is associated with weight loss. Diagnostic evaluations, including endoscopy, laboratory tests, and gastric-emptying testing are normal. High-resolution gastric electrophysiology mapping with simultaneous patient symptom profiling is recommended for further evaluation.

Description of Procedure (0868T)

A nurse prepares the test system, which involves unboxing the disposables and arranging them on a bedside table, preparing the bed and chair, confirming the reader and computer hardware are charged, reviewing the procedure documentation, logging into the proprietary computer system, and entering patient,

clinical, meal, and test procedure details. After the patient has fasted for 6 hours or more, bring the patient to the procedure room and position on the bed. The nurse explains the test procedure to the fasted patient; measures the anatomical features of the patient (height, weight, xiphoid process to umbilicus, xiphoid process to anterior superior iliac spine, and waist circumference at umbilicus level); and enters those values into the proprietary computer system. Prepare the patient's skin, place an array of 64 high-sensitivity electrodes on the abdomen, and attach the reader to the array. Obtain a 30-minute fasted baseline recording. The patient eats a standardized meal in ≤10 minutes, and continue obtaining data for a 4-hour post-prandial period. Prompt the patient to log her symptoms every 15 minutes for the duration of the test, while collecting high-resolution gastric electrophysiology data. At the end of the procedure, remove the electrode array from the patient. Upload the data for review by the physician, who interprets the results and generates a report.

● **0869T** Injection(s), bone-substitute material for bone and/or soft tissue hardware fixation augmentation, including intraoperative imaging guidance, when performed

▶(Do not report 0869T in conjunction with 0707T)◀

Rationale

Category III code 0869T has been established for reporting the injection of bone-substitute material for bone and/or soft tissue hardware fixation augmentation. An exclusionary parenthetical note has been added restricting the use of code 0869T with code 0707T.

Prior to 2025, Category III code 0707T was the only CPT code that described the injection of bone-substitute material. For code 0707T, the bone-substitute material is injected into a subchondral defect and is typically performed to reduce chronic bone pain and other changes due to osteoarthritis. The injection is performed with imaging guidance and arthroscopic assistance for joint visualization. The procedure described in code 0869T differs in that the bone-substitute material is injected to reinforce the bone prior to affixing hardware in the affected area.

Clinical Example (0869T)

A 70-year-old male, who is undergoing rotator cuff repair, is noted to have deficient proximal humeral bone at the optimal site(s) for rotator cuff suture anchor placement and undergoes intraoperative injection of bone substitute into the bone deficient area(s) immediately before the suture anchor placement.

▲ = Revised code   ● = New code   ▶◀ = Contains new or revised text   ✛ = Duplicate PLA test   ↕ = Category I PLA   American Medical Association   **161**

Category III   0042T-0713T

Description of Procedure (0869T)

During a rotator cuff repair, it is determined that the quality of the proximal humeral bone is deficient at the point(s) of optimal suture anchor placement. Carry out reinforcement of the bone with a bone substitute by first identifying the optimal position of the bone-substitute delivery system entry portal using a spinal needle. Introduce an outer drill cannula following the spinal needle trajectory to penetrate the humeral head to the desired depth. Remove the obturator, and put the appropriate inner cannula in place to deliver the bone substitute. Mix the components of the bone substitute and inject into the area of the proposed suture anchor placement, taking care to avoid intra-articular extravasation. Remove the injection system.

● **0870T**   Implantation of subcutaneous peritoneal ascites pump system, percutaneous, including pump-pocket creation, insertion of tunneled indwelling bladder and peritoneal catheters with pump connections, including all imaging and initial programming, when performed

▶(Do not report 0870T in conjunction with 49082, 49083, 49405, 49406, 49418, 51100, 51101, 51102, 76942, 76989, 77002, 0871T, 0872T, 0873T, 0874T, 0875T)◀

● **0871T**   Replacement of a subcutaneous peritoneal ascites pump, including reconnection between pump and indwelling bladder and peritoneal catheters, including initial programming and imaging, when performed

▶(Do not report 0871T in conjunction with 49082, 49083, 75984, 76998, 77002, 0870T, 0873T, 0874T, 0875T)◀

● **0872T**   Replacement of indwelling bladder and peritoneal catheters, including tunneling of catheter(s) and connection with previously implanted peritoneal ascites pump, including imaging and programming, when performed

▶(Do not report 0872T in conjunction with 49082, 49083, 49405, 49406, 49418, 51100, 51101, 51102, 75984, 76942, 76989, 76998, 77002, 0870T, 0873T, 0874T, 0875T)◀

▶(For single-catheter replacement, report 0872T with modifier 52)◀

● **0873T**   Revision of a subcutaneously implanted peritoneal ascites pump system, any component (ascites pump, associated peritoneal catheter, associated bladder catheter), including imaging and programming, when performed

▶(Do not report 0873T in conjunction with 0870T, 0871T, 0872T, 0874T, 0875T)◀

● **0874T**   Removal of a peritoneal ascites pump system, including implanted peritoneal ascites pump and indwelling bladder and peritoneal catheters

▶(Do not report 0874T in conjunction with 0870T, 0871T, 0872T, 0873T, 0875T)◀

● **0875T**   Programming of subcutaneously implanted peritoneal ascites pump system by physician or other qualified health care professional

▶(Do not report 0875T in conjunction with 0870T, 0871T, 0872T, 0873T)◀

Rationale

Category III codes 0870T-0875T have been established to report the implantation, replacement, revision, programming, and removal of a peritoneal ascites pump system. In addition, parenthetical notes have been added to provide directions regarding the intended reporting for these codes.

These services may be performed for patients with refractory or recurrent ascites due to liver cirrhosis.

Code 0870T involves the implantation of an ascites pump system to alleviate symptoms of recurrent ascites, including the placement of all components needed for treatment using this service. Code 0901T is used to report a pump-system replacement that is pumping inadequately. Code 0872T identifies the replacement of a catheter to address certain issues, such as blockage. Code 0873T is used to report revising the pump system. Code 0874T is used to report surgical removal of the pump system once the procedure has been completed. Code 0875T is used to identify programming adjustments of the parameters postimplantation.

In accordance with the establishment of codes 0870T-0875T, an exclusionary parenthetical note has been added following these codes to provide instruction on their appropriate reporting with the addition of a cross-reference parenthetical note following code 0872T. This includes restrictions in reporting services that are already included (eg, reporting programming [0875T] in conjunction with implantation services [0870T], because the implantation inherently includes initial programming).

Clinical Example (0870T)

A 66-year-old male, who has a long-standing nonalcoholic steatohepatitis that has evolved to liver cirrhosis, presents with recurrent ascites over the last year, despite the use of diuretics and lifestyle modifications. The frequency of paracentesis has increased over the past months, decreasing the patient's quality of life. The patient is found to be a suitable candidate for implantation of the ascites pump system.

Description of Procedure (0870T)

The physician locates and prepares the surgical site above the symphysis pubis and below the palpable bladder dome. Using ultrasound guidance, create a 1- to 2-cm incision with the introducer/needle attached to a small syringe. Remove the syringe from the needle, then insert the guidewire through the needle into the bladder. Remove the introducer/needle, dilate the opening to accept an 18F peel-away introducer, and remove the dilator and guidewire. Introduce the bladder catheter through the introducer until the cuff touches the top of the introducer. Split the sheath while continuing to slide the catheter down over the rod until the cuff is positioned below the skin level. Remove both the introducer and the rod, and ensure the coil resides completely in the bladder. Allow the bladder to drain to verify the correct placement. Using non-resorbable sutures, anchor the catheter to prevent migration, cut the tubing next to the fitting, and remove the fitting. Clamp the bladder catheter.

Placement of the Peritoneal Catheter

Locate and prepare the skin at the surgical site slightly lateral to the midline and just above the umbilicus. Prepare the peritoneal catheter and insert the stylet. Use Doppler ultrasound to avoid any large vessels. Cut the pigtail catheter between the two cuffs distally to the bend and close to the second cuff and attach the connector and blue extension tube. Fixate the catheters to the connector using sutures. Create an incision of approximately 1 cm through the skin. Introduce the needle into the peritoneal space at an oblique angle in a caudal direction and pass the guidewire through the needle. Dilate the opening using 10F and 14F dilators. Insert the 18F peel-away introducer and remove the dilator and guidewire. Insert stylet into the peritoneal catheter and introduce a catheter through the peel-away introducer as far as the catheter cuff. Split the sheath while sliding the catheter down over the stylet until the cuff is positioned at skin level. Remove the stylet and verify the free flow of ascitic fluid. Use a purse string suture through the fascia to reduce the chance of leakage.

Placement and Connection of Ascites Pump

Make a transverse incision of 5- to 6-cm in length beneath the coastal margin. Using blunt dissection, create the pump pocket. Implant the pump above the abdominal wall fascia. Verify the function of each catheter by injecting and aspirating fluid. If fluid is present in the abdomen/bladder, fluid should flow spontaneously from the catheters. Using the ascites pump as a guide, trim the length of the bladder and peritoneal catheters to fit. Allow sufficient slack to slide the ascites pump into the pocket and for normal movement of the upper body but not too much because

it can lead to "kinking." Insert the cut ends of the catheters into the catheter locking cap of the ascites pump. Push the catheters fully onto the ascites pump nipples using the catheter locking cap to determine the correct orientation. Test the pump and then lock the catheters in place. Slide the ascites pump into the pump pocket and verify that the catheters are not kinked or bent. Place subcutaneous non-resorbable sutures deep into the pocket and through the ascites pump fixation holes to prevent migration. Perform a multilayer closure of the pump pocket, ensuring that neither the ascites pump nor the catheters cross the line of the initial incision. Perform a multilayer closure of the bladder and peritoneal catheter implantation site incisions. Perform initial pump programming.

Clinical Example (0871T)

A 67-year-old male received an implanted ascites pump system. The patient has not presented with any clinical characteristics to indicate an increase in ascites volume 18 months postimplantation; however, the pressure-sensor data indicates that the system is not pumping the adequate/programmed ascites volume, and the patient is confirmed to be a suitable candidate for a pump replacement.

Description of Procedure (0871T)

Open the pump pocket and remove the fixation suture. Disengage the catheters from the ascites pump. After the new pump fixation, reconnect the catheters, and close the incision. Program the new pump.

Clinical Example (0872T)

A 66-year-old male had an ascites pump system implanted 12 months ago. Based on the patient's pump data, the speed of the pump motor is increasing, resulting in a rapid depletion of the battery. Based on the patient's clinical signs (ie, weight gain), and upon discussion with the ascites pump system engineer, it is confirmed that debris is lodged in the catheter, requiring catheter replacement.

Description of Procedure (0872T)

If a catheter is blocked, open the corresponding catheter incision and place a new catheter, and then cut off and remove the distal part of the old catheter. Reconnect the tubing with the catheter extension connector and secure with a non-resorbable suture. Perform multilayer incision closure and pump reprogramming.

Clinical Example (0873T)

A 64-year-old male, who previously received an implanted ascites pump system within the last 12 months, fell on the floor, resulting in a loss of pump

Category III 0042T-0713T

stability within the pocket. Imaging confirms a shift in the pump positioning. The patient is found to be a suitable candidate for revision and repositioning of the pump.

Description of Procedure (0873T)

Reopen the placement incision and dissect tissues to the pump pocket to reposition the pump, or reopen the incision to access the implanted catheters for manipulation. Close the incision in multilayered sutures. Reprogram the pump if indicated.

Clinical Example (0874T)

A 68-year-old male is 23 months postimplantation of an ascites pump system, and ascites production has halted. The patient has been found to no longer require the use of the ascites pump system and is confirmed to be a candidate for pump system removal.

Description of Procedure (0874T)

Open the pump pocket via an incision of the skin. Cut the sutures that fixed the ascites pump. Remove the ascites pump from the pocket. Dissection of the tissue from the fixation discs will be required. Make an incision in the suprapubic area, and locate the bladder catheter and fixation suture. Cut the fixation suture and ensure all suture material is removed. Locate the cuff and ensure it is freed from tissue. Cut the bladder catheter and pull the distal part out of the bladder. Cut the bladder catheter at the ascites pump side and pull the tubing out via the suprapubic incision. Make an incision at the location of the initial implantation for the peritoneal catheter and locate the cuff. Cut the fixation suture (if sutured) and ensure all suture material is removed. Close all incisions.

Clinical Example (0875T)

A 67-year-old male receives an implanted ascites pump system, and 6 months postimplantation, the patient is accumulating ascites despite the pump data indicating that the programmed volume has been reached. The patient is found to need a higher-volume setting, requiring reprogramming of new pump parameters.

Description of Procedure (0875T)

Link the programming software with the patient's implanted ascites pump system through the smart charger, enabling it to communicate with the ascites pump. Assess the parameters (eg, operating time, ascites volume, pump performance, fluid-transport parameters, charging profile) and change as necessary. Create or amend the new program setting for the ascites pump system, including the daily pump volumes and

scheduled-times for pump activation (eg, start/stop times, pauses, etc).

● **0876T** Duplex scan of hemodialysis fistula, computer-aided, limited (volume flow, diameter, and depth, including only body of fistula)

▶(Do not report 0876T in conjunction with 76376, 76377, 90940, 90951-90966, 93990)◀

▶(For duplex scan of hemodialysis access, including arterial inflow and venous outflow, use 93990)◀

Rationale

Category III code 0876T has been established for reporting a computer-aided limited (volume flow, diameter, and depth, including only the fistula body) duplex scan of a hemodialysis fistula.

Patients who receive dialysis often undergo a procedure to create an arteriovenous hemodialysis fistula (AVF) for dialysis access. A period of several weeks follows the AVF procedure to allow the fistula to mature to an adequate level for hemodialysis use. Before 2025, there was no CPT code to describe a radiologic evaluation that is limited to the fistula body to assess the level of maturation. Instead, code 93990 is reported for a duplex scan of a hemodialysis access to evaluate its performance, including arterial inflow, body of access, and venous outflow. Code 0876T differs from code 93990 in that it describes a duplex scan of the AVF prior to use for hemodialysis. Furthermore, the scan is limited to the evaluation of only the fistula body, including volume flow, diameter, and depth.

An exclusionary parenthetical note following code 0876T has been added, restricting its use with codes 76376, 76377, 90951-90966, and 93990. A cross-reference parenthetical note has been added following code 0876T directing users to code 93990 for the duplex scan of hemodialysis access, including arterial inflow and venous outflow.

Clinical Example (0876T)

A 68-year-old male, who has end-stage renal disease, is being dialyzed through a central venous catheter. An arteriovenous fistula was constructed 6 weeks ago and is being monitored for useability for dialysis. A limited duplex scan of the fistula is indicated to assess fistula flow and size.

Description of Procedure (0876T)

On the order from a physician, a staff member with minimal training performs the service using a specialized

★ = Telemedicine　◀ = Add-on code　✚ = Add-on code　✗ = FDA approval pending　# = Resequenced code　⊘ = Modifier 51 exempt

diagnostic ultrasound imaging machine with integrated computer-aided processing software. First, move the transducer along the arm until an echogenic implantable vessel marker device, which was previously placed approximately 3-cm distal to the anastomosis on the outflow vein, is located. This marker allows computer-aided calculation of volume flow. When the center of the marker device is found via B-mode imaging, collect a volume scan using the three-dimensional ultrasound to measure the volume flow through the fistula and the diameter and depth at that location. Move the transducer so that it is imaging the body of the fistula. Collect a volume scan to measure the diameter and depth along a segment within the body of the fistula. Move the transducer toward the venous outflow, and collect another volume scan for diameter and depth measurements. Repeat this step again to capture the entire body of the fistula. The physician reviews the volume-flow and anatomic measurements (diameter and depth) generated by the computer. The data informs the physician's interpretation of indicating the maturation status. The physician determines an appropriate course of action and dictates a report.

● **0877T** Augmentative analysis of chest computed tomography (CT) imaging data to provide categorical diagnostic subtype classification of interstitial lung disease; obtained without concurrent CT examination of any structure contained in previously acquired diagnostic imaging

▶(Do not report 0877T in conjunction with 71250, 71260, 71270, 71275)◀

● **0878T** obtained with concurrent CT examination of the same structure

▶(Use 0878T in conjunction with 71250, 71260, 71270, 71271, 71275, when evaluating same organ, tissue, or target structure)◀

● **0879T** radiological data preparation and transmission

● **0880T** physician or other qualified health care professional interpretation and report

Rationale

Four Category III codes (0877T-0880T) have been established to report augmentative analysis of chest computed tomography (CT) to provide categorical diagnostic subtype classification of interstitial lung disease. In these services, the algorithm completes the analysis without manual processing. The physician or other qualified health professional (QHP) interprets the algorithm's output in the context of the individual patient's clinical data (eg, laboratory results, lung function tests) and issues a report. A core difference between these codes and other existing codes (eg, 0721T and 0722T) is

that this algorithm's output is categorical (eg, qualitative, supportive or non-supportive of idiopathic pulmonary fibrosis) rather than quantitative.

Code 0877T describes the qualitative analysis of chest CT imaging data, utilizing augmentative analysis to assess and provide diagnostic subtype classification of interstitial lung disease, and is obtained without concurrent CT examination of any structure contained in previously acquired diagnostic imaging. This is reported as a categorical result (eg, supportive of idiopathic pulmonary fibrosis diagnosis). An exclusionary parenthetical note has been added following code 0877T to preclude the reporting of this code with codes 71250, 71260, 71270, and 71275.

Code 0878T is intended to report an augmentative analysis of chest CT data to provide a categorical diagnostic subtype classification of interstitial lung disease when obtained with a concurrent CT examination of the same structure. A conditional inclusionary parenthetical note has been added following code 0878T to enable reporting it with codes 71250, 71260, 71270, 71271, and 71275 when evaluating the same organ, tissue, or target structure.

Code 0879T only identifies the radiological data preparation and transmission. Code 0880T is used to report physician or other QHP interpretation and report.

Clinical Example (0877T)

A 65-year-old male, who has a chronic cough, had a laboratory panel for inflammatory biomarkers, pulmonary function testing, and a high-resolution pulmonary computed tomography (CT) scan with an indeterminate pattern that was inconclusive for idiopathic pulmonary fibrosis. The physician or other qualified health care professional orders computerized, machine-learning analysis of the pulmonary CT imaging data to provide categorical subtype classification of interstitial lung disease.

Description of Procedure (0877T)

Upon receipt of the necessary images, subject the data to computerized, machine-learning analysis of thousands of features and feature combinations along with the biomarker laboratory review to evaluate for patterns compatible with specific lung fibrosis diagnoses. The system output represents qualitative, categorical output with a classification of the lung fibrosis diagnosis based on historical comparators to multidisciplinary, assigned diagnoses. The output provides the qualitative classification with reported sensitivity and specificity metrics from various populations.

Clinical Example (0878T)

A 65-year-old male, who has a chronic cough, had a laboratory panel for inflammatory biomarkers, pulmonary function testing, and a high-resolution pulmonary computed tomography (CT) scan with an indeterminate pattern that was inconclusive for idiopathic pulmonary fibrosis. The physician or other qualified health care professional orders computerized, machine-learning analysis of the pulmonary CT imaging data to provide categorical subtype classification of interstitial lung disease.

Description of Procedure (0878T)

Upon receipt of the necessary images, subject the data to computerized, machine-learning analysis of thousands of features and feature combinations along with the biomarker laboratory review to evaluate for patterns compatible with specific lung fibrosis diagnoses. The system output represents qualitative, categorical output with a classification of the lung fibrosis diagnosis based on historical comparators to multidisciplinary, assigned diagnoses. The output provides the qualitative classification with reported sensitivity and specificity metrics from various populations.

Clinical Example (0879T)

A 65-year-old male, who has a chronic cough, had a laboratory panel for inflammatory biomarkers, pulmonary function testing, and a high-resolution pulmonary computed tomography (CT) scan with an indeterminate pattern that was inconclusive for idiopathic pulmonary fibrosis. The physician or qualified health care professional orders computerized, machine-learning analysis of the pulmonary CT imaging data to provide categorical subtype classification of interstitial lung disease.

Description of Procedure (0879T)

The radiology technician extracts the necessary data on the patient's pulmonary CT and uploads the necessary images into the software program.

Clinical Example (0880T)

A 65-year-old male, who has a chronic cough, had a laboratory panel for inflammatory biomarkers, pulmonary function testing, and a high-resolution pulmonary computed tomography (CT) scan with an indeterminate pattern that was inconclusive for idiopathic pulmonary fibrosis. The physician or other qualified health care professional orders computerized, machine-learning analysis of the pulmonary CT imaging data to provide categorical subtype classification of interstitial lung disease.

Description of Procedure (0880T)

The ordering physician or other qualified health care professional interprets the categorical result with reference to the sensitivity and specificity of the result in the context of the patient's clinical presentation.

● **0881T**   Cryotherapy of the oral cavity using temperature regulated fluid cooling system, including placement of an oral device, monitoring of patient tolerance to treatment, and removal of the oral device

▶(Use 0881T in conjunction with 96409, 96413, 96416, when chemotherapy is also performed)◀

▶(Do not report 0881T more than once per chemotherapy session)◀

Rationale

Category III code 0881T has been established to report oral cavity cryotherapy using a temperature-regulated fluid cooling system, including the placement of an oral device, monitoring of patient tolerance to treatment, and removal of the oral device. An instructional and conditional exclusionary note has been added to provide additional reporting instructions.

This procedure involves administering cryotherapy with a temperature-regulated oral cooling treatment during chemotherapy infusion therapy for a patient diagnosed with diseases such as lymphoma to reduce potential complications associated with oral mucositis.

In accordance with its establishment, a conditional exclusionary parenthetical note following code 0881T has been added to restrict reporting the procedure more than once per session.

In addition, an instructional cross-reference parenthetical note has been added following code 0881T to instruct users to report this service in conjunction with chemotherapy code 96409, 96413, or 96416 when chemotherapy is also provided.

Clinical Example (0881T)

A 62-year-old female, who is diagnosed with lymphoma, presents for chemotherapy infusion therapy.

Description of Procedure (0881T)

The physician conducts a clinical assessment and orders cryotherapy using a temperature-regulated oral cooling treatment during administration of chemotherapy. Place an appropriately sized mouthpiece in the patient's mouth before the chemotherapy session. Periodically assess patient tolerance to the cryotherapy. Remove the mouthpiece device at the conclusion of the treatment and inspect the oral cavity.

+● 0882T   Intraoperative therapeutic electrical stimulation of peripheral nerve to promote nerve regeneration, including lead placement and removal, upper extremity, minimum of 10 minutes; initial nerve (List separately in addition to code for primary procedure)

▶(Use 0882T in conjunction with 64702, 64704, 64708, 64713, 64718, 64719, 64721, 64831, 64834, 64835, 64836, 64856, 64857, 64892, 64893, 64895, 64896, 64897, 64898, 64905, 64910, 64911, 64912)◀

+● 0883T   each additional nerve (List separately in addition to code for primary procedure)

▶(Use 0883T in conjunction with 0882T)◀

Rationale

Codes 0882T and 0883T have been established to report intraoperative therapeutic electrical stimulation of peripheral nerves. Parenthetical notes have also been added to provide reporting instructions.

Code 0882T describes a therapeutic electrical stimulation of a peripheral nerve during an operation. It is an add-on code that may only be reported in conjunction with a primary procedure. If an additional nerve is treated, then add-on code 0883T may be reported to identify each additional nerve treated. Parenthetical notes following each code provide instructions regarding the primary procedures for which each of these codes may be additionally reported.

For this procedure, leads are placed at the location where nerve healing is needed. The placement uses a non-implantable device that is removed subsequent to the treatment during the operation. As noted in the descriptor, the procedure is intended to promote regeneration of nerves of the upper extremity and should be reported only if stimulation of 10 minutes or more is performed.

Clinical Example (0882T)

A 55-year-old female presents with increasing episodes of numbness and tingling, as well as weakness in the hand. Prior electrodiagnostic testing confirmed ulnar neuropathy at the cubital tunnel. Symptoms are no longer controlled by conservative treatments of physical therapy and splinting, and increasing levels of hand weakness are affecting activities of daily living. In conjunction with the surgical treatment repair, the physician opts to perform intraoperative therapeutic electrical stimulation of the peripheral nerve [**Note:** This is an add-on code. Only consider the additional work

related to intraoperative therapeutic electrical stimulation of the peripheral nerve.]

Description of Procedure (0882T)

Immediately following the surgical treatment or repair of a single injured nerve, the physician places the lead on or around the nerve proximal to the site of decompression or repair, connects the lead to the stimulator, and initiates the delivery of the therapy to the nerve by turning on the stimulator. The physician periodically monitors the system for adequate connection and delivery of stimulation. At the conclusion of the therapy delivery, the physician removes the lead from the nerve, taking care to ensure that tension is released before suturing the surgical site in layers.

Clinical Example (0883T)

A 23-year-old male presents with continued arm paralysis and loss of sensation, persisting from a previous traumatic accident 4 months ago. Clinical examination and electrodiagnostic testing confirm areas of injury in the median and radial nerves. Repeat examination at 6 months post-injury shows little to no progression of recovery of motor or sensory function, with the patient unable to complete many activities of daily living. In conjunction with surgical treatment or repair of the injured nerve, the physician opts to perform intraoperative therapeutic electrical stimulation of the additional peripheral nerves. [**Note:** This is an add-on code. Only consider the additional work related to treating additional nerves using intraoperative therapeutic electrical stimulation of peripheral nerve.]

Description of Procedure (0883T)

The physician places the lead on or around the nerve proximal to the site of decompression or repair, connects the lead to the stimulator, and initiates the delivery of the therapy to the subsequent nerve by turning on the stimulator. The physician periodically monitors the system for adequate connection and delivery of stimulation. At the conclusion of therapy delivery, the physician removes the lead from the nerve, taking care to ensure that tension is released before suturing the surgical site in layers.

● 0884T   Esophagoscopy, flexible, transoral, with initial transendoscopic mechanical dilation (eg, nondrug-coated balloon) followed by therapeutic drug delivery by drug-coated balloon catheter for esophageal stricture, including fluoroscopic guidance, when performed

▶(Do not report 0884T in conjunction with 43191, 43195, 43196, 43200, 43213, 43214, 43220, 43226, 76000)◀

● **0885T**   Colonoscopy, flexible, with initial transendoscopic mechanical dilation (eg, nondrug-coated balloon) followed by therapeutic drug delivery by drug-coated balloon catheter for colonic stricture, including fluoroscopic guidance, when performed

▶(Do not report 0885T in conjunction with 45378, 45386, 76000, 0886T)◀

▶(For endoscopic balloon dilation of multiple strictures during the same procedure, use 0885T with modifier 59 for each additional stricture dilated)◀

● **0886T**   Sigmoidoscopy, flexible, with initial transendoscopic mechanical dilation (eg, nondrug-coated balloon) followed by therapeutic drug delivery by drug-coated balloon catheter for colonic stricture, including fluoroscopic guidance, when performed

▶(Do not report 0886T in conjunction with 45300, 45303, 45330, 45340, 76000, 0885T)◀

▶(For endoscopic balloon dilation of multiple strictures during the same procedure, use 0886T with modifier 59 for each additional stricture dilated)◀

Rationale

For CPT 2025, three new Category III codes (0884T-0886T) have been established to report endoscopic drug-coated gastrointestinal balloon procedures. In addition, parenthetical notes have been provided for the procedures.

These new codes report a two-step procedure performed at the same setting—an initial transendoscopic mechanical dilation followed by therapeutic drug delivery by drug-coated balloon catheter for either esophageal or colonic stricture. All three procedures include fluoroscopic guidance, when performed. However, they differ in that code 0884T describes a flexible transoral esophagoscopy, code 0885T describes a flexible colonoscopy, and code 0886T describes a flexible sigmoidoscopy.

Exclusionary parenthetical notes have been established in multiple locations to restrict separate reporting of endoscopy and fluoroscopic imaging.

Following codes 0885T and 0886T, parenthetical notes have been established to provide instruction for reporting multiple strictures.

Clinical Example (0884T)

A 58-year-old male, who has a history of severe reflux esophagitis and previous benign esophageal stricture disease refractory to previous balloon dilation, now presents with recurrent difficulty swallowing solid food and an Ogilvie dysphagia score of 3. The esophagram demonstrates a recurrent, tight 1-cm-long stricture. To minimize the possibility of stricture recurrence, the

patient elects for flexible esophagoscopy with initial esophageal stricture dilation by a nondrug-coated balloon catheter followed by dilation with a drug-coated balloon (DCB) catheter to achieve therapeutic drug delivery into the stricture scar tissue.

Description of Procedure (0884T)

Position the patient in the operating room. The physician performs a flexible esophagoscopy to the level of the stricture. Pass a guidewire beyond the stricture and pass a nondrug-coated balloon catheter over the guidewire and through the lumen of the stricture. Dilate the stricture in the standard fashion, and then remove the nondrug-coated catheter. The physician then selects the appropriate DCB catheter so that the balloon diameter is slightly greater or equal to the diameter of the predilated channel and long enough to extend beyond the stricture. Under endoscopic vision, position the DCB appropriately and leave it in place for one minute to allow hydration of the drug coating. Using a mixture of saline and contrast and an inflation device, slowly inflate the balloon to approximately one atmosphere of pressure over 30 seconds until the desired balloon diameter is achieved and left in place for 10 minutes to allow the paclitaxel to penetrate the scar tissue. Visually check the position of the balloon or check by fluoroscopy to confirm that the balloon has achieved its full diameter along the stricture. After the secondary drug delivery is complete, deflate and remove the DCB and the endoscope.

Clinical Example (0885T)

A 42-year-old female, who has a long history of Crohn's disease of the large bowel, presents with worsening abdominal bloating and pain over the past 3 weeks consistent with intermittent large bowel obstruction. Barium study shows a solitary 3-cm transverse colon stricture. To minimize the possibility of stricture recurrence, the patient elects for a colonoscopy with initial colonic stricture dilation by a nondrug-coated balloon catheter followed by dilation with a drug-coated balloon (DCB) catheter to achieve drug delivery into the stricture scar tissue.

Description of Procedure (0885T)

Position the patient in the operating room. The physician performs a flexible colonoscopy to the level of the stricture. Pass a guidewire beyond the stricture and pass a nondrug-coated balloon catheter over the guidewire and through the lumen of the stricture. Dilate the stricture in the standard fashion, and then remove the nondrug-coated catheter. The physician then selects the appropriate DCB catheter so that the balloon diameter is slightly greater or equal to the diameter of the predilated channel and long enough to extend beyond the stricture. Under endoscopic vision, position the DCB appropriately and leave it in place for one minute to allow hydration of the drug coating. Using a mixture of saline and contrast and an inflation device, slowly inflate the balloon to approximately one atmosphere of pressure over 30 seconds until the desired balloon diameter is achieved and left in place for 10 minutes to allow the paclitaxel to penetrate the scar tissue. Visually check the position of the balloon or check by fluoroscopy to confirm that the balloon has achieved its full diameter along the stricture. After the drug delivery is complete, deflate and remove the DCB and the endoscope.

Clinical Example (0886T)

A 76-year-old male, who previously underwent a sigmoid colectomy for localized sigmoid diverticulitis, presents with abdominal cramping and constipation due to recurrent benign strictures at the anastomotic site refractory to previous balloon dilations. To minimize the possibility of stricture recurrence, the patient elects for a flexible sigmoidoscopy with initial stricture dilation by a nondrug-coated balloon catheter followed by dilation with a drug-coated balloon (DCB) catheter to achieve drug delivery into the stricture scar tissue.

Description of Procedure (0886T)

Position the patient in the operating room. The physician performs a flexible sigmoidoscopy to the level of the stricture. Pass a guidewire beyond the stricture and pass a nondrug-coated balloon catheter over the guidewire and through the lumen of the stricture. Dilate the stricture in the standard fashion, and then remove the nondrug-coated catheter. The physician then selects the appropriate DCB catheter so that the balloon diameter is slightly greater or equal to the diameter of the predilated channel and long enough to extend beyond the stricture. Under endoscopic vision, position the DCB appropriately and leave it in place for one minute to allow hydration of the drug coating. Using a mixture of saline and contrast and an inflation device, slowly inflate the balloon to approximately one atmosphere of pressure over 30 seconds until the desired balloon diameter is achieved and left in place for 10 minutes to allow the paclitaxel to penetrate the scar tissue. Visually check the position of the balloon or check by fluoroscopy to confirm that the balloon has achieved its full diameter along the stricture. After the drug delivery is complete, deflate and remove the DCB and the endoscope.

+● **0887T**   End-tidal control of inhaled anesthetic agents and oxygen to assist anesthesia care delivery (List separately in addition to code for primary procedure)

▶(Use 0887T in conjunction with 00100-01999)◀

Rationale

Add-on Category III code 0887T has been established for reporting end-tidal control of inhaled anesthetic agents and oxygen to assist anesthesia care delivery. An inclusionary parenthetical note has been added following code 0887T instructing its use in conjunction with codes 00100-01999.

Code 0887T describes the use of a device that assists the delivery of anesthesia with end-tidal control of the inhaled anesthetic agents and oxygen using computer software based on the target end-tidal concentrations of oxygen and anesthetic agent plus total gas flow, which are determined and entered into the computer-aided device by the anesthesia provider.

Clinical Example (0887T)

A 65-year-old male patient undergoes abdominal surgery under general anesthesia with end-tidal control of inhaled anesthetic agents and oxygen to assist anesthesia care delivery. [**Note:** This is an add-on code. Only consider the additional practice expense of anesthesia delivery.]

Description of Procedure (0887T)

Initiate the end-tidal control of inhaled anesthetic agents and oxygen to assist the anesthesia care delivery procedure after the placement of a controlled airway. The physician or other qualified health care professional determines the target end-tidal concentrations of oxygen and anesthetic agent plus total gas flow and switches the machine from manual administration to clinician-administered semi-closed loop delivery, and adjusts the inhaled anesthetic agents and oxygen. Throughout the surgery, the physician or other qualified health care professional uses the interface to adjust the expired gas targets and gas flow.

● **0888T**   Histotripsy (ie, non-thermal ablation via acoustic energy delivery) of malignant renal tissue, including imaging guidance

Rationale

Code 0888T has been established for reporting histotripsy of malignant renal tissue. Histotripsy is a noninvasive, real-time image-guided (ie, nonionizing radiation, mechanical destruction) acoustic energy beam therapy that destroys tissue at a subcellular level. The code includes the necessary imaging guidance to perform the procedure.

Clinical Example (0888T)

A 66-year-old male, who has been diagnosed with renal cell carcinoma with a lesion of ≤ 3 cm, is not a surgical candidate and is intolerant of other therapies. Histotripsy is performed.

Description of Procedure (0888T)

A complex simulation–aided field setting is performed to determine where the site of treatment will enter the body. Perform dose calculations, which include depth, time, and inhomogeneity factors. Use specific treatment devices to reduce patient motion and to protect both intervening and non-targeted tissue from damage. Position the patient, and then deliver histotripsy to the tumor.

● **0889T**   Personalized target development for accelerated, repetitive high-dose functional connectivity MRI–guided theta-burst stimulation derived from a structural and resting-state functional MRI, including data preparation and transmission, generation of the target, motor threshold–starting location, neuronavigation files and target report, review and interpretation

▶(Report 0889T once per personalized target development)◀

▶(Do not report 0889T in conjunction with 70551, 70552, 70553, 70554, 70555, for the same session)◀

▶(Do not report 0889T in conjunction with 77022)◀

● **0890T**   Accelerated, repetitive high-dose functional connectivity MRI–guided theta-burst stimulation, including target assessment, initial motor threshold determination, neuronavigation, delivery and management, initial treatment day

▶(Report 0890T once on the first day of the course of treatment)◀

▶(Do not report 0890T in conjunction with 77022)◀

● **0891T**   Accelerated, repetitive high-dose functional connectivity MRI–guided theta-burst stimulation, including neuronavigation, delivery and management, subsequent treatment day

▶(Do not report 0891T in conjunction with 77022)◀

● **0892T**   Accelerated, repetitive high-dose functional connectivity MRI–guided theta-burst stimulation, including neuronavigation, delivery and management, subsequent motor threshold redetermination with delivery and management, per treatment day

▶(Do not report 0892T in conjunction with 77022)◀

▶(Do not report 0892T in conjunction with 0890T, 0891T on the same day)◀

▶(If a significant, separately identifiable evaluation and management, medication management, or psychotherapy service is performed, the appropriate E/M or psychotherapy code may be reported in addition to 0890T, 0891T, 0892T. E/M activities directly related to cortical mapping, motor-threshold determination, delivery and management of accelerated, repetitive high-dose functional connectivity MRI–guided theta-burst stimulation are not separately reported)◀

Rationale

Four Category III codes (0889T-0892T) have been established to report personalized target development for accelerated, repetitive high-dose functional connectivity magnetic resonance imaging (MRI)–guided theta-burst stimulation. In addition, three parenthetical notes have been added or revised to further clarify the appropriate reporting of these codes in the Other Psychiatric Services or Procedures subsection in the Medicine section. A number of exclusionary and cross-reference parenthetical notes have also been added to accommodate the addition of the new codes.

Codes 0889T-0892T discern the use of MRI to identify/ assess and treat targeted brain structures using accelerated, repetitive high-dose functional connectivity theta-burst stimulation for the treatment of conditions, such as depression, resistant depression, and bipolar disorders. Similar to transcranial magnetic stimulation, this service is noninvasive and involves passing an electrical current through a magnetic coil placed superficial to the scalp. This produces a high-intensity magnetic field that passes through the scalp, skull, and meninges to excite neuronal tissue. Repeated, shortened-duration excitation (ie, theta-burst stimulation) that is accelerated and used on a specific MRI-identified brain region is identified as "accelerated, repetitive high-dose functional connectivity MRI-guided theta-burst stimulation" and represents the action that causes/actuates the treatment for these procedures.

These codes are used to both identify the target areas that need to be treated within the brain, as well as to treat the areas of interest. In order to perform the accelerated, repetitive high-dose functional connectivity MRI-guided theta-burst stimulation procedure, personalized targets need to be generated for each patient by using the baseline structural and resting-state MRI scans. Using that information, segments are mapped for probability as the tissue of interest, algorithms are used to determine the placement of coils for treatments, personalized targets are developed, and other services are provided as identified by code 0889T. These services include data preparation and transmission, generation of the target, determination of the motor threshold starting

★ = Telemedicine   ◀ = Add-on code   ✚ = Add-on code   ⁄ = FDA approval pending   # = Resequenced code   ⊘ = Modifier 51 exempt

locations, neuronavigation, and review and interpretation of the data.

The treatment is performed over a number of days and during multiple sessions each day. Code 0890T is used to identify the initial day of motor threshold determination, neuronavigation, delivery, and management. If additional, subsequent treatment sessions are necessary, code 0891T may be reported for each subsequent treatment day. If a subsequent motor threshold redetermination with delivery and management is necessary, code 0892T is used to identify the motor threshold redetermination.

To provide users with instructions and clarify usage, various parenthetical notes have been added, including:

1. instructional parenthetical notes that direct users regarding the number of times that a personalized target development (0889T) or initial treatment day service (0890T) may be reported;

2. exclusionary parenthetical notes to restrict reporting of overlapping services (such as MRI guidance procedures that are inherently included as part of the service and restrictions regarding reporting the service represented by code 0892T in conjunction with other delivery and management services [0890T, 0891T]); and

3. an instructional parenthetical note regarding appropriate reporting for evaluation and management (E/M) services.

Instructions have also been updated or added following the therapeutic repetitive transcranial magnetic stimulation services (90867-90869) to restrict reporting these treatments together because the services are mutually exclusive.

Clinical Example (0889T)

A 50-year-old female, who has a history of major depressive disorder with unsuccessful results from using pharmacologic treatment with three separate antidepressant medications from two different chemical classes, is referred for accelerated, repetitive high-dose functional connectivity magnetic resonance imaging (MRI)–guided theta-burst stimulation.

Description of Procedure (0889T)

The technician extracts the MRI data from the medical records system, which contains the previously performed structural and functional brain MRI scans, and transmits the necessary MRI images after de-identification for processing to identify the brain location (target) where the transcranial magnetic stimulator should be placed for treatment. The processing software inspects the MRI images to ensure they are of sufficient quality. The functional units of the individual's brain are identified, and the software

determines which functional unit is of optimal size, shape, location, and network properties to serve as a target for treating the patient. An analyst reviews the treatment target, navigation landmark locations, motor-threshold starting location, navigation and neuronavigation file, and creates a report. The navigation files to allow neuronavigation to the appropriate target are created. Notify the physician that the report and navigation file are ready for review. The physician reviews and interprets the targeting report and schedules the patient for treatment.

Clinical Example (0890T)

A 35-year-old female, who has a history of major depressive disorder with unsuccessful results from using pharmacologic treatment with three separate antidepressant medications from two different chemical classes, is referred for accelerated, repetitive high-dose functional connectivity magnetic resonance imaging (MRI)–guided theta-burst stimulation.

Description of Procedure (0890T)

Seat the patient in a treatment chair. The physician performs a brief interview to determine the patient's mental status and ability to proceed with the procedure. The physician selects the patient's targeting information, motor-threshold (MT) starting location, and neuronavigation file from the secure cloud. Place a fiducial marker on the patient's head and align the tracking camera. Register the neuronavigation system to the individual patient's target using computer assistance. Using the computer-assisted neuronavigation system, the physician identifies the MT, which is the location of the stimulating coil that results in movement of the hand muscle with the lowest-stimulation intensity, and places the stimulating coil over the patient's personalized target. The computer then calculates the treatment intensity based on the MT and the distance from the coil to the treatment target. Select the stimulus frequency, intensity, number of stimuli, and inter-stimulus interval treatment parameters. Activate the neurostimulator and perform an initial 10-minute session of accelerated, repetitive high-dose functional connectivity MRI-guided theta-burst stimulation.

During the treatment session, closely monitor the patient to ensure the coil remains in the optimal location and orientation to the treatment target. Monitor the patient for comfort and tolerability, and adjust treatment intensity to mitigate discomfort. After 10 minutes, the neurostimulator turns off and a 50-minute intersession interval occurs before the start of the next treatment. Monitor the patient during her resting period before the next treatment session. Review and document a treatment summary.

Category III 0042T-0713T

Clinical Example (0891T)

A 46-year-old male, who has a history of major depressive disorder with unsuccessful results from using pharmacologic treatment with three separate antidepressant medications from two different chemical classes, is referred for accelerated, repetitive high-dose functional connectivity magnetic resonance imaging (MRI)–guided theta-burst stimulation.

Description of Procedure (0891T)

Seat the patient in a treatment chair. The physician performs a brief interview to determine the patient's mental status and ability to proceed with the procedure. The physician selects the patient's targeting information, motor-threshold starting location, and neuronavigation file from the secure cloud. Place a fiducial marker on the patient's head and align the tracking camera. Register the neuronavigation system to the individual patient's target using computer assistance. Select the stimulus frequency, intensity, number of stimuli, and inter-stimulus interval treatment parameters. Activate the neurostimulator and perform an initial 10-minute session of accelerated, repetitive high-dose functional connectivity MRI-guided theta-burst stimulation. During the treatment session, closely monitor the patient to ensure the coil remains in the optimal location and orientation to the treatment target. Monitor the patient for comfort and tolerability, and adjust treatment intensity to mitigate discomfort. After 10 minutes, the neurostimulator turns off and a 50-minute intersession interval occurs before the start of the next treatment. Monitor the patient during his resting period before the next treatment session. Review and document a treatment.

Clinical Example (0892T)

A 65-year-old female, who has a history of major depressive disorder with unsuccessful results from using pharmacologic treatment with three separate antidepressant medications from two different chemical classes, is referred for accelerated, repetitive high-dose functional connectivity magnetic resonance imaging (MRI)–guided theta-burst stimulation.

Description of Procedure (0892T)

Seat the patient in a treatment chair. The physician performs a brief interview to determine the patient's mental status and ability to proceed with the procedure. The physician selects the patient's targeting information, motor-threshold (MT) starting location, and neuronavigation file from the secure cloud. Place a fiducial marker on the patient's head and align the tracking camera. Register the neuronavigation system to

the patient's target using computer assistance. Using the computer-assisted neuronavigation system, the physician identifies the MT, which is the location of the stimulating coil that results in movement of the hand muscle with the lowest-stimulation intensity, and places the stimulating coil over the patient's personalized target. The computer then calculates the treatment intensity based on the MT and the distance from the coil to the treatment target. Select the stimulus frequency, intensity, number of stimuli, and inter-stimulus interval treatment parameters. Activate the neurostimulator and perform an initial 10-minute session of accelerated, repetitive high-dose functional connectivity MRI-guided theta-burst stimulation. During the treatment session, closely monitor the patient to ensure the coil remains in the optimal location and orientation to the treatment target. Monitor the patient for comfort and tolerability, and adjust treatment intensity to mitigate discomfort. After 10 minutes, the neurostimulator turns off and a 50-minute intersession interval occurs before the start of the next treatment. Monitor the patient during her resting period before the next treatment session. Review and document a treatment summary.

● **0893T** Noninvasive assessment of blood oxygenation, gas exchange efficiency, and cardiorespiratory status, with physician or other qualified health care professional interpretation and report

Rationale

New Category III code 0893T has been established to report a noninvasive assessment of blood oxygenation, gas-exchange efficiency, and cardiorespiratory status with a physician or other QHP interpretation and report. The new procedure provides multiple measurements simultaneously on the efficiency of pulmonary gas exchange, blood oxygenation sufficiency, and ventilation adequacy from a single patient test procedure. The procedure provides the clinical information needed to support the diagnosis, prognosis, and treatment of chronic and acute infections (eg, pneumonia) to respiratory diseases (eg, chronic obstructive pulmonary disease, pulmonary edema, pulmonary embolism).

Clinical Example (0893T)

A 68-year-old male patient presents with unexplained dyspnea and a cardiac history. The patient undergoes a cardiac panel to assess acute coronary syndrome (ACS). A noninvasive pulmonary gas-exchange assessment was performed for differential diagnosis. The patient's alveolar-arterial oxygen difference was 65 mmHg despite an oxygen saturation of 94% in room air. The ACS diagnosis could not account for this severe gas-exchange impairment and a chest computed tomography (CT) scan was ordered to confirm pulmonary embolism (PE). The CT scan was positive for PE.

Description of Procedure (0893T)

Gas-exchange analysis can be performed by a physician or other qualified health care professional. The procedure is performed in the emergency department for triage or diagnosis support based on admitted hospital patients for treatment–effectiveness confirmation or discharge readiness, or in outpatient settings to help guide treatment and care escalation decisions. Place an integrated pulse oximeter on the patient's finger and a nose clip on the patient's nose, and ask the patient to breathe through a mouthpiece that collects side-stream gas samples of the ambient air and the patient's breath. The patient normally breathes through the mouthpiece at tidal volume, and the procedure ends automatically once steady state breathing has been detected, typically under 2 minutes.

● **0894T** Cannulation of the liver allograft in preparation for connection to the normothermic perfusion device and decannulation of the liver allograft following normothermic perfusion

● **0895T** Connection of liver allograft to normothermic machine perfusion device, hemostasis control; initial 4 hours of monitoring time, including hourly physiological and laboratory assessments (eg, perfusate temperature, perfusate pH, hemodynamic parameters, bile production, bile pH, bile glucose, biliary bicarbonate, lactate levels, macroscopic assessment)

+● **0896T** each additional hour, including physiological and laboratory assessments (eg, perfusate temperature, perfusate pH, hemodynamic parameters, bile production, bile pH, bile glucose, biliary bicarbonate, lactate levels, macroscopic assessment) (List separately in addition to code for primary procedure)

▶(Use 0896T in conjunction with 0895T)◀

Rationale

For CPT 2025, three new Category III codes (0894T-0896T) have been established to report normothermic liver perfusion services. In addition, a parenthetical note has been added to specify reporting for the add-on code.

Normothermic liver perfusion services involve the cannulation and surgical preparation of the liver allograft with subsequent removal of the cannula (decannulation) following normothermic perfusion and the connection of the liver allograft to the normothermic perfusion device.

These new codes identify the different services performed or needed for the procedure. Code 0894T identifies the placement of cannulation, including any effort necessary to prepare the liver for connection to the normothermic device. Because decannulation is always performed, the procedure inherently includes this service as well. Code 0895T reports the connection of the liver allograft to the normothermic perfusion device. Because perfusion monitoring time varies considerably between donor allografts, code 0896T is used to report each additional hour of service. An add-on parenthetical note has been added following code 0896T to direct users that it may be used in conjunction with code 0895T for the additional hours of normothermic perfusion provided.

Clinical Example (0894T)

The transplant surgeon evaluates a cadaver-donor whole-liver allograft and determines that the allograft requires surgical preparation and cannulation in preparation for normothermic perfusion to sustain the functionality of the allograft before transplantation.

Description of Procedure (0894T)

Following standard backbench whole-liver graft preparation, prepare the liver allograft for normothermic machine perfusion. Cannulate the allograft using a specific technique involving careful suturing of the supra-hepatic inferior vena cava and inserting and securing of the cannulae into the hepatic artery, portal vein, and inferior vena cava. Spend significant time positioning and angulating each cannula. Take care to prime the cannulae with colloid to ensure all air is expelled before connecting the liver allograft to the normothermic machine perfusion device. After normothermic perfusion, perform decannulation of the liver allograft in preparation for the allograft transplant. Note that liver allograft preparation is significantly different and distinct from standard backbench work.

Clinical Example (0895T)

The liver transplant surgeon has assessed a cadaver-donor whole-liver allograft and determined that it requires normothermic perfusion to sustain its functionality before transplantation. Following cannulation, connect the liver allograft to the perfusion system, and commence the initial 4 hours of perfusion.

Description of Procedure (0895T)

Transfer the liver allograft to the normothermic perfusion device. Fit the cannulae to the connectors on the primed perfusion circuit. Further prime the tubing and cannulae, taking care to exclude air. Commence perfusion. At 15 minutes, take a perfusate sample to

Category III 0042T-0713T

determine a blood glucose reading (82945). Enter the value into the perfusion device. Visually inspect the organ. Initiate additional interventions (typically sodium bicarbonate) or attention to hemostasis if required. Carefully inspect the organ to ensure adequate global perfusion and rectify any hemostatic imbalance. Make hourly physiological and laboratory assessments, such as perfusate temperature; perfusate pH; hemodynamic parameters; bile production; bile pH; bile glucose; biliary bicarbonate; lactate levels; and macroscopic assessment.

Clinical Example (0896T)

The liver transplant surgeon has assessed a cadaver-donor whole-liver allograft and determined that the allograft requires normothermic perfusion to sustain the functionality of the allograft before transplant. After 4 hours of initial perfusion, the surgeon determines that additional normothermic perfusion is required. [**Note:** This is an add-on code. Only consider the additional work related to cannulation of the liver allograft.]

Description of Procedure (0896T)

After the initial 4 hours of normothermic perfusion, visually inspect the liver allograft to determine if the allograft meets the criteria for transplant. Take biochemical readings again. Initiate additional interventions (typically sodium bicarbonate) or attention to hemostasis if required. At least every 4 hours, take a perfusate sample to determine a blood glucose reading (82945), and enter the value into the perfusion device. Make hourly physiological and laboratory assessments, such as perfusion temperature; perfusate pH; hemodynamic parameters; bile production; bile pH; bile glucose; biliary bicarbonate; lactate levels; and macroscopic assessment.

● **0897T** Noninvasive augmentative arrhythmia analysis derived from quantitative computational cardiac arrhythmia simulations, based on selected intervals of interest from 12-lead electrocardiogram and uploaded clinical parameters, including uploading clinical parameters with interpretation and report

▶(Do not report 0897T in conjunction with 93000, 93005, 93010, when performed on the same day)◀

Rationale

Category III code 0897T has been established for reporting arrhythmia analysis derived from quantitative computational cardiac arrhythmia simulations based on selected intervals of interest from a 12-lead ECG and uploaded clinical parameters.

Before 2025, there were no CPT codes that described augmentative analysis of cardiac arrhythmias. An ECG (not reported separately) is performed in the procedure described in code 0897T. The ECG is uploaded into a software system with the patient's arrhythmia characteristics. The system processes the ECG and the patient characteristics, localizing areas of the heart that may require further investigation based on the uploaded data. The software system generates an output report, and the physician interprets the output and provides a written report. This service is augmentative because of the system's analysis and quantification of the data from the ECG and the patient's characteristics providing clinically meaningful output for interpretation by the physician. A conditional exclusionary parenthetical note has been added that restricts the use of code 0897T with ECG codes 93000, 93005, and 93010 when performed on the same day.

Clinical Example (0897T)

A 59-year-old female who has frequent premature ventricular complexes (PVCs) continues to experience symptoms of palpitations despite antiarrhythmic therapy. Given the frequency of her PVCs, the physician decides to seek a more comprehensive understanding of the arrhythmia.

Description of Procedure (0897T)

A physician records a 12-lead electrocardiogram (ECG) from the patient with frequent PVCs and tachycardia-mediated cardiomyopathy during a new patient clinic visit. The physician reviews the medical record and collects information about the left ventricular dilation, myocardial scar location, and previous ablations. The physician also reviews the patient's cardiac computed tomography imaging to further understand the ventricular disease locations. The physician inputs the data into the software system and uploads the ECG. The physician identifies two distinct PVC morphologies and analyzes both using the system. The software processes the ECG, personalizes the output based on the input patient characteristics, and localizes both PVC origins. Then the system generates a report highlighting areas for further investigation in the left ventricle (LV), including the mid-lateral LV wall and apical posteroseptal LV regions. The physician refers the patient for targeted therapy at a center specializing in LV PVC ablation.

● **0898T** Noninvasive prostate cancer estimation map, derived from augmentative analysis of image-guided fusion biopsy and pathology, including visualization of margin volume and location, with margin determination and physician interpretation and report

★=Telemedicine ◀=Add-on code ✚=Add-on code ✔=FDA approval pending #=Resequenced code ⊘=Modifier 51 exempt

►(Do not report 0898T in conjunction with 76376, 76377)◄

Rationale

New Category III code 0898T has been established to report noninvasive prostate cancer estimation mapping.

Code 0898T describes the augmentative analysis of data, such as image-guided fusion biopsy, to better visualize the location and extent of cancer (ie, margin volume and location, with margin determination) in the prostate. The artificial intelligence (AI) produces a "cancer-estimation map" that is clinically meaningful to the physician's determination of the optimal location and size of the margin and treatment recommendation.

An exclusionary parenthetical has been added to preclude the reporting of code 0898T with codes 76376 and 76377 because a three-dimensional (3D) rendering for MRI and ultrasound are both excluded from use in conjunction with this procedure.

Clinical Example (0898T)

A 68-year-old male previously presented to undergo magnetic resonance imaging (MRI) of the pelvis and a transperineal MR/ultrasound-guided fusion biopsy of the prostate. A localized prostatic tumor was identified and confirmed, with a Gleason grade group ≥2. The physician orders a cancer-estimation map.

Description of Procedure (0898T)

The physician uploads the required data from the patient's medical record, picture archiving and communication system, and/or other medical devices to the secure, cloud-based platform. The data includes previously acquired and interpreted (separately reported) MRI images, fusion biopsy core locations, and pathology data.

Once the data inputs are received and validated in the platform, initiate the cancer estimation–map algorithm to conduct the analysis in several steps. The algorithm first integrates the data to classify the probability of cancer at each voxel in the images. It then generates a cancer-estimation map with default margins designed to maximize the encapsulation confidence score while minimizing margin size. Next, the algorithm displays the margin alongside the cancer estimation map, both overlaid onto the original MRI. An encapsulation confidence score (the likelihood that all clinically significant cancer is encapsulated within the margin) is also calculated for the margin.

Make the MRI image, overlaid with the cancer-estimation map, available to the ordering physician through an interactive cloud-based viewer. The ordering

physician can visualize the tumor in three dimension and can further modify the margin using the cloud-based viewing tool. As the physician adjusts the margin by selecting a different cancer estimation–map threshold, the algorithm recalculates a new encapsulation confidence score. The physician performs all the margin calculations in a single session, which allows the physician to determine the optimal location and size of the margin and treatment recommendation and to complete the case. The physician generates a report and files it in the patient's record.

+● 0899T   Noninvasive determination of absolute quantitation of myocardial blood flow (AQMBF), derived from augmentative algorithmic analysis of the dataset acquired via contrast cardiac magnetic resonance (CMR), pharmacologic stress, with interpretation and report by a physician or other qualified health care professional (List separately in addition to code for primary procedure)

►(Use 0899T in conjunction with 75563)◄

►(Do not report 0899T in conjunction with 0900T)◄

►(For AQMBF with PET, use 78434)◄

►(For AQMBF with SPECT, use 0742T)◄

+● 0900T   Noninvasive estimate of absolute quantitation of myocardial blood flow (AQMBF), derived from assistive algorithmic analysis of the dataset acquired via contrast cardiac magnetic resonance (CMR), pharmacologic stress, with interpretation and report by a physician or other qualified health care professional (List separately in addition to code for primary procedure)

►(Use 0900T in conjunction with 75563)◄

►(Do not report 0900T in conjunction with 0899T)◄

►(For AQMBF with PET, use 78434)◄

►(For AQMBF with SPECT, use 0742T)◄

Rationale

Add-on Category III codes 0899T and 0900T have been established for reporting the noninvasive determination of absolute quantitation of myocardial blood flow (AQMBF) using augmentative and assistive algorithmic analysis. In addition, guidelines have been revised and added in the Heart subsection of the Radiology section with the addition of a parenthetical note. Parenthetical notes have also been added to the Category III section to clarify the intended reporting of these new codes.

Codes 0899T and 0900T are intended to provide additional information to diagnose the causes of myocardial ischemia (ie, a lack of blood to the heart) and its extent and severity in patients. It does this by using a noninvasive method to provide an AQMBF and analyze

Category III 0042T-0713T

myocardial blood flow reserves to stratify risk for patients who have acute chest pain and no known coronary artery disease. This method is used in conjunction with other procedures to identify blood-flow problems and determine the cause of the ischemia.

Code 0899T uses an augmentative algorithm to analyze and/or quantify data from contrast magnetic resonance (CMR) and pharmacologic stressing of the heart. As an add-on code, this procedure is intended to be used in addition to other procedures that may reveal vital information regarding blood flow within the heart, such as cardiac MRI (75563), which provides CMR imaging information regarding the morphology and function of the heart. This is further exemplified within the parenthetical note, stating that code 75563 should be used with code 0899T. (**Note:** For definitions regarding AI analysis [ie, assistive, augmentative], refer to Appendix S in the codebook.)

Code 0900T is also an add-on code that provides a different aspect of AQMBF because this procedure uses assistive algorithmic analysis of the dataset. For this service, the "machine" detects clinically relevant data but does not analyze the data or generate any conclusions. Differentiating the services in this way allows for specificity regarding the type of AI provided for the services.

The services identified by codes 0899T and 0900T are mutually exclusive and may not be reported together. This is clarified by the exclusionary parenthetical instructions that follow each code, which restrict users from reporting them together.

Other parenthetical notes provide cross-reference direction within the Category III section to users regarding the appropriate codes to report for AQMBF performed with positron emissions tomography (PET) (78434) and single proton-emission computed tomography (SPECT) (0742T). An additional parenthetical note has been included within the Radiology section to direct users to use one of the new codes in conjunction with code 75563 for a CMR.

In addition, a sentence that notes "only one add-on code for flow velocity can be reported per session" has been deleted from the Radiology guidelines to provide users with clarity and flexibility for the use of CMR procedures because other add-on codes may be used during their provision. For example, there are instances in which patients with both valvular heart disease and suspected coronary artery disease may require diagnostic information that could be obtained from CMR imaging of velocity flow mapping (ie, add-on code 75565). Removal of this guideline instruction provides the flexibility to report all services that may be provided.

Clinical Example (0899T)

A 72-year-old male, who has atypical chest pain, intermediate probability of coronary artery disease, and moderate renal failure, presents with progressive chest pain after a coronavirus 2019 vaccination. Cardiac enzymes are elevated. Stress cardiac magnetic resonance (CMR) with quantified myocardial blood flow is performed to assess the presence and severity of any underlying coronary artery disease before any planned high-risk intervention. [**Note:** This is an add-on code. Only consider the additional work related to CMR absolute quantitation of myocardial blood flow {AQMBF}.]

Description of Procedure (0899T)

Under the direction of the physician, following cardiovascular stress, the radiological technologist collects perfusion CMR data in a manner that allows AQMBF. Perform data quality control (QC) to be analyzed by a dedicated software. The software may automatically locate blood pool and myocardial margins and/or apply filters. The interpreting physician either validates the QC (eg, the bolus duration, peak, and plateau waveforms) or decides it is not valid before the algorithmic analysis of data, which is ultimately adjusted and confirmed by the physician. The physician reviews, affirms, and interprets the final numeric output for AQMBF (typically in ml/g/min). The final report includes static visual dynamic perfusion image data.

Clinical Example (0900T)

A 68-year-old female, who has a history of prior radiation therapy for breast cancer, presents with dyspnea and atypical chest pain. A stress perfusion cardiac magnetic resonance (CMR) with quantified myocardial blood flow is performed to estimate the presence and severity of any underlying coronary artery disease and, with other diagnostic information, is used to determine the presence and possible etiologies of cardiomyopathy. [**Note:** This is an add-on code. Only consider the additional work related to CMR absolute quantitation of myocardial blood flow {AQMBF}.]

Description of Procedure (0900T)

Under the direction of the physician, following cardiovascular stress, the radiological technologist collects perfusion CMR data in a manner that allows AQMBF. Perform data quality control (QC) to be analyzed by a dedicated software. The interpreting physician affirms the QC (eg, the bolus duration, peak, and plateau waveforms). The software identifies areas of noise and blood pool and myocardial margins before the algorithmic processing of data, which is ultimately adjusted and confirmed by the physician. The physician reviews and interprets the final numeric output for

AQMBF (typically in ml/g/min). The final report includes static visual dynamic perfusion image data.

0901T   Code is out of numerical sequence. See 0222T-0235T

● **0902T**   QTc interval derived by augmentative algorithmic analysis of input from an external, patient-activated mobile ECG device

▶(Do not report 0902T in conjunction with 93000, 93005, 93010, 93040, 93041, 93042)◀

Rationale

Category III code 0902T has been established to report a QTc interval derived by augmentative algorithmic analysis. A parenthetical note has been added to preclude the reporting of code 0902T with codes 93000, 93005, 93010, 93040, 93041, and 93042.

This code describes the use of an augmentative algorithm to derive the QTc from mobile electrocardiogram (ECG) data. Specifically, code 0902T describes the procedure of analyzing the 30 seconds of ECG data/tracing that is measured from a six-lead mobile ECG. The algorithmic output is QT and RR interval information. Using these two parameters, QTc is calculated using the standard QT correction formulae. An exclusionary parenthetical note has been included to restrict the reporting of other ECG services.

Clinical Example (0902T)

A 66-year-old male who has atrial fibrillation is prescribed an antiarrhythmic drug (AAD) that can cause prolonged QT. The patient is a candidate for an outpatient AAD loading because his appropriate baseline heart rate and uncorrected QT interval are <450ms and serum electrolytes are normal, and no type III drug-related proarrhythmia risk factors are present. Serial acquisition of electrocardiograms (ECGs) is planned for the algorithmic derivation of QTc to assess for QT prolongation.

Description of Procedure (0902T)

Analyze 30 seconds of electrocardiographic data acquired from an ambulatory ECG device for QTc interval measurements. The service computes a representative ECG beat, which is then analyzed using various algorithms to compute the QT interval. In addition, the service uses algorithms to compute the RR-interval, which is used in a mathematical formula to generate the corrected QTc. Include the QTc and electrocardiographic tracing in the report.

● **0903T**   Electrocardiogram, algorithmically generated 12-lead ECG from a reduced-lead ECG; with interpretation and report

▶(Do not report 0903T in conjunction with 93000, 93005, 93010, 0904T, 0905T)◀

● **0904T**   tracing only

▶(Do not report 0904T in conjunction with 93000, 93005, 93010, 0903T, 0905T)◀

● **0905T**   interpretation and report only

▶(Do not report 0905T in conjunction with 93000, 93005, 93010, 0903T, 0904T)◀

Rationale

Three new Category III codes (0903T-0905T) have been established to report a 12-lead ECG from a reduced-lead ECG. This means, for example, that an eight-lead ECG may be processed by the algorithm to yield a 12-lead ECG result. Code 0903T identifies the complete service of producing the ECG recording and providing an interpretation and report. If only tracing or interpretation and report are provided as individual services, then code 0904T or 0905T may be reported to identify the specific service that was provided. Exclusionary parenthetical notes have been included to restrict reporting any of the new services in conjunction with each other or with other ECG services.

Clinical Example (0903T)

A 72-year-old female is experiencing chest pain. An algorithmically generated 12-lead electrocardiogram (ECG) is ordered because conventional 12-lead ECG systems are not readily available.

Description of Procedure (0903T)

With the patient in the supine position, the health care professional attaches the electrode to the cable and places the electrodes into position. Activate the mobile device and enter patient data. The system software records and mathematically derives leads I, II, III, aVR, aVF, aVL, v4, and v2 (or v1). Machine-learning algorithms synthesize the remaining chest leads. The system generates a 12-lead data output that the physician interprets and subsequently generates a report.

Clinical Example (0904T)

A 72-year-old female is experiencing chest pain. An algorithmically generated 12-lead electrocardiograms (ECGs) is ordered because conventional 12-lead ECG systems are not readily available.

Description of Procedure (0904T)

With the patient in the supine position, the health care professional attaches the electrode to the cable and places the electrodes into position. Activate the mobile device and enter patient data. The system software records and mathematically derives leads I, II, III, aVR, aVF, aVL, v4, and v2 (or v1). Machine-learning algorithms synthesize the remaining chest leads. The system generates a 12-lead data output that the physician interprets and subsequently generates a report.

Clinical Example (0905T)

A 72-year-old female is experiencing chest pain. An algorithmically generated 12-lead electrocardiograms (ECGs) is ordered because conventional 12-lead ECG systems are not readily available.

Description of Procedure (0905T)

A physician interprets an assistive, algorithmically synthesized 12-lead ECG and subsequently generates a report.

▶For purposes of reporting 0906T, 0907T for concurrent optical and magnetic stimulation (COMS) therapy, the treatment area is limited to 50 sq cm of skin-surface area per application.◀

● **0906T** Concurrent optical and magnetic stimulation (COMS) therapy, wound assessment and dressing care; first application, total wound(s) surface area less than or equal to 50 sq cm

+● **0907T** each additional application, total wound(s) surface area less than or equal to 50 sq cm (List separately in addition to code for primary procedure)

▶(Use 0907T in conjunction with 0906T)◀

Rationale

Category III codes 0906T and 0907T have been established for reporting concurrent optical and magnetic stimulation (COMS) therapy, wound assessment, and dressing care. New guidelines have been added to define the treatment area as it applies to codes 0906T and 0907T.

Before the establishment of codes 0906T and 0907T, wound treatment was reported with codes, such as 97010, 97026, 97032, 97605-97608, and 97610. However, no codes existed to describe wound treatment using combined, concurrent optical and magnetic stimulation. COMS therapy may be used to treat wounds such as diabetic foot ulcers. The therapy is administered with the use of a device that provides optical stimulation for cell proliferation using low-energy light-emitting diodes and,

concurrently, provides magnetic stimulation for tissue perfusion by generating pulses of magnetic fields. Code 0906T is reported for the first application, with a total wound(s) surface area of less than or equal to 50 sq cm. Code 0907T is an add-on code reported with code 0906T for each additional application of COMS therapy, also with a total wound(s) surface area less than or equal to 50 sq cm. Wound assessment and dressing care are included in codes 0906T and 0907T.

Clinical Example (0906T)

A 67-year-old male, who has type 2 diabetes and chronic arterial insufficiency, presents with a nonhealing neuropathic diabetic ulcer on the right plantar forefoot. The patient is referred for concurrent optical and magnetic stimulation therapy.

Description of Procedure (0906T)

Remove existing bandages and thoroughly assess and clean the ulcer and periwound area. Ensure adequate hemostasis is achieved. Maneuver the patient's leg and foot to allow optimal positioning of the therapy device to the ulcer. Mount the therapy device to the patient coupler and position the therapy device–patient coupler against and directly over the patient's ulcer. Secure the therapy device–patient coupler in place using a hook-and-loop fixation strap. Initiate therapy. Remove the fixation strap and the therapy device-patient coupler when therapy is complete. Apply new wound dressings. Provide post-care instructions for ulcer cleansing and dressing changes.

Clinical Example (0907T)

A 67-year-old male, who has type 2 diabetes and chronic arterial insufficiency, has a nonhealing neuropathic diabetic ulcer on the left plantar forefoot that requires concurrent optical and magnetic stimulation therapy. [**Note:** This is an add-on code for the additional work related to an additional application of concurrent optical and magnetic stimulation {COMS} therapy, wound{s} surface area of less than or equal to 50 sq cm. The work related to the first application of COMS therapy is reported separately as the primary procedure and not included in the work of this add-on code.]

Description of Procedure (0907T)

Following the first application of COMS therapy, treat an additional wound by removing the bandage and cleansing the wound and periwound area. Place and secure the COMS therapy device at the patient's wound in position with a hook-and-loop fixation strap. Perform therapy and remove the device and strap when therapy is complete. Apply new wound dressings over the wound.

Category III 0042T-0713T

- **0908T**   Open implantation of integrated neurostimulation system, vagus nerve, including analysis and programming, when performed

  ▶(Do not report 0908T in conjunction with 64553, 64568, 0909T, 0910T, 0911T, 0912T)◀

- **0909T**   Replacement of integrated neurostimulation system, vagus nerve, including analysis and programming, when performed

  ▶(Do not report 0909T in conjunction with 64570, 0908T, 0910T, 0911T, 0912T)◀

- **0910T**   Removal of integrated neurostimulation system, vagus nerve

  ▶(Do not report 0910T in conjunction with 64570, 0908T, 0909T)◀

- **0911T**   Electronic analysis of implanted integrated neurostimulation system, vagus nerve; without programming by physician or other qualified health care professional

  ▶(Do not report 0911T in conjunction with 95970, 95971, 95972, 0908T, 0909T, 0912T)◀

- **0912T**   with simple programming by physician or other qualified health care professional

  ▶(Do not report 0912T in conjunction with 95970, 95971, 95972, 0908T, 0909T, 0911T)◀

Rationale

Codes 0908T-0912T have been established to report open implantation (0908T), replacement (0909T), removal (0910T), and electronic analysis (0911T, 0912T) of integrated neurostimulator systems for the vagus nerve. New parenthetical notes have also been added in the Extracranial Nerves, Peripheral Nerves, and Autonomic Nervous System subsection and the Category III section to accommodate the provision of instructions regarding the intended use of these codes.

Similar to other open integrated neurostimulator services, new codes have been included within the code set to specifically identify services for the use of integrated neurostimulators for the vagus nerve. As is true of other vagus nerve implantation and replacement procedures, programming performed during the procedure is inherently included as part of the service. As a result, language that specifies "programming" has been included in codes 0908T and 0909T. In addition, to further confirm the restriction of separate reporting of programming services for integrated neurostimulator systems of the vagus nerve (0911T, 0912T), exclusionary parenthetical notes have been included in the Category III section to restrict reporting implantation and replacement services in conjunction with programming performed on the same

date. This includes the exclusion of codes 64553 and 64568 because the vagus nerve is a cranial nerve. It also excludes reporting any other codes that may overlap with those inherently included within the new codes.

Clinical Example (0908T)

A 50-year-old female continues to experience painful and swollen joints in the hands and wrists with periodic flare-ups despite being on conventional and biologic disease-modifying antirheumatic drugs. She undergoes an open procedure to implant an integrated vagus nerve neurostimulator system.

Description of Procedure (0908T)

After the induction of general anesthesia, make an incision on the left side of the neck at the C4-C6 level over the sternocleidomastoid muscle. Carefully dissect soft tissue and fascia until the carotid sheath is exposed. Make a careful circumferential dissection of the surrounding tissue within the carotid sheath to expose the vagus nerve while minimizing manipulation of the nerve, carotid artery, or jugular vein. Confirm with a surgical ruler that at least 3 cm of nerve segment, free of branches, has been exposed to allow for manipulation and insertion of the positioning device and integrated neurostimulator. Hold the silicone positioning device open flat using curved forceps or similar surgical instruments to minimize its profile for positioning. Insert the positioning device under the vagus nerve, minimally touching the nerve. Once the positioning device is in place under the nerve, release the forceps to allow it to close around the vagus nerve. Insert the integrated neurostimulator device into the positioning device in the correct orientation and close the positioning device around the neurostimulator. Then suture and close the positioning device, taking care not to pull on the device or nerve. Visually confirm accurate device placement to ensure that the vagus nerve is not constricted by the positioning device or the integrated neurostimulator. Close the musculature, fascia, and skin with standard surgical closure and close the skin incision using cosmetic-closure techniques.

Clinical Example (0909T)

A 66-year-old female, who has an integrated vagus nerve neurostimulator, undergoes a procedure to replace the device because of the end of battery life.

Description of Procedure (0909T)

After the induction of general anesthesia, make an incision on the left ventral surface of the neck, and dissect the fascia and musculature to expose the positioning device. Remove the suture holding the positioning device, and hold the device open using curved forceps. Remove the neurostimulator from the positioning device, and inspect the positioning device for any damage. Replace it if the positioning device is damaged. Place a new neurostimulator inside the positioning device using forceps, and allow the positioning device to close around the vagus nerve and the new neurostimulator. Then suture and close the positioning device again, taking care not to pull on the device or nerve. Visually confirm accurate device placement and nerve positioning, and close the musculature, fascia, and skin with cosmetic-closure techniques.

Clinical Example (0910T)

A 63-year-old female who has an implanted integrated vagus nerve neurostimulator is not seeing improvement in her disease activity and continues to experience swollen and tender joints. She undergoes a procedure to remove the device.

Description of Procedure (0910T)

After the induction of general anesthesia, make a transverse incision on the left ventral surface of the neck, and incise the fascia and musculature to expose the positioning device. Remove the suture holding the implant in place and remove the neurostimulator from the positioning device. Cut the silicone positioning device in half and remove each half separately. Close the musculature, fascia, and skin with cosmetic-closure techniques.

Clinical Example (0911T)

A 45-year-old female, who has an implanted integrated vagus nerve neurostimulation system, returns to the clinic for device analysis without programming.

Description of Procedure (0911T)

Verify the patient-specific data in the programming application. Place the programming charger around the patient's neck, close the magnetic latch in the front, and connect the neurostimulator to the programming application. Perform electronic analysis of the implanted integrated neurostimulator (eg, dosing strength, schedule, battery health). Ensure that the parameters are captured in the patient's record. Remove the programming charger from the patient's neck without changing any program settings.

Clinical Example (0912T)

A 52-year-old patient who has an implanted integrated vagus nerve neurostimulation system returns to the clinic for a simple device programming.

Description of Procedure (0912T)

Verify the patient-specific data in the programming application. Place the programming charger around the patient's neck, close the magnetic latch in the front, and connect the neurostimulator to the programming application. Perform electronic analysis of the implanted integrated neurostimulator (eg, dosing strength, schedule, battery health). Change dose strength up or down on the programming application and then test for a minimum of 15 seconds to ensure the selected dose does not cause patient discomfort. Once optimal dosing is achieved, save it as a new prescription in the programming application, which is automatically communicated to the implanted device through the programming charger worn around the patient's neck. Save the program and remove the programming charger from the patient's neck.

▶Transcatheter Therapeutic Drug Delivery by Intracoronary Drug-Delivery Balloon◀

▶Codes 0913T, 0914T describe percutaneous coronary revascularization services by intracoronary antiproliferative drug delivery, performed for occlusive disease of the coronary vessels (major coronary arteries, coronary artery branches) using drug-delivery balloon (eg, drug-coated, drug-eluting) for intracoronary antiproliferative drug delivery. Code 0913T includes the work of accessing and selectively catheterizing the vessel, coronary angiography and intracoronary imaging (eg, intracoronary ultrasound, intracoronary optical coherence tomography) to guide the intervention, traversing the lesion, radiological supervision and interpretation directly related to the intervention(s) performed, closure of the arteriotomy when performed through the access sheath, and imaging performed to document completion of the intervention in addition to the intervention(s) performed. Code 0914T is an add-on code and includes only the coronary angiography and intracoronary imaging (eg, intracoronary ultrasound, intracoronary optical coherence tomography) to guide the additional intervention, traversing the additional lesion, and radiological supervision and interpretation directly related to the intervention(s) performed on the additional lesion. Codes 0913T, 0914T include mechanical dilation by nondrug-delivery balloon angioplasty followed by therapeutic drug delivery by drug-delivery balloon. Code 0913T may not be reported with 92920, 92924, 92928, 92933, 92937, 92941, 92943, 92973, 92978 for percutaneous coronary interventions (PCI) on the same target lesion in the same major coronary artery or graft as the drug-delivery balloon intervention. For drug delivery by intracoronary drug-delivery balloon (eg, drug-coated, drug-eluting) performed on a separate target lesion in the same major coronary artery or graft, 0914T may be reported for the separate target lesion in conjunction with 92920, 92924, 92928, 92933, 92937, 92941, 92943 for the first target lesion. For PCI in other major coronary arteries, see the appropriate PCI codes (92920, 92924, 92928, 92933, 92937, 92941, 92943, 0913T).

Diagnostic coronary angiography codes (93454, 93455, 93456, 93457, 93458, 93459, 93460, 93461) and injection procedure codes (93563, 93564) should not be used with percutaneous coronary revascularization services by intracoronary antiproliferative drug-delivery balloon services (0913T, 0914T) to report:

1. Contrast injections, angiography, roadmapping, and/ or fluoroscopic guidance for the coronary intervention,

2. Vessel measurement for the coronary intervention, or

3. Postcoronary intervention angiography, as this work is captured in the percutaneous coronary revascularization services by intracoronary antiproliferative drug-delivery balloon codes (0913T, 0914T).

Diagnostic angiography performed at the time of a coronary interventional procedure may be separately reportable, if:

1. No prior catheter-based coronary angiography study is available, and a full-diagnostic study is performed, and a decision to intervene is based on the diagnostic angiography, or

2. A prior study is available, but as documented in the medical record:

   a. The patient's condition with respect to the clinical indication has changed since the prior study, or

   b. The prior study provides inadequate visualization of the anatomy and/or pathology, or

   c. There is a clinical change during the procedure that requires new evaluation outside the target area of intervention.

Diagnostic coronary angiography performed at a separate session from an interventional procedure is separately reportable.◄

● **0913T** Percutaneous transcatheter therapeutic drug delivery by intracoronary drug-delivery balloon (eg, drug-coated, drug-eluting), including mechanical dilation by nondrug-delivery balloon angioplasty, endoluminal imaging using intravascular ultrasound (IVUS) or optical coherence tomography (OCT) when performed, imaging supervision, interpretation, and report, single major coronary artery or branch

▶(Do not report 0913T in conjunction with 92920, 92924, 92928, 92933, 92937, 92941, 92943, 92973, 92978, for interventions on the same target lesion in the same major coronary artery or graft as the target lesion treated with drug-delivery balloon intervention)◄

✚● **0914T** Percutaneous transcatheter therapeutic drug delivery by intracoronary drug-delivery balloon (eg, drug-coated, drug-eluting) performed on a separate target lesion from the target lesion treated with balloon angioplasty, coronary stent placement or coronary atherectomy, including mechanical dilation by nondrug-delivery balloon angioplasty, endoluminal imaging using intravascular ultrasound (IVUS) or optical coherence tomography (OCT) when performed, imaging supervision, interpretation, and report, single major coronary artery or branch (List separately in addition to code for percutaneous coronary stent or atherectomy intervention)

▶(Use 0914T in conjunction with 92920, 92924, 92928, 92933, 92937, 92941, 92943)◄

Rationale

For the CPT 2025, two Category III codes (0913T, 0914T) have been established to report percutaneous coronary intervention by therapeutic drug delivery as a new treatment for coronary artery disease. In addition to the two new codes, a new subsection heading titled "Transcatheter Therapeutic Drug Delivery by Intracoronary Drug-Delivery Balloon" and guidelines have been established to instruct users on the correct use of these codes. Other guidelines and parenthetical notes have been added and revised throughout the code set to accommodate the addition of the new codes and subsection.

These procedures differ from traditional coronary angioplasty, which centers around the mechanical dilation of an artery that may be accompanied by the insertion of a stent. The new codes focus on antiproliferative drug delivery directly into the coronary vessels using a balloon as the delivery mechanism.

To accommodate the addition of these codes, a new subsection and new guidelines have been added to provide instruction for users. This includes what services are inherently included (ie, always performed and therefore not separately reported) for both services in general, services that are included for each specific service, what restricts reporting, and other intervention methods.

Both codes 0913T and 0914T include all the services identified within the guidelines and code descriptors: mechanical dilation; catheterization to access the vessel and lesion; delivery of the drug to maintain patency of the vessel; and all imaging to guide and perform the procedure. Code 0913T is used for a single major coronary artery or branch of that artery, and add-on code 0914T is used for treatment of a separately targeted lesion done for a separate intervention. An exclusionary parenthetical note following code 0913T exemplifies this intent. In

Category III 0042T-0713T

addition, an instructional parenthetical note following code 0914T directs the use of this add-on code in conjunction with other coronary interventions.

Other parenthetical notes throughout the code set have been added or revised to convey the same instruction. This includes parenthetical notes instructing when the new codes may be reported in conjunction with other interventions (ie, when both are performed on different lesions) or when to restrict reporting, such as when the procedures are mutually exclusive (ie, when balloon drug delivery is chosen as the intervention method instead of another intervention method such as angioplasty or atherectomy for that lesion).

Clinical Example (0913T)

A 67-year-old male, who has a history of diabetes and underwent drug-eluting stent (DES) of the left anterior descending (LAD) artery 6 months ago, now presents with escalating angina. Coronary angiography demonstrates a focal 80% in-stent stenosis at the DES site. Drug-delivery balloon treatment with intravascular imaging of the in-stent restenosis is recommended.

Description of Procedure (0913T)

Obtain arterial access. Position a guide catheter in the left main coronary artery, and under fluoroscopic guidance, advance a steerable guidewire into the LAD artery, across and distal to the stenotic segment. Perform an intracoronary ultrasound of the target vessel. Assess the morphology of the stenotic lesion, measure the length of the stenotic lesion within the stent, and determine the reference vessel diameters of the coronary artery. Perform lesion preparation using traditional balloon angioplasty, typically involving repeated balloon inflations, deflations, and reinflation at progressively higher pressures to mechanically dilate the vessel to gain maximal lumen area before therapeutic drug delivery by balloon. Perform intracoronary ultrasound imaging again to confirm adequate mechanical lesion preparation within the stent and ensure no significant stenoses proximal to the target lesion would compromise the drug-delivery balloon coating during delivery. Calculate the precise measurement of the drug-delivery balloon treatment area and select an appropriate-sized drug-delivery balloon to ensure contact with the vessel wall. Advance the drug-delivery balloon to the stenotic lesion while preventing delamination of the drug-coating. Hold the inflated drug-delivery balloon in place during the drug-delivery transfer process, continuously occluding blood flow. Assess patient vitals, including chest pain, electrocardiogram, hemodynamics, and blood pressure, for signs of ischemia or arrhythmia, which may occur during the purposeful prolonged continuous occlusion of the vessel by the inflated drug-delivery balloon. Confirm

vessel patency following the completion of the drug-transfer process, and withdraw the drug-delivery balloon. Perform intravascular imaging and angiography confirmation, remove the guidewire, and close the arterial access site. Send the patient to the recovery area.

Clinical Example (0914T)

A 76-year-old male, who has obesity, presents with accelerated angina consistent with acute coronary syndrome. Coronary angiography demonstrates multiple 80% lesions at the ostium and distal segment of the circumflex coronary artery. Proximal lesion stent placement and distal lesion drug-coated balloon treatment are performed guided by intravascular imaging. [**Note:** This is an add-on code. Only consider the additional work related to the percutaneous transcatheter therapeutic drug delivery by intracoronary drug-delivery balloon {eg, drug- coated, drug-eluting}.]

Description of Procedure (0914T)

Following coronary stent placement (separately reported), perform an intracoronary ultrasound of the target vessel. Assess the morphology of the stenotic lesion, measure the length of the stenotic lesion within the stent, and determine the reference vessel diameters of the coronary artery. Perform lesion preparation using traditional balloon angioplasty, typically involving repeated balloon inflations, deflations, and reinflation at progressively higher pressures to mechanically dilate the vessel to gain maximal lumen area before therapeutic drug delivery by balloon. Perform intracoronary ultrasound imaging again to confirm adequate mechanical lesion preparation within the stent and ensure no significant stenoses proximal to the target lesion would compromise the drug-delivery balloon coating during delivery. Calculate precise measurement of the drug-delivery balloon treatment area and select an appropriate-sized drug-delivery balloon to ensure contact with the vessel wall. Advance the drug-delivery balloon to the stenotic lesion while preventing delamination of the drug-coating. Hold the inflated drug-delivery balloon in place during the drug-delivery transfer process, continuously occluding blood flow. Assess patient vitals, including chest pain, electrocardiogram, hemodynamics, and blood pressure, for signs of ischemia or arrhythmia, which may occur during the purposeful prolonged continuous occlusion of the vessel by the inflated drug-delivery balloon. Confirm vessel patency following the completion of the drug-transfer process, and withdraw the drug-delivery balloon. Perform intravascular imaging and angiography confirmation.

★ = Telemedicine   ◀ = Add-on code   ✚ = Add-on code   ✗ = FDA approval pending   # = Resequenced code   ⊘ = Modifier 51 exempt

►Cardiac Contractility Modulation-Defibrillation◄

►A cardiac contractility modulation-defibrillation (CCM-D) system combines cardiac contractility modulation (CCM) for symptom relief from chronic heart failure with defibrillation protection against sudden cardiac arrhythmia into a single therapy. A CCM-D system consists of a pulse generator and two transvenous electrodes (leads): one defibrillation lead and one pacemaker lead. An implantable CCM-D system's electrodes (leads) are placed transvenously under fluoroscopic guidance. One right ventricular pacing lead is placed on the high septum and a second defibrillation lead is placed in the mid-septum. The pulse generator is implanted in a subcutaneous pocket in the pectoral region.

A CCM-D differs from a CCM system (0408T-0418T). A CCM system consists of a pulse generator and two ventricular pacemaker electrodes (leads) and does not include a defibrillator component. Do not report CCM-D services in conjunction with 0408T-0418T. All services associated with CCM-D implantation, revision, extraction, and follow-up should be reported utilizing Category III codes 0915T-0931T. Do not report CCM-D services with existing Category I codes for pacemaker and defibrillator services (33206-33275).

All catheterization and imaging guidance required to complete a CCM-D procedure are included in the work of each code. Contractility evaluation and programming of sensing and therapeutic parameters (0926T, 0927T) are performed each time a pulse generator or lead is implanted or replaced and cannot be reported separately.

For the implantation of a CCM-D system (generator plus dual leads), report 0915T. If only a pulse generator is implanted without insertion of transvenous electrodes, report 0916T for the implantation or 0923T for the removal and replacement. When CCM-D leads are placed without insertion of a pulse generator, report 0917T for a single-lead insertion or 0918T when both leads are inserted.

In certain circumstances, relocation of the skin pocket is required and is reported using 0925T. Skin pocket relocation includes all services associated with the initial pocket (eg, opening the pocket, incision and drainage of hematoma or abscess if performed, and any closure performed), in addition to the creation of a new pocket for the new generator to be placed.◄

● **0915T** Insertion of permanent cardiac contractility modulation-defibrillation system component(s), including fluoroscopic guidance, and evaluation and programming of sensing and therapeutic parameters; pulse generator and dual transvenous electrodes/leads (pacing and defibrillation)

● **0916T** pulse generator only

● **0917T** single transvenous lead (pacing or defibrillation) only

● **0918T** dual transvenous leads (pacing and defibrillation) only

►(Do not report 0915T, 0916T, 0917T, 0918T in conjunction with 33206-33275, 0926T, 0927T, 0931T)◄

►(Do not report 0916T, 0917T, 0918T in conjunction with 0915T)◄

● **0919T** Removal of a permanent cardiac contractility modulation-defibrillation system component(s); pulse generator only

►(Do not report 0919T in conjunction with 33206-33275, 0915T, 0916T, 0923T, 0925T, 0926T, 0927T, 0931T)◄

● **0920T** single transvenous pacing lead only

● **0921T** single transvenous defibrillation lead only

● **0922T** dual (pacing and defibrillation) transvenous leads only

►(Do not report 0920T, 0921T, 0922T in conjunction with 33206-33275, 0926T, 0927T, 0931T)◄

● **0923T** Removal and replacement of permanent cardiac contractility modulation-defibrillation pulse generator only

►(Do not report 0923T in conjunction with 33206-33275, 0915T, 0916T, 0919T, 0925T, 0926T, 0927T, 0931T)◄

● **0924T** Repositioning of previously implanted cardiac contractility modulation-defibrillation transvenous electrode(s)/lead(s), including fluoroscopic guidance and programming of sensing and therapeutic parameters

►(Do not report 0924T in conjunction with 33206-33275, 0915T, 0926T, 0927T, 0931T)◄

● **0925T** Relocation of skin pocket for implanted cardiac contractility modulation-defibrillation pulse generator

►(Do not report 0925T in conjunction with 10140, 10180, 11042, 11043, 11044, 11045, 11046, 11047, 13100, 13101, 13102, 33206-33275, 0915T, 0916T, 0919T, 0923T, 0931T)◄

● **0926T** Programming device evaluation (in person) with iterative adjustment of the implantable device to test the function of the device and select optimal permanent programmed values with analysis, including review and report, implantable cardiac contractility modulation-defibrillation system

►(Do not report 0926T in conjunction with 33206-33275, 0915T, 0916T, 0917T, 0918T, 0919T, 0920T, 0921T, 0922T, 0923T, 0924T, 0927T, 0930T, 0931T)◄

● **0927T** Interrogation device evaluation (in person) with analysis, review, and report, including connection, recording, and disconnection, per patient encounter, implantable cardiac contractility modulation-defibrillation system

►(Do not report 0927T in conjunction with 33206-33275, 0915T, 0916T, 0917T, 0918T, 0919T, 0920T, 0921T, 0922T, 0923T, 0924T, 0926T, 0930T, 0931T)◄

- **0928T** Interrogation device evaluation (remote), up to 90 days, cardiac contractility modulation-defibrillation system with interim analysis and report(s) by a physician or other qualified health care professional

  ▶(Do not report 0928T in conjunction with 33206-33275)◀

- **0929T** Interrogation device evaluation (remote), up to 90 days, cardiac contractility modulation-defibrillation system, remote data acquisition(s), receipt of transmissions, technician review, technical support, and distribution of results

  ▶(Do not report 0929T in conjunction with 33206-33275)◀

- **0930T** Electrophysiologic evaluation of cardiac contractility modulation-defibrillator leads, including defibrillation-threshold evaluation (induction of arrhythmia, evaluation of sensing and therapy for arrhythmia termination), at time of initial implantation or replacement with testing of cardiac contractility modulation-defibrillator pulse generator

  ▶(Do not report 0930T in conjunction with 33206-33275, 0931T)◀

- **0931T** Electrophysiologic evaluation of cardiac contractility modulation-defibrillator leads, including defibrillation-threshold evaluation (induction of arrhythmia, evaluation of sensing and therapy for arrhythmia termination), separate from initial implantation or replacement with testing of cardiac contractility modulation-defibrillator pulse generator

  ▶(Do not report 0931T in conjunction with 33206-33275, 0915T-0927T, 0930T)◀

Rationale

Seventeen Category III codes (0915T-0931T) have been established to report cardiac contractility modulation-defibrillation (CCM-D) services. A new subsection with guidelines have been added in the Category III section titled "Cardiac Contractility Modulation-Defibrillation," and existing guidelines in the Pacemaker or Implantable Defibrillator subsection have been revised to direct users to report the new codes. In addition, multiple parenthetical notes have been added and revised throughout the code set to accommodate these new codes and subsection.

The existing CPT codes within the code set identify either pacemaker services or defibrillator services and include all work necessary for the placement, removal, repositioning, and programming (when separately performed) of any and all components that compose these devices. Codes 0915T-0931T are different because they represent cardiac contractility modulation and cardiac defibrillation. As a result, the work required for these devices is different, and the new Category III codes have been included to

enable separate reporting for CCM-D from existing pacemaker services and defibrillator services for the heart.

The changes include: (1) codes for the placement of the complete or individual components of CCM-D (0915T-0918T); (2) efforts involved in reporting the removal of any or all components (0919T-0922T); (3) efforts to replace only the pulse generator (0923T); (4) efforts for repositioning the previously implanted transvenous electrode(s)/lead(s), which includes any guidance and programming of sensing and therapeutic parameters needed to treat the patient (0924T); (5) relocation of the pulse generator skin pocket (0925T); (6) programming, with iterative adjustment and function testing of the device performed independently of the initial device placement (0926T); (7) in-person (0927T), remote (0928T) or remote with technical support (0929T) device interrogation evaluation; and (8) electrophysiologic evaluation of the CCM-D defibrillation-threshold performed either at the time of the initial implantation or replacement (0930T) or performed separately from the initial implantation or replacement (0931T).

Introductory guidelines have been established to define CCM-D services, identify components of the CCM-D device, and assist users in understanding the work included and how to report these services. This includes specific instruction regarding services that are inherently included, such as catheterization, imaging guidance, and specific programming. It also includes a description of all work associated with skin pocket relocation (0925T).

Multiple exclusionary parenthetical notes have been included throughout the section to restrict reporting redundant or otherwise excluded services. This includes instruction that restricts reporting electrophysiologic evaluation of CCM-D for defibrillation-threshold evaluation in conjunction with any pacemaker services. However, the exclusionary parenthetical note following code 0930T does not restrict reporting code 0915T because defibrillation-threshold evaluation is not always performed on the same day.

Clinical Example (0915T)

A 65-year-old male presents with stage C heart failure with an ejection fraction of 35% and without indication for cardiac resynchronization therapy. He is scheduled for a new cardiac contractility modulation-defibrillation system implantation.

Description of Procedure (0915T)

Monitor, prepare, and sedate the patient. Inject local anesthetic, and make an incision below either the right or left clavicle. Create a device pocket. Access the venous system. Insert the implantable cardioverter-defibrillator and pacing leads into the venous system and pass into the right ventricle under fluoroscopic guidance. Position the leads, test for appropriate function, and reposition if needed. Attach a cardiac contractility modulation-defibrillation generator to the leads. Place the pulse generator and leads in the device pocket. Test the leads through the generator. Close the incision and dress the wound.

Clinical Example (0916T)

A 65-year-old female presents for a cardiac contractility modulation-defibrillation (CCM-D) system implantation. The patient has existing therapy-delivery leads; however, the pulse generator device was previously removed to allow for radiation-therapy delivery, and it needs to be implanted.

Description of Procedure (0916T)

Monitor, prepare, and sedate the patient. Inject local anesthetic, and make an incision below either the right or left clavicle. Create a device pocket, and access and uncap the leads. Attach the CCM-D generator to the leads. Place the pulse generator and leads in the device pocket. Test the leads through the generator. Close the incision and dress the wound.

Clinical Example (0917T)

A 65-year-old male, who has a cardiac contractility modulation-defibrillation (CCM-D) system, presents with the CCM-D's system whose right ventricular pacing electrode no longer functions properly and requires a new electrode implant.

Description of Procedure (0917T)

Monitor, prepare, and sedate the patient. Inject local anesthetic, and make an incision below either the right or left clavicle. Then make an incision in the area of the existing device pocket. Open the device pocket and access the venous system. Insert and pass the right ventricular lead into the right ventricle under fluoroscopic guidance. Position the lead, test for appropriate function, and reposition if needed. Attach the existing CCM-D generator to the leads. Place the pulse generator and leads in the device pocket. Test the leads through the generator. Close the incision and dress the wound.

Clinical Example (0918T)

A 65-year-old male, who has a cardiac contractility modulation-defibrillation (CCM-D) system, was assessed and it was noted that neither leads functioned properly and two new leads will need to be inserted.

Description of Procedure (0918T)

Monitor, prepare, and sedate the patient. Inject local anesthetic, and make an incision below either the right or left clavicle. Then make an incision in the area of the existing device pocket. Open the device pocket and access the venous system. (Note that the removal of the two defective leads is reported separately and is not part of the services of code 0918T.) Sequentially insert and pass two leads into the right ventricle under fluoroscopic guidance. Position the leads, test for appropriate function, and reposition if needed. Connect the new leads to the existing CCM-D generator.

Clinical Example (0919T)

A 65-year-old male who has a cardiac contractility modulation-defibrillation system presents to have the generator removed for radiation-therapy delivery to the pectoral region in which the device resides.

Description of Procedure (0919T)

Monitor, prepare, and sedate the patient. Inject local anesthetic. Make an incision in the area of the existing device pocket. Remove the generator from the device pocket and disconnect the leads. Close the incision and dress the wound.

Clinical Example (0920T)

A 65-year-old male, who has a cardiac contractility modulation-defibrillation system, presents with a right ventricular pacing lead that has malfunctioned and requires extraction.

Description of Procedure (0920T)

Monitor, prepare, and sedate the patient. Inject local anesthetic. Make an incision in the area of the existing device pocket. Disconnect the pacing lead from the generator, and extract and remove from the heart and venous system. Close the incision and dress the wound.

Clinical Example (0921T)

A 65-year-old male, who has a cardiac contractility modulation-defibrillation system, presents with a right ventricular defibrillation lead that has malfunctioned and requires extraction.

Description of Procedure (0921T)

Monitor, prepare, and sedate the patient. Inject local anesthetic. Make an incision in the area of the existing device pocket. Disconnect the defibrillation lead from the generator, and extract and remove from the heart and venous system. Close the incision and dress the wound.

▲ = Revised code   ● = New code   ▶◀ = Contains new or revised text   ✷ = Duplicate PLA test   ↕ = Category I PLA   American Medical Association   **185**

Category III 0042T-0713T

Clinical Example (0922T)

A 65-year-old male, who a cardiac contractility modulation-defibrillation system, presents with both right ventricular leads (pacing and defibrillation) that have malfunctioned and require extraction.

Description of Procedure (0922T)

Monitor, prepare, and sedate the patient. Inject local anesthetic. Make an incision in the area of the existing device pocket. Then disconnect the pacing and defibrillation leads from the generator, and extract and remove both leads from the heart and venous system. Close the incision and dress the wound.

Clinical Example (0923T)

A 65-year-old male who has a cardiac contractility modulation-defibrillation system presents with a generator that needs to be replaced because of the end of battery life.

Description of Procedure (0923T)

Monitor, prepare, and sedate the patient. Inject local anesthetic. Make an incision in the area of the existing device pocket. Then remove the generator from the device pocket and disconnect the leads. Insert a new generator and connect to the leads. Close the incision and dress the wound.

Clinical Example (0924T)

A 65-year-old male who has a cardiac contractility modulation-defibrillation (CCM-D) system presents with a right ventricular pacing electrode that has dislodged and requires repositioning.

Description of Procedure (0924T)

Monitor, prepare, and sedate the patient. Inject local anesthetic. Make an incision in the area of the existing device pocket. Then remove the generator from the device pocket and disconnect the leads. Under fluoroscopic guidance, retract the fixation mechanism of the pacing lead, if required, and place a stylet in the lumen of the lead. Reposition the lead in the right ventricle, test for appropriate function, and reposition again if necessary. Attach a CCM-D generator to the leads. Place the pulse generator and leads in the device pocket. Test the leads through the generator. Close the incision and dress the wound.

Clinical Example (0925T)

A 65-year-old male, who has a cardiac contractility modulation-defibrillation system, presents with a device pocket that requires relocation because of the patient's significant weight loss.

Description of Procedure (0925T)

Monitor, prepare, and sedate the patient. Inject local anesthetic. Make an incision in the area of the existing device pocket. Then remove the generator from the device pocket and disconnect the leads. Create a new device pocket. Attach a CCM-D generator to the leads. Place the pulse generator and leads in the device pocket. Test the leads through the generator. Close the incision and dress the wound.

Clinical Example (0926T)

A 65-year-old male, who has a cardiac contractility modulation-defibrillation (CCM-D) system, presents to the office for a routine follow-up to assess device functionality.

Description of Procedure (0926T)

Seat and connect the patient to external electrocardiogram (ECG) monitoring equipment. Position the telemetry wand from the programmer over the CCM-D device and establish telemetry. The physician or other qualified health care professional performs tests on sensing and therapeutic CCM-D parameters. If necessary, make and document permanent programming changes to the CCM-D device. Discontinue telemetry between the CCM-D device and programmer. Disconnect the patient if he is connected to an external ECG monitoring equipment.

Clinical Example (0927T)

A 65-year-old male, who has a cardiac contractility modulation-defibrillation (CCM-D) system, presents to the operating room for an unrelated procedure, and the operator wishes to confirm device settings.

Description of Procedure (0927T)

Position the telemetry wand from the programmer over the CCM-D device, and establish telemetry. The physician or other qualified health care professional confirms the programmed parameters for the device. Discontinue telemetry between the CCM-D device and programmer.

★=Telemedicine ◀=Add-on code ✛=Add-on code ⁄=FDA approval pending #=Resequenced code ⊘=Modifier 51 exempt

Clinical Example (0928T)

A 65-year-old male, who has a cardiac contractility modulation-defibrillation system, is monitored with interrogation device evaluations (remote) of the pulse generator from the patient's home for device functionality and performance.

Description of Procedure (0928T)

The physician or other qualified health care professional (QHP) either obtains the report prepared by a device follow-up professional or logs into the online remote follow-up portal and selects the appropriate patient. The physician or other QHP assesses the findings. If any abnormalities are observed, the physician or other QHP arranges for the appropriate programming changes to be made.

Clinical Example (0929T)

A 65-year-old male, who has a cardiac contractility modulation-defibrillation system, is monitored with interrogation device evaluations (remote) of the pulse generator from the patient's home for device functionality and performance.

Description of Procedure (0929T)

A device follow-up professional logs into the online remote follow-up portal and selects the appropriate patient. The device follow-up professional acquires all data required to assess the functionality of the device, including any stored diagnostics. The device follow-up professional prepares the material in a format that enables a physician or other qualified health care professional to review them.

Clinical Example (0930T)

A 65-year-old male, who has an ischemic cardiomyopathy and heart failure, undergoes the implantation of a cardiac contractility modulation device. After implantation, while still in the operating room, the decision is made to perform a defibrillation efficacy assessment to ensure appropriate sensing of ventricular fibrillation and termination through the device.

Description of Procedure (0930T)

Patient is sedated while he is still in the operating room for the implant or replacement of the cardiac contractility modulation therapy device. Induce ventricular fibrillation through the device. Allow the device to detect the tachycardia and then deliver defibrillation energy to terminate the arrhythmia. Perform external defibrillation if the device

unsuccessfully terminates the arrhythmia. To assess device reliability, multiple inductions of ventricular fibrillation and defibrillation may be necessary.

Clinical Example (0931T)

A 65-year-old male, who has an ischemic cardiomyopathy and heart failure, underwent implantation of a cardiac contractility modulation device 6 months ago. There has been a change in the defibrillation lead impedance, and the decision has been made to perform defibrillation efficacy testing to ensure detection reliability and treatment of ventricular fibrillation through the device.

Description of Procedure (0931T)

Sedate the patient. Induce ventricular fibrillation through the device. Allow the device to detect the tachycardia and then deliver defibrillation energy to terminate the arrhythmia. Perform external defibrillation if the device unsuccessfully terminates the arrhythmia. To assess device reliability, multiple inductions of ventricular fibrillation and defibrillation may be necessary.

● **0932T** Noninvasive detection of heart failure derived from augmentative analysis of an echocardiogram that demonstrated preserved ejection fraction, with interpretation and report by a physician or other qualified health care professional

▶(Use 0932T in conjunction with a concurrent echocardiography [separately reported] or a previously performed transthoracic echocardiography [ie, 93306, 93307, 93308, 93350, 93351])◀

Rationale

Category III code 0932T has been established to report noninvasive detection of heart failure derived from augmentative analysis of an ECG that demonstrated preserved ejection fraction (pEF), with interpretation and report by a physician or other QHP.

This procedure uses an AI platform to analyze ECG data to assess heart failure with preserved ejection fraction. pEF is a type of heart failure that occurs when the heart's left ventricle pumps less blood than the body needs, despite a normal or near-normal EF of at least 50%. The ventricle is unable to fill with blood properly during the diastolic (filling) phase because it is too stiff to relax. The analysis allows physicians or other QHPs to accurately identify patients with this type of heart failure by analyzing the ECG data and providing a probability score.

A cross-reference parenthetical note following code 0932T has been added to provide instructions that it may be separately reported from a concurrently performed ECG procedure or previously performed transthoracic echocardiography (ie, 93306-93308, 93350, 93351) when these separate procedures are performed.

Clinical Example (0932T)

A 67-year-old female presents with dyspnea and hypertension. The physician or other qualified health care professional (QHP) orders an echocardiogram to evaluate potential heart failure. Upon interpreting the echocardiogram and reviewing the patient's symptoms and history, the ejection fraction (EF) is measured at 58%; thus, excluding heart failure with reduced EF. The physician or other QHP orders noninvasive detection of heart failure derived from analysis of an echocardiogram with preserved EF.

Description of Procedure (0932T)

The physician, other QHP, or clinical staff uploads the echocardiogram's apical 4-chamber view onto a secure cloud-based platform. The platform receives the data and performs several steps to provide an assessment of heart failure, including (i) automatically preprocessing each apical 4-chamber view; (ii) generating a convolutional neural network to derive a final prediction score based on a quantitative probability threshold; and (iii) calculating the probability of the classification. Machine output includes a standard message capture that is appended to the original echocardiogram. The image displays the provided apical 4-chamber view with the patient's vitals (age, sex, height, weight, and heart rate) along with one of the following outputs: (a) is suggestive of heart failure; (b) is not suggestive of heart failure; or (c) did not meet the pre-defined artificial intelligence certainty threshold. The physician or other QHP reviews the probability score, reassesses the previously acquired echocardiogram with the patient's history, interprets the findings, and documents a report.

● **0933T** Transcatheter implantation of wireless left atrial pressure sensor for long-term left atrial pressure monitoring, including sensor calibration and deployment, right heart catheterization, transseptal puncture, imaging guidance, and radiological supervision and interpretation

▶(Do not report 0933T in conjunction with 33289, 36013, 36014, 36015, 75741, 75743, 75746, 76000, 93451, 93453, 93456, 93457, 93460, 93461, 93568, 93569, 93573, 93593, 93594, 93596, 93597, 93598)◀

▶(For implantation of a wireless pulmonary artery pressure sensor, use 33289)◀

● **0934T** Remote monitoring of a wireless left atrial pressure sensor for up to 30 days, including data from daily uploads of left atrial pressure recordings, interpretation(s) and trend analysis, with adjustments to the diuretics plan, treatment paradigm thresholds, medications or lifestyle modifications, when performed, and report(s) by a physician or other qualified health care professional

▶(Report 0934T only once per 30 days)◀

▶(Do not report 0934T, if monitoring period is less than 16 days)◀

▶(Do not report 0934T in conjunction with 93264)◀

▶(For remote monitoring of an implantable wireless pulmonary artery pressure sensor, use 93264)◀

Rationale

Category III codes 0933T and 0934T have been established to report the transcatheter implantation of a wireless left atrial pressure sensor (0933T) and the remote service for measuring and monitoring left atrial pressures (0934T). In addition, parenthetical notes have been added to reflect the addition of the new codes.

Code 0933T is intended to report the implantation of a wireless left atrial pressure sensor in patients with persistent symptoms of heart failure. Implantation involves transcatheter placement of the sensor using right heart catheterization to access the left atrium and includes transseptal puncture. The procedure also includes the deployment of the sensor and any necessary imaging guidance and radiological supervision and interpretation. The procedure represented by code 0934T involves continuous monitoring and interpretation of left atrial pressure data from a wireless left atrial pressure sensor in patients with, for example, heart failure, preserved left ventricular EF, and mild renal insufficiency, allowing for adjustments in treatment based on trends and changes in pressure readings.

In accordance with the establishment of codes 0933T and 0934T, cross-reference parenthetical notes have been added following codes 33289 and 93264; cross-reference and exclusionary parenthetical notes have been added following codes 0933T and 0934T; and the Surgery and Medicine sections instruct users regarding the frequency of reporting; services that are inherently included as part of the service; and how to report other similar services.

Clinical Example (0933T)

A 67-year-old male, who had previous multiple hospitalizations for decompensated heart failure and persistent New York Heart Association functional classification III symptoms, was identified as a patient eligible to receive an implantable left atrial pressure monitoring device.

Description of Procedure (0933T)

Perform implant calibration before the implantation. While the implant remains in sterile conditions, implement an offset update, if needed. Prepare the patient per standard catheterization laboratory practice for right heart catheterization with wedge pressure measurements. Under visualization, obtain percutaneous venous access through the right femoral vein and perform transseptal puncture within the fossa ovalis. Replace the transseptal sheath with a 12-French vessel introducer sheath over an access guidewire. Verify the position across the fossa ovalis and flush the delivery system continuously through both flushing ports. Connect the delivery system to the sheath, insert it until it reaches the stopper, and then retract the system. Using echocardiography and fluoroscopy, insert the delivery system until the implant is revealed in the left atrium. Retract and anchor the distal disc in the left septum. Rotate and anchor the proximal disc into the right atrium. Verify the position using echocardiography and fluoroscopy. Remove the delivery system and obtain hemostasis per standard of care.

Clinical Example (0934T)

A 69-year-old male, who has heart failure, preserved left ventricular ejection fraction, and mild renal insufficiency with an implanted left atrial pressure (LAP) monitoring system, undergoes continued monitoring.

Description of Procedure (0934T)

The physician interprets data and analyzes trends and changes in daily and mean LAP readings, including trends and changes in LAP waveform, from daily uploaded data during the 30-day period. Evaluate symptomatic and asymptomatic events with abnormal LAP, and make any necessary adjustments in the diuretics plan, treatment paradigm thresholds, and/or medications or lifestyle modifications, as needed.

● **0935T**   Cystourethroscopy with renal pelvic sympathetic denervation, radiofrequency ablation, retrograde ureteral approach, including insertion of guide wire, selective placement of ureteral sheath(s) and multiple conformable electrodes, contrast injection(s), and fluoroscopy, bilateral

▶(Do not report 0935T in conjunction with 52000, 52005, 76000, 0338T, 0339T)◀

Rationale

New Category III code 0935T has been established to report cystourethroscopy with renal pelvic sympathetic denervation. To support the addition of this new code, two parenthetical notes have been revised and added in the Cystoscopy, Urethroscopy, Cystourethroscopy subsection in the Urinary System section to clarify the appropriate reporting of this new code.

Code 0935T describes treatment for conditions such as uncontrolled hypertension by renal nerve denervation. This is accomplished by ablating the afferent and efferent nerve fibers located in the renal pelvis that affect hypertension. A cystoscopy accesses the renal pelvis and delivers radiofrequency energy directly inside the pelvis, where afferent and efferent nerve fibers also exist. This accesses nerves beyond those that may be treated when the treatment is administered through vascular access of the adjacent afferent and efferent nerve fibers that are the focus of the treatment.

To support the addition of this new code, two parenthetical notes have been added to restrict reporting other cystourethroscopy (52000, 52005), imaging (76000), and denervation (0338T, 0339T) procedures. In addition, an existing exclusionary parenthetical note following code 52000 has been revised to list additional codes that include cystourethroscopy (57240, 57260, 57265, 0935T).

Clinical Example (0935T)

A 72-year-old female, who has a two-year history of hypertension, was initially placed on two antihypertensive medications but has become progressively refractory to treatment. Despite maximum dosing and the addition of a third medication, her recent mean 24-hour blood pressure (BP) monitoring shows a systolic BP of 170 mm Hg and diastolic BP of 110 mm Hg. After discussing further options, she decides to proceed with renal pelvic sympathetic denervation.

Description of Procedure (0935T)

Take the patient to the operating room and the urologist places her in the lithotomy position. Pass a cystoscope into the bladder and pass a guidewire up the right ureter and into the renal pelvis. Pass an 8-French ureteral sheath with obturator over the guidewire and position it at the level just below the ureteropelvic junction. Remove the obturator and inject contrast to demonstrate the renal pelvis. Pass the ablation device through the sheath into the renal pelvis and deploy it. The device consists of four spherical electrodes on a nitinol helix that is designed to expand into the renal pelvis and abut the urothelial lining while also monitoring surface temperatures. After fluoroscopic confirmation of the

Category III   0042T-0713T

device's correct position, connect the device to the low-power, radiofrequency generator, which delivers up to 30 watts of power via the ablative device. Activate radiofrequency ablation and deliver energy by increasing the temperature to 60°C and maintaining that temperature for the required ablation period. Upon completion of the ablation, remove the device and sheath and perform the exact same procedure on the contralateral side. After both sides are treated, take the patient to the recovery room.

● **0936T** Photobiomodulation therapy of retina, single session

▶(For bilateral procedure, report 0936T with modifier 50)◀

Rationale

Category III code 0936T has been established to report photobiomodulation therapy of the retina. This procedure involves photobiomodulation treatment for patients who have conditions, such as dry age-related macular degeneration and vision loss, and includes all the therapy necessary for a single session.

A parenthetical note has been added to provide instructions regarding how to report the service when it is performed on both eyes.

In accordance with the establishment of code 0936T, a cross-reference parenthetical note has been added following code 67729 to direct users to the new code.

Clinical Example (0936T)

A 67-year-old female patient presents with dry age-related macular degeneration in both eyes. The patient has some vision loss.

Description of Procedure (0936T)

Seat the patient in front of the light-delivery system in the physician's office. Treat the eye with photobiomodulation for 4 to 5 minutes.

● **0937T** External electrocardiographic recording for greater than 15 days up to 30 days by continuous rhythm recording and storage; including recording, scanning analysis with report, review and interpretation by a physician or other qualified health care professional

● **0938T** recording (including connection and initial recording)

● **0939T** scanning analysis with report

● **0940T** review and interpretation by a physician or other qualified health care professional

▶(Report 0937T, 0938T, 0939T, 0940T for each 30-day period of service)◀

▶(Do not report 0938T, 0939T, 0940T in conjunction with 0937T)◀

▶(Do not report 0937T, 0938T, 0939T, 0940T in conjunction with 93224, 93225, 93226, 93227, 93228, 93229, 93241, 93242, 93243, 93244, 93245, 93246, 93247, 93248, 93268, 93270, 93271, 93272, 99091, 99453, 99454, for the same monitoring period)◀

Rationale

New codes and parenthetical notes have been added and existing parenthetical notes have been revised to accommodate reporting external electrocardiographic recording services of greater than 15 to 30 days by continuous rhythm recording and storage.

Codes 0937T-0940T have been established for reporting external electrocardiographic recording services that last more than 15 days and may record up to 30 days continuously. These new codes are important, because services identified by other codes within the code set may only be used for external electrocardiographic device recordings that last for a shorter period of time (eg, devices that record up to 48 hours [93224]). In addition, other services may include more than just electrocardiographic recording services, such as concurrent computerized real-time data analysis and remote attendance surveillance that may be patient- or ECG-triggered (eg, 93228) and are therefore not appropriate for reporting these non-monitored services. Externally worn ambulatory cardiac monitoring devices present challenges for monitoring that do not exist for long-term monitoring services. Shorter-term, external devices use electroconductive gel and adhesives for the electrodes that limit the total potential monitoring time that a patient may wear the device due to the eventual development of skin irritation. Improvements in technology regarding the electrodes that may be used for these external electrocardiographic monitoring devices have extended the time that these devices may be used and, therefore, enable extended data collection for the analysis of cardiovascular issues that may exist.

Code 0937T identifies the complete external electrocardiographic monitoring service and includes recording, scanning analysis with report, and review and interpretation by the physician or other QHP. Codes 0938T-0940T are used to report these services independently. Because code 0937T describes the complete service, it may not be reported separately from any of its component services. As a result, exclusionary parenthetical notes that follow codes 0937T-0940T restrict reporting the component codes (0938T-0940T) in conjunction with the complete service (0937T). In addition, because electrocardiographic monitoring services are commonly mutually exclusive, parenthetical notes have been added and other parenthetical notes revised throughout the code set to restrict reporting the new codes in conjunction with other codes that either describe different types of electrocardiographic monitoring or that already include it as part of the service. Finally, because these external electrocardiographic recording services identify cardiac monitoring that may occur over a 30-day period, an instructional parenthetical note directs users to report these codes only once during that period.

Clinical Example (0937T)

A 72-year-old female presents with a prior neurologic ischemic episode but no prior history of atrial fibrillation. The physician decides to proceed with long-term (greater than 15 days, up to 30 days) external electrocardiographic recording to evaluate for possible paroxysmal atrial fibrillation.

Description of Procedure (0937T)

Clinical staff applies the monitor on the patient's arm and verifies/records the initial signal quality. Provide the patient with education regarding the ongoing monitoring instructions that include marking (tagging) events and caring for the device. Perform an electrocardiogram (ECG) recording for 30 days by continuous recording and storage. The device periodically transmits the full-disclosure ECG recordings to a secure computing cloud for algorithmic assessment. An independent technician performs a comprehensive analysis of the ECG signal data and creates a summary report. The physician reviews and interprets the report, including (1) heart rate trends (minimum, maximum, average); (2) tabular summary of supraventricular and ventricular ectopy; (3) tachyarrhythmia and bradyarrhythmia verified by the technician; and (4) symptomatic events identified (tagged) by the patient to assess the heart rhythm at those times.

Clinical Example (0938T)

A 72-year-old female presents with a prior neurologic ischemic episode but no prior history of atrial fibrillation. The physician decides to proceed with long-term (greater than 15 days, up to 30 days) external electrocardiographic recording to evaluate for possible paroxysmal atrial fibrillation.

Description of Procedure (0938T)

A cardiovascular technician applies the monitor on the patient's arm and verifies/records the initial signal quality. Provide the patient with education regarding ongoing monitoring instructions that include marking

(tagging) events and caring for the device. Perform an electrocardiogram (ECG) recording for 30 days by continuous rhythm recording and storage. The device periodically transmits the full-disclosure ECG recordings to a secure computing cloud for algorithmic assessment.

Clinical Example (0939T)

A 72-year-old female presents with a prior neurologic ischemic episode but no prior history of atrial fibrillation. The physician decides to proceed with long-term (greater than 15 days and up to 30 days) external electrocardiographic recording to evaluate for possible paroxysmal atrial fibrillation.

Description of Procedure (0939T)

Perform an electrocardiographic recording for 30 days by continuous rhythm recording and storage by the device. An independent technician performs a comprehensive analysis of the electrocardiogram signal data and creates a summary report.

Clinical Example (0940T)

A 72-year-old female presents with a prior neurologic ischemic episode but no prior history of atrial fibrillation. The physician decides to proceed with long-term (greater than 15 days up to 30 days) external electrocardiographic recording to evaluate for possible paroxysmal atrial fibrillation.

Description of Procedure (0940T)

The physician reviews and interprets the report, including (1) heart rate trends (minimum, maximum, average); (2) tabular summary of supraventricular and ventricular ectopy; (3) tachyarrhythmias and bradyarrhythmias verified by the technician; and (4) symptomatic events identified (tagged) by the patient to assess the heart rhythm at those times.

● 0941T   Cystourethroscopy, flexible; with insertion and expansion of prostatic urethral scaffold using integrated cystoscopic visualization

▶(For insertion of permanent urethral stent, use 52282)◀

▶(For placement of temporary prostatic urethral stent, use 53855)◀

● 0942T   with removal and replacement of prostatic urethral scaffold

● 0943T   with removal of prostatic urethral scaffold

▶(Do not report 0943T in conjunction with 0942T)◀

▶(Do not report 0941T, 0942T, 0943T in conjunction with 52000, 52282, 52310, 52315, 52441, 52442, 53855)◀

Category III 0042T-0713T

Rationale

Category III codes 0941T-0943T have been established for reporting prostatic urethral scaffold procedures performed via flexible cystourethroscopy. A prostatic urethral scaffold is an implant placed in the prostatic urethra and expanded to an appropriate size to hold the prostatic urethra open, which may relieve pressure and lower urinary symptoms in conditions such as benign prostatic hypertrophy.

Code 0941T is reported for the insertion and expansion of the prostatic urethral scaffold using integrated cystoscopic visualization. Cross-reference parenthetical notes have been added following code 0941T that direct users to code 52282 for insertion of a permanent urethral stent and to code 53855 for placement of a temporary prostatic urethral stent. Code 0942T is reported for removal and replacement, and code 0943T is reported for removal without replacement. Code 0943T should not be reported with code 0942T. Codes 0941T-0943T should not be reported with code 52000, 52282, 52310, 52315, 52441, 52442, or 53855. Exclusionary parenthetical notes have been added.

Clinical Example (0941T)

A 66-year-old male, who is suffering from mild-to-moderate prostatic obstruction, has an elevated International Prostate Symptom Score, a low-peak urinary flow rate, and elevated post-void residual volume. His prostate volume is 42 grams without a median lobe component, and he responded insufficiently to watchful waiting and/or medical therapy. The patient is scheduled for implantation of an expandable prostatic urethral scaffold.

Description of Procedure (0941T)

Prepare and drape the patient in a dorsal lithotomy position. Prepare and drape the penis. Insert a flexible cystourethroscope into the meatus and advance to the patient's bladder neck. The physician selects the appropriate size expandable scaffold based on the anatomic cystoscopic characterization. Position the delivery-system balloon within the bladder to ensure proper position between the bladder neck and verumontanum and inflate with air. While continuously applying light tension, the physician pulls the delivery system's handle trigger repeatedly until it stops to deploy the expandable scaffold into the prostatic urethra. The physician may reverse direction and retract the implant several times to ensure accurate positioning, as necessary. Once the position is final and placement is confirmed, release the implant, deflate the balloon, and undock and remove the delivery system from the cystoscope.

Clinical Example (0942T)

A 66-year-old male, who is suffering from continued or worsening mild-to-moderate lower urinary tract symptoms and was implanted with an expandable prostatic urethral scaffold to treat his prostatic outlet obstruction, now requires its removal and reintervention because of cystoscopic evidence of unsupported tissue in which a different scaffold size or position is indicated. The patient is scheduled for removal and replacement of the expandable prostatic urethral scaffold.

Description of Procedure (0942T)

Prepare and drape the patient in the dorsal lithotomy position. Prepare and drape the penis. Using a transurethral approach, insert either a rigid sheath or flexible cystoscope. To remove, grasp the scaffold under direct visualization and pull it into the working channel of the sheath. Remove the sheath from the patient once the scaffold is fully within the sheath.

Insert a flexible cystourethroscope into the meatus and advance to the patient's bladder neck. The physician selects the appropriate size expandable scaffold based on the anatomic cystoscopic characterization. Position the delivery-system balloon within the bladder to ensure proper position between the bladder neck and verumontanum and inflate with air. While continuously applying light tension, the physician pulls the delivery system's handle trigger repeatedly until it stops to deploy the expandable scaffold into the prostatic urethra. The physician may reverse direction and retract the implant several times to ensure accurate positioning, as necessary. Once the position is final and placement is confirmed, release the implant, deflate the balloon, and undock and remove the delivery system from the cystoscope.

Clinical Example (0943T)

A 66-year-old male, who is suffering from continued or worsening mild-to-moderate lower urinary tract symptoms and was implanted with an expandable prostatic urethral scaffold to treat his prostatic outlet obstruction, is scheduled for removal of the expandable scaffold because of the lack of improvement, patient preference, or an unrelated cause (ie, recent bladder cancer diagnosis).

Description of Procedure (0943T)

Prepare and drape the patient in the dorsal lithotomy position. Prepare and drape the penis. Using a transurethral approach, insert either a rigid sheath or flexible cystoscope. To remove, grasp the scaffold under direct visualization and pull it into the working channel of the sheath. Remove the sheath from the patient once the scaffold is fully within the sheath.

▶Code 0944T describes three-dimensional (3D) contour simulation of liver lesion(s) performed by a physician or other qualified health care professional to create model probe pathways and locations, as well as to perform simulated volumetric calculations of the ablation cavity, overlaying of proposed ablation volumes on computed tomography (CT) imaging of the liver, and post-ablation volume comparisons requiring pre- and post-procedure CT imaging and guidance. A 3D contour simulation is separate and distinct from intraoperative imaging guidance and other pre-procedure imaging that are typically performed prior to image-guided liver microwave ablation procedures. Code 0944T is reported once per microwave ablation session, regardless of the number of distinct tumors ablated.◀

● **0944T**   3D contour simulation of target liver lesion(s) and margin(s) for image-guided percutaneous microwave ablation

▶(Report 0944T once per liver microwave ablation procedure)◀

▶(Do not report 0944T in conjunction with 76376, 76377)◀

Rationale

Category III code 0944T has been established to report a 3D contour simulation of liver lesion(s) and margin(s) for image-guided percutaneous microwave ablation. In addition, guidelines and two parenthetical notes have been added to provide instructions regarding the code and how it should be reported.

This procedure involves creating a 3D simulation to evaluate and plan microwave ablation of liver lesions in a patient with, for example, stage IV colorectal cancer metastases. The accompanying guidelines provide education regarding the service and the important elements needed for performing the procedure. This includes instruction regarding the separate, distinct nature of the 3D contour simulation "from intraoperative imaging guidance and other pre-procedure imaging that are typically performed prior to image-guided liver microwave ablation procedures."

The guidelines also direct users to report the procedure only once, regardless of the number of tumors ablated. This is also noted in the parenthetical note that follows code 0944T.

The second exclusionary parenthetical note following code 0944T restricts the use of code 0944T in conjunction with ultrasound imaging (76376, 76377).

Clinical Example (0944T)

A 61-year-old male, who has stage IV colorectal cancer metastases, has a diagnostic computed tomography imaging that demonstrates two suspicious lesions in the right lobe of his liver. Following a discussion at a multidisciplinary tumor board, the patient is referred for an evaluation for microwave ablation. Due to the complex locations of the lesions within the liver, three-dimensional (3D) simulation is ordered and performed to ensure the ability to satisfactorily treat tumors while limiting damage/risk to adjacent organs.

Description of Procedure (0944T)

Diagnostic cross-sectional imaging to identify the presence of tumors is typically performed before the simulation and separately reported. To create a 3D simulation, review advanced imaging scans and upload the most appropriate study into a local workstation. From the chosen study, the physician generates multi-planar and 3D volume renderings to further identify the target lesion(s). Transfer this dataset to an ablation simulation system on the same workstation. Within the ablation simulation system, the physician then segments and contours the target lesion(s) while reviewing each target in multi-planar reformatted views. Identify adjacent critical structures (eg, vessels, bowel, bile ducts) to ensure their safety is accounted for during an ablation simulation. Create a probe trajectory and placement plan based on the anticipated number of probes and access pathway. The physician reviews the simulated placement and trajectory of all probes in multiplanar reformatted views. After satisfactory simulated probe placement, create an ablation zone simulation based on lesion size/location and modifying parameters, such as desired margin, probe type, and ablation energy settings/duration, when applicable. If this initial simulation suffers from insufficient degrees of freedom, there are further iterative refinements in probe placement/trajectory and ablation zone simulations, which are performed as needed until the creation and evaluation process results in a satisfactory plan that generates sufficient ablation margins while sparing critical structures. The physician reviews and confirms that the simulated ablation plan is stored so that it can be referenced and carried out during the subsequent ablation procedure.

+● **0945T**   Intraoperative assessment for abnormal (tumor) tissue, in-vivo, following partial mastectomy (eg, lumpectomy) using computer-aided fluorescence imaging (List separately in addition to code for primary procedure)

▶(Use 0945T in conjunction with 19301)◀

▶(Report 0945T once per procedure)◀

▶(Do not report 0945T in conjunction with 88172, 0546T)◀

Rationale

Category III code 0945T has been established to report an intraoperative assessment of abnormal tumor tissue for partial mastectomy. In addition, parenthetical notes have been added to provide users with instructions regarding reporting the code.

This procedure involves using a handheld probe and fluorescence imaging to assess intraoperative margins for tumor cells following a lumpectomy in a patient who has stage II invasive ductal carcinoma and ductal carcinoma in situ. The surgeon uses the probe to scan the lumpectomy cavity, identify and resect regions with suspected residual cancer, and repeat scanning until no positive fluorescence signals are observed.

Accordingly, a cross-reference parenthetical note following codes 19301 and 0945T has been added, along with an exclusionary parenthetical note following code 0945T, to instruct users on the correct use of code 0945T. Because this is an add-on code, a parenthetical note has been added to direct users to the mastectomy procedure with which this service is intended to be reported (19301). In addition, parenthetical notes provide instruction regarding the number of times the procedure may be reported and restrict services that are mutually excluded (eg, use of cytopathology to identify remaining suspected cancerous tissue [88172]).

A parenthetical note within the Mastectomy Procedures subsection directs users to code 0945T when the new procedure is additionally performed.

Clinical Example (0945T)

A 64-year-old female, who is diagnosed with stage II invasive ductal carcinoma and ductal carcinoma in situ, is scheduled for a breast-conserving surgery (also known as lumpectomy). [**Note:** This is an add-on code. Only consider the additional work of intraoperative margin assessment for tumor cells using fluorescence imaging following excision.]

Description of Procedure (0945T)

Bring the cart and console of the margin detection system and the sterilized handheld probe into the operative room. Place the handheld probe, calibration plates, and sterile covers in the sterile field. Following aseptic procedures, connect the cables from the probe to the cart and console, install the calibration plates, and initialize the system following the instructions for use. After completing the initialization, remove and discard the calibration plates, install the sterile cover over the probe, and leave the probe idle in the sterile field. The surgeon completes the standard-of-care lumpectomy by resecting the main specimen and, if needed, cavity

shaves guided by visual inspection, palpation, intraoperative X-ray imaging of the main specimen, or by any other standard-of-care procedure practiced at the institution. Once the lumpectomy procedure is completed, the surgeon introduces the handheld probe into the lumpectomy cavity, ensuring that the viewing window of the probe is in contact with the tissue. The surgeon records one image from six different cavity orientations used by the patient-calibrated cancer-detection software to set the patient's baseline fluorescence intensity; signals above this threshold are considered to contain suspected regions of cancer. Then, the surgeon uses the probe to scan the lumpectomy while observing the display. When the display shows a region suspected to contain residual cancer (displayed as red on the computer screen), the surgeon identifies this orientation, removes the probe from the lumpectomy cavity, and resects a cavity shave from that orientation. Repeat scanning the cavity until no more positive fluorescence signal is observed in the display. This concludes the use of the optical imaging agent during the surgery. The surgeon then proceeds to complete the lumpectomy procedure per the institution's standard of care.

● **0946T** Orthopedic implant movement analysis using paired computed tomography (CT) examination of the target structure, including data acquisition, data preparation and transmission, interpretation and report (including CT scan of the joint or extremity performed with paired views)

▶(Do not report CT scan of the extremity or joint obtained separately)◀

Rationale

Category III code 0946T has been established to report CT-guided orthopedic implant movement analysis using a paired CT method.

Orthopedic implant movement analysis is a procedure that uses paired CT examination of the target structure CT. In this procedure, two CT scans are acquired at an endpoint of possible movements, such as maximal internal and external rotation for a hip examination or maximal flexion and extension over the relevant segment for a spine examination. A physician uses these two induced-displacement CT volumes to perform an implant movement analysis to identify whether there is a loose implant or pseudarthrosis and to see exactly how and where the implant is moving.

The procedure includes data acquisition, preparation, and transmission. As noted in the descriptor, provision of the report and paired CT views of the joint or extremity are also inherently included as part of the service. As a result,

Category III   0042T-0713T

an exclusionary parenthetical note has been added
following code 0946T to instruct users not to separately
report the CT scan of the extremity or joint.

Clinical Example (0946T)

A 60-year-old female experiences left knee pain
following a total left knee arthroplasty. She undergoes
diagnostic radiography to enable comparison to
postoperative images, and the result is inconclusive. As
the patient remains symptomatic, she is referred for
orthopedic implant movement analysis.

Description of Procedure (0946T)

The physician obtains two computed tomography
images and reviews them for induced displacement.
Import the images into the orthopedic implant
movement-analysis software. The physician identifies the
anatomy to include in the overlay. Determine the
presence or absence of movement and quantify any
movement. Create a video file and report the findings.

● **0947T**   Magnetic resonance image guided low intensity focused
ultrasound (MRgFUS), stereotactic blood-brain barrier
disruption using microbubble resonators to increase the
concentration of blood-based biomarkers of target,
intracranial, including stereotactic navigation and frame
placement, when performed

Rationale

Category III code 0947T has been established to report a
MRgFUS for blood-brain barrier disruption. This is a noninvasive method of combining conventional diagnostic
MRI scanning with low intensity–focused ultrasound
delivery with microbubble resonators to identify
intracranial tumors and areas of interest around the tumor.
Because this procedure is noninvasive (ie, does not
involve invasive needle brain biopsy), it is different from
other methods for blood-brain barrier disruption.

Clinical Example (0947T)

A 71-year-old male presents with a history of high-grade
glioma. He underwent repeat magnetic resonance
imaging (MRI) scans with and without contrast, which
revealed increasing contrast enhancement within the
right temporal lobe with significant, moderate
surrounding T2-hyperintensity, concerning for
pseudoprogression vs tumor progression and mass effect.
MR image–guided low intensity–focused ultrasound
(MRgFUS), stereotactic blood-brain barrier disruption
using microbubble resonators is ordered to help
distinguish pseudoprogression from tumor progression.

Description of Procedure (0947T)

Take the patient to the MRgFUS suite awake, alert, and
hemodynamically stable. Place and secure the
appropriate lines, then place the water bolus membrane
over his head, and position him supinely on the MRI
machine. Immobilize his head using the dental mold
apparatus. Position and connect the transducer and then
fill the water bolus with the degassed water. Check the
patient's comfort and breathing. Next, acquire and fuse
the MR registration imaging with the pre-procedure
MRI. The sonication planning maps relevant brain
regions across the tumor and peri-tumoral regions where
a subsequent evaluation of the enhanced biomarkers
retrieved from the procedure helps discern between true
vs pseudoprogression. Sonication targets include 10
shapes with 25 to 32 subspots covering the regions
planned. Initiate the microbubble infusion at 5ul/kg/
min. Set the acoustic power at 30 watts, the sonication
time per target to 180 seconds, and the sonication
(cavitation) dose at 0.8 volts. Perform the sonications
sequentially with real-time acoustic emissions and MRI
T2* monitoring. Ensure the patient remains comfortable
throughout the procedure, which is completed in 55
minutes. Following completion, stop the microbubble
infusion and remove the patient's head from the
transducer, membrane, and head immobilization
apparatus. Draw and collect blood from an intravenous
catheter per the specifications from the treating
physician for subsequent analysis as relevant. Test the
patient, and if found to be neurologically unchanged,
perform a post-procedure MRI to complete the brain
tumor imaging sequences and assess other changes.

Notes

Appendix O

Summary of Additions, Deletions, and Revisions

The summary of changes shows the actual changes that have been made to the code descriptors.

New codes appear with a bullet (●) and are indicated as "Code added." Revised codes are preceded with a triangle (▲). Within revised codes, or if a code symbol has been deleted, the deleted language and code symbol appear with a ~~strikethrough~~, while new text appears <u>underlined</u>.

The ⚡ symbol is used to identify codes for vaccines that are pending FDA approval. The # symbol is used to identify codes that have been resequenced. CPT add-on codes are annotated by the ✚ symbol. The ⊘ symbol is used to identify codes that are exempt from the use of modifier 51. The ★ symbol is used to identify codes that may be used for reporting telemedicine services. The ✣ symbol is used to identify a proprietary laboratory analyses (PLA) test that has an identical descriptor as another PLA test. A PLA code that satisfies Category I code criteria and has been accepted by the CPT Editorial Panel is annotated with the ↕ symbol. The ◀ symbol is used to identify codes that may be used to report audio-only telemedicine services when appended by modifier 93 (**see Appendix T**).

Proprietary Name and Clinical Laboratory or Manufacturer	Alpha-Numeric Code	Code Descriptor
Administrative Codes for Multianalyte Assays with Algorithmic Analyses (MAAA)		
	●0020M	Code added
Category I Codes for Multianalyte Assays with Algorithmic Analyses (MAAA)		
	●81515	Code added
	●81558	Code added
Proprietary Laboratory Analyses (PLA)		
~~INFINITI® Neural Response Panel, PersonalizeDx Labs, AutoGenomics Inc~~	~~0078U~~	~~Pain management (opioid-use disorder) genotyping panel, 16 common variants (ie, *ABCB1, COMT, DAT1, DBH, DOR, DRD1, DRD2, DRD4, GABA, GAL, HTR2A, HTTLPR, MTHFR, MUOR, OPRK1, OPRM1*), buccal swab or other germline tissue sample, algorithm reported as positive or negative risk of opioid-use disorder~~
~~ADEXUSDx hCG Test, NOWDiagnostics, NOWDiagnostics~~	~~0167U~~	~~Gonadotropin, chorionic (hCG), immunoassay with direct optical observation, blood~~
~~Afirma Xpression Atlas, Veracyte, Inc, Veracyte, Inc~~	~~0204U~~	~~Oncology (thyroid), mRNA, gene expression analysis of 593 genes (including *BRAF, RAS, RET, PAX8,* and *NTRK*) for sequence variants and rearrangements, utilizing fine needle aspirate, reported as detected or not detected~~
3D Predict Glioma, KIYATEC®, Inc	▲0248U	Oncology ~~(brain)~~, spheroid cell culture in a<u>3D</u> microenvironment, 12<u>-</u>drug panel, ~~tumor~~ <u>brain- or brain metastasis</u> response prediction for each drug

(Continued on page 198)

Appendix O

Proprietary Name and Clinical Laboratory or Manufacturer	Alpha-Numeric Code	Code Descriptor
MeMed BV®, MeMed Diagnostics, Ltd, MeMed Diagnostics, Ltd	▲0351U	Infectious disease (bacterial or viral), biochemical assays, tumor necrosis factor-related apoptosis-inducing ligand (TRAIL), interferon gamma-induced protein-10 (IP-10), and C-reactive protein, serum, <u>or venous whole blood,</u> algorithm reported as likelihood of bacterial infection
~~Xpert® Xpress MVP, Cepheid®~~	~~0352U~~	~~Infectious disease (bacterial vaginosis and vaginitis), multiplex amplified probe technique, for detection of bacterial vaginosis-associated bacteria (BVAB-2, Atopobium vaginae, and Megasphera type 1), algorithm reported as detected or not detected and separate detection of Candida species (C. albicans, C. tropicalis, C. parapsilosis, C. dubliniensis), Candida glabrata/Candida krusei, and trichomonas vaginalis, vaginal-fluid specimen, each result reported as detected or not detected~~
~~Xpert® CT/NG, Cepheid®~~	~~0353U~~	~~Infectious agent detection by nucleic acid (DNA), Chlamydia trachomatis and Neisseria gonorrhoeae, multiplex amplified probe technique, urine, vaginal, pharyngeal, or rectal, each pathogen reported as detected or not detected~~
~~PreTect HPV-Proofer' 7, GenePace Laboratories, LLC, PreTech~~	~~0354U~~	~~Human papilloma virus (HPV), high-risk types (ie, 16, 18, 31, 33, 45, 52 and 58) qualitative mRNA expression of E6/E7 by quantitative polymerase chain reaction (qPCR)~~
NavDx®, Naveris, Inc, Naveris, Inc	▲0356U	Oncology (oropharyngeal <u>or anal</u>), evaluation of 17 DNA biomarkers using droplet digital PCR (ddPCR), cell-free DNA, algorithm reported as a prognostic risk score for cancer recurrence
~~Spectrum PGT-M, Natera, Inc, Natera, Inc~~	~~0396U~~	~~Obstetrics (pre-implantation genetic testing), evaluation of 300000 DNA single-nucleotide polymorphisms (SNPs) by microarray, embryonic tissue, algorithm reported as a probability for single-gene germline conditions~~
MyProstateScore 2.0, LynxDX, LynxDX	▲0403U	Oncology (prostate), mRNA, gene expression profiling of 18 genes, first-catch ~~post-digital rectal examination~~ urine ~~(or processed first-catch urine)~~, algorithm reported as percentage of likelihood of detecting clinically significant prostate cancer
~~GENETWORx UTI with ABR, RCA Laboratory Services LLC d/b/a GENETWORx, GENETWORx~~	~~0416U~~	~~Infectious agent detection by nucleic acid (DNA), genitourinary pathogens, identification of 20 bacterial and fungal organisms, including identification of 20 associated antibiotic-resistance genes, if performed, multiplex amplified probe technique, urine~~
	●0420U	Code added
	●0421U	Code added
	●0422U	Code added
	●0423U	Code added
	●0424U	Code added

★=Telemedicine   ◄=Audio-only   ✚=Add-on code   ✗=FDA approval pending   #=Resequenced code   ⊘=Modifier 51 exempt

Proprietary Name and Clinical Laboratory or Manufacturer	Alpha-Numeric Code	Code Descriptor
	●0425U	Code added
	●0426U	Code added
	✛●0427U	Code added
	●0428U	Code added
	●0429U	Code added
	●0430U	Code added
	●0431U	Code added
	●0432U	Code added
	●0433U	Code added
	●0434U	Code added
	●0435U	Code added
	●0436U	Code added
	●0437U	Code added
	●0438U	Code added
	●0439U	Code added
	●0440U	Code added
	●0441U	Code added
	●0442U	Code added
	●0443U	Code added
	●0444U	Code added
	●0445U	Code added
	●0446U	Code added
	●0447U	Code added
	●0448U	Code added
	●0449U	Code added
	●0450U	Code added
	●0451U	Code added
	●0452U	Code added
	●0453U	Code added
	✖●0454U	Code added
	●0455U	Code added
	●0456U	Code added
	●0457U	Code added
	●0458U	Code added
	●0459U	Code added
	●0460U	Code added
	●0461U	Code added
	●0462U	Code added
	●0463U	Code added
	●0464U	Code added
	●0465U	Code added

(*Continued on page 200*)

▲ = Revised code   ● = New code   ▶ ◀ = Contains new or revised text   ✖ = Duplicate PLA test   ↕ = Category I PLA   American Medical Association   **199**

Proprietary Name and Clinical Laboratory or Manufacturer	Alpha-Numeric Code	Code Descriptor
	●0466U	Code added
	●0467U	Code added
	●0468U	Code added
	●0469U	Code added
	●0470U	Code added
	●0471U	Code added
	●0472U	Code added
	●0473U	Code added
	●0474U	Code added
	●0475U	Code added
	●0476U	Code added
	●0477U	Code added
	●0478U	Code added
	●0479U	Code added
	●0480U	Code added
	●0481U	Code added
	●0482U	Code added
	●0483U	Code added
	●0484U	Code added
	●0485U	Code added
	●0486U	Code added
	●0487U	Code added
	●0488U	Code added
	●0489U	Code added
	●0490U	Code added
	●0491U	Code added
	●0492U	Code added
	●0493U	Code added
	●0494U	Code added
	●0495U	Code added
	●0496U	Code added
	●0497U	Code added
	●0498U	Code added
	●0499U	Code added
	●0500U	Code added
	●0501U	Code added
	●0502U	Code added
	●0503U	Code added
	●0504U	Code added
	●0505U	Code added
	●0506U	Code added

★=Telemedicine   ◀=Audio-only   ✚=Add-on code   ✗=FDA approval pending   #=Resequenced code   ⃠=Modifier 51 exempt

Proprietary Name and Clinical Laboratory or Manufacturer	Alpha-Numeric Code	Code Descriptor
	●0507U	Code added
	●0508U	Code added
	●0509U	Code added
	●0510U	Code added
	●0511U	Code added
	●0512U	Code added
	●0513U	Code added
	●0514U	Code added
	●0515U	Code added
	●0516U	Code added
	●0517U	Code added
	●0518U	Code added
	●0519U	Code added
	●0520U	Code added

Appendix O

Multianalyte Assays with Algorithmic Analyses and Proprietary Laboratory Analyses

The following list includes three types of CPT codes:

1. Multianalyte assays with algorithmic analyses (MAAA) administrative codes
2. Category I MAAA codes
3. Proprietary laboratory analyses (PLA) codes

1. Multianalyte assays with algorithmic analyses (MAAAs) are procedures that utilize multiple results derived from assays of various types, including molecular pathology assays, fluorescent in situ hybridization assays and non-nucleic acid based assays (eg, proteins, polypeptides, lipids, carbohydrates). Algorithmic analysis using the results of these assays as well as other patient information (if used) is then performed and reported typically as a numeric score(s) or as a probability. MAAAs are typically unique to a single clinical laboratory or manufacturer. The results of individual component procedure(s) that are inputs to the MAAAs may be provided on the associated laboratory report, however these assays are not reported separately using additional codes. MAAAs, by nature, are typically unique to a single clinical laboratory or manufacturer.

The list includes a proprietary name and clinical laboratory or manufacturer in the first column, an alpha-numeric code in the second column and code descriptor in the third column. The format for the code descriptor usually includes (in order):

- Disease type (eg, oncology, autoimmune, tissue rejection),
- Chemical(s) analyzed (eg, DNA, RNA, protein, antibody),
- Number of markers (eg, number of genes, number of proteins),
- Methodology(s) (eg, microarray, real-time [RT]-PCR, in situ hybridization [ISH], enzyme linked immunosorbent assays [ELISA]),
- Number of functional domains (if indicated),
- Specimen type (eg, blood, fresh tissue, formalin-fixed paraffin-embedded),
- Algorithm result type (eg, prognostic, diagnostic),
- Report (eg, probability index, risk score).

MAAA procedures that have been assigned a Category I code are noted in the list below and additionally listed in the Category I MAAA section (81500-81599). The Category I MAAA section introductory language and associated parenthetical instruction(s) should be used to govern the appropriate use for Category I MAAA codes. If a specific MAAA procedure has not been assigned a Category I code, it is indicated as a four-digit number followed by the letter M.

When a specific MAAA procedure is not included in either the list below or in the Category I MAAA section, report the analysis using the Category I MAAA unlisted code (81599). The codes below are specific to the assays identified in Appendix O by proprietary name. In order to report an MAAA code, the analysis performed must fulfill the code descriptor **and**, if proprietary, must be the test represented by the proprietary name listed in Appendix O. When an analysis is performed that may potentially fall within a specific descriptor, however the proprietary name is not included in the list below, the MAAA unlisted code (81599) should be used.

Additions in this section may be released tri-annually (or quarterly for PLA codes) via the AMA CPT website to expedite dissemination for reporting. See the Introduction section of the CPT code set for a complete list of the dates of release and implementation.

These administrative codes encompass all analytical services required for the algorithmic analysis (eg, cell lysis, nucleic acid stabilization, extraction, digestion, amplification, hybridization and detection) in addition to the algorithmic analysis itself, when applicable. Procedures that are required prior to cell lysis (eg, microdissection, codes 88380 and 88381) should be reported separately.

★=Telemedicine ◀=Audio-only ✚=Add-on code ✗=FDA approval pending #=Resequenced code ⃠=Modifier 51 exempt

The codes in this list are provided as an administrative coding set to facilitate accurate reporting of MAAA services. The minimum standard for inclusion in this list is that an analysis is generally available for patient care. The AMA has not reviewed procedures in the administrative coding set for clinical utility. The list is not a complete list of all MAAA procedures.

2. Category I MAAA codes are included below along with their proprietary names. These codes are also listed in the Pathology and Laboratory section of the CPT code set (81490-81599).

3. PLA codes created in response to the Protecting Access to Medicare Act (PAMA) of 2014 are listed along with their proprietary names. These codes are also located at the end of the Pathology and Laboratory section of the CPT code set. In some instances, the descriptor language of PLA codes may be identical, which are differentiated only by the listed propriety names.

The accuracy of a PLA code is to be maintained by the original applicant, or the current owner of the test kit or laboratory performing the proprietary test.

A new PLA code is required when:

1. Additional nucleic acid (DNA or RNA) and/or protein analysis(es) are added to the current PLA test, or

2. The name of the PLA test has changed in association with changes in test performance or test characteristics.

The addition or modification of the therapeutic applications of the test require submission of a code change application, but it may not require a new code number.

Proprietary Name and Clinical Laboratory or Manufacturer	Alpha-Numeric Code	Code Descriptor
Administrative Codes for Multianalyte Assays with Algorithmic Analyses (MAAA)		
ASH FibroSURE™, BioPredictive S.A.S	0002M	Liver disease, ten biochemical assays (ALT, A2-macroglobulin, apolipoprotein A-1, total bilirubin, GGT, haptoglobin, AST, glucose, total cholesterol and triglycerides) utilizing serum, prognostic algorithm reported as quantitative scores for fibrosis, steatosis and alcoholic steatohepatitis (ASH)
NASH FibroSURE™, BioPredictive S.A.S	0003M	Liver disease, ten biochemical assays (ALT, A2-macroglobulin, apolipoprotein A-1, total bilirubin, GGT, haptoglobin, AST, glucose, total cholesterol and triglycerides) utilizing serum, prognostic algorithm reported as quantitative scores for fibrosis, steatosis and nonalcoholic steatohepatitis (NASH)
ScoliScore™ Transgenomic	0004M	Scoliosis, DNA analysis of 53 single nucleotide polymorphisms (SNPs), using saliva, prognostic algorithm reported as a risk score
HeproDX™, GoPath Laboratories, LLC	0006M	Oncology (hepatic), mRNA expression levels of 161 genes, utilizing fresh hepatocellular carcinoma tumor tissue, with alpha-fetoprotein level, algorithm reported as a risk classifier
NETest, Wren Laboratories, LLC	0007M	Oncology (gastrointestinal neuroendocrine tumors), real-time PCR expression analysis of 51 genes, utilizing whole peripheral blood, algorithm reported as a nomogram of tumor disease index
NeoLAB™ Prostate Liquid Biopsy, NeoGenomics Laboratories	0011M	Oncology, prostate cancer, mRNA expression assay of 12 genes (10 content and 2 housekeeping), RT-PCR test utilizing blood plasma and urine, algorithms to predict high-grade prostate cancer risk

(Continued on page 204)

Proprietary Name and Clinical Laboratory or Manufacturer	Alpha-Numeric Code	Code Descriptor
Cxbladder™ Detect, Pacific Edge Diagnostics USA, Ltd	0012M	Oncology (urothelial), mRNA, gene expression profiling by real-time quantitative PCR of five genes (*MDK, HOXA13, CDC2 [CDK1], IGFBP5,* and *CXCR2*), utilizing urine, algorithm reported as a risk score for having urothelial carcinoma
Cxbladder™ Monitor, Pacific Edge Diagnostics USA, Ltd	0013M	Oncology (urothelial), mRNA, gene expression profiling by real-time quantitative PCR of five genes (*MDK, HOXA13, CDC2 [CDK1], IGFBP5,* and *CXCR2*), utilizing urine, algorithm reported as a risk score for having recurrent urothelial carcinoma
—	(0014M has been deleted) (For multianalyte assay with algorithmic analysis [MAAA] for liver disease using analysis of 3 biomarkers, use 81517)	—
Adrenal Mass Panel, 24 Hour, Urine, Mayo Clinic Laboratories (MCL), Mayo Clinic	0015M	Adrenal cortical tumor, biochemical assay of 25 steroid markers, utilizing 24-hour urine specimen and clinical parameters, prognostic algorithm reported as a clinical risk and integrated clinical steroid risk for adrenal cortical carcinoma, adenoma, or other adrenal malignancy
Decipher Bladder, Veracyte Labs SD	0016M	Oncology (bladder), mRNA, microarray gene expression profiling of 219 genes, utilizing formalin-fixed paraffin-embedded tissue, algorithm reported as molecular subtype (luminal, luminal infiltrated, basal, basal claudin-low, neuroendocrine-like)
Lymph2Cx, Mayo Clinic Arizona Molecular Diagnostics Laboratory	0017M	Oncology (diffuse large B-cell lymphoma [DLBCL]), mRNA, gene expression profiling by fluorescent probe hybridization of 20 genes, formalin-fixed paraffin-embedded tissue, algorithm reported as cell of origin (Do not report 0017M in conjunction with 0120U)
Pleximark™, Plexision, Inc	0018M	Transplantation medicine (allograft rejection, renal), measurement of donor and third-party-induced CD154+T-cytotoxic memory cells, utilizing whole peripheral blood, algorithm reported as a rejection risk score (Do not report 0018M in conjunction with 81560, 85032, 86353, 86821, 88184, 88185, 88187, 88230, 88240, 88241)
SOMAmer®, SomaLogic	0019M	Cardiovascular disease, plasma, analysis of protein biomarkers by aptamer-based microarray and algorithm reported as 4-year likelihood of coronary event in high-risk populations

★ = Telemedicine   ◀ = Audio-only   ✚ = Add-on code   ✗ = FDA approval pending   # = Resequenced code   ⊘ = Modifier 51 exempt

Proprietary Name and Clinical Laboratory or Manufacturer	Alpha-Numeric Code	Code Descriptor
▶Epignostix CNS Tumor Methylation Classifier, Heidelberg Epignostix GmbH◀	●0020M	▶Oncology (central nervous system), analysis of 30000 DNA methylation loci by methylation array, utilizing DNA extracted from tumor tissue, diagnostic algorithm reported as probability of matching a reference tumor subclass◀
Category I Codes for Multianalyte Assays with Algorithmic Analyses (MAAA)		
Vectra®, Labcorp	81490	Autoimmune (rheumatoid arthritis), analysis of 12 biomarkers using immunoassays, utilizing serum, prognostic algorithm reported as a disease activity score (Do not report 81490 in conjunction with 86140)
AlloMap®, CareDx, Inc	#81595	Cardiology (heart transplant), mRNA, gene expression profiling by real-time quantitative PCR of 20 genes (11 content and 9 housekeeping), utilizing subfraction of peripheral blood, algorithm reported as a rejection risk score
Corus® CAD, CardioDx, Inc	81493	Coronary artery disease, mRNA, gene expression profiling by real-time RT-PCR of 23 genes, utilizing whole peripheral blood, algorithm reported as a risk score
PreDx Diabetes Risk Score™, Tethys Clinical Laboratory	81506	Endocrinology (type 2 diabetes), biochemical assays of seven analytes (glucose, HbA1c, insulin, hs-CRP, adiponectin, ferritin, interleukin 2-receptor alpha), utilizing serum or plasma, algorithm reporting a risk score (Do not report 81506 in conjunction with constituent components [ie, 82728, 82947, 83036, 83525, 86141], 84999 [for adopectin], and 83520 [for interleukin 2-receptor alpha])
Harmony™ Prenatal Test, Ariosa Diagnostics	81507	Fetal aneuploidy (trisomy 21, 18, and 13) DNA sequence analysis of selected regions using maternal plasma, algorithm reported as a risk score for each trisomy (Do not report 81228, 81229, 88271 when performing genomic sequencing procedures or other molecular multianalyte assays for copy number analysis)

(Continued on page 206)

▲ = Revised code   ● = New code   ▶◀ = Contains new or revised text   ✕ = Duplicate PLA test   ↑↓ = Category I PLA   American Medical Association   **205**

Proprietary Name and Clinical Laboratory or Manufacturer	Alpha-Numeric Code	Code Descriptor
No proprietary name and clinical laboratory or manufacturer. Maternal serum screening procedures are well-established procedures and are performed by many laboratories throughout the country. The concept of prenatal screens has existed and evolved for over 10 years and is not exclusive to any one facility.	81508	Fetal congenital abnormalities, biochemical assays of two proteins (PAPP-A, hCG [any form]), utilizing maternal serum, algorithm reported as a risk score (Do not report 81508 in conjunction with 84163, 84702)
	81509	Fetal congenital abnormalities, biochemical assays of three proteins (PAPP-A, hCG [any form], DIA), utilizing maternal serum, algorithm reported as a risk score (Do not report 81509 in conjunction with 84163, 84702, 86336)
	81510	Fetal congenital abnormalities, biochemical assays of three analytes (AFP, uE3, hCG [any form]), utilizing maternal serum, algorithm reported as a risk score (Do not report 81510 in conjunction with 82105, 82677, 84702)
	81511	Fetal congenital abnormalities, biochemical assays of four analytes (AFP, uE3, hCG [any form], DIA) utilizing maternal serum, algorithm reported as a risk score (may include additional results from previous biochemical testing) (Do not report 81511 in conjunction with 82105, 82677, 84702, 86336)
	81512	Fetal congenital abnormalities, biochemical assays of five analytes (AFP, uE3, total hCG, hyperglycosylated hCG, DIA) utilizing maternal serum, algorithm reported as a risk score (Do not report 81512 in conjunction with 82105, 82677, 84702, 86336)
Aptima® BV Assay, Hologic, Inc	81513	Infectious disease, bacterial vaginosis, quantitative real-time amplification of RNA markers for Atopobium vaginae, Gardnerella vaginalis, and Lactobacillus species, utilizing vaginal-fluid specimens, algorithm reported as a positive or negative result for bacterial vaginosis
BD MAX™ Vaginal Panel, Becton Dickinson and Company	81514	Infectious disease, bacterial vaginosis and vaginitis, quantitative real-time amplification of DNA markers for Gardnerella vaginalis, Atopobium vaginae, Megasphaera type 1, Bacterial Vaginosis Associated Bacteria-2 (BVAB-2), and Lactobacillus species (L. crispatus and L. jensenii), utilizing vaginal-fluid specimens, algorithm reported as a positive or negative for high likelihood of bacterial vaginosis, includes separate detection of Trichomonas vaginalis and/or Candida species (C. albicans, C. tropicalis, C. parapsilosis, C. dubliniensis), Candida glabrata, Candida krusei, when reported (Do not report 81514 in conjunction with 87480, 87481, 87482, 87510, 87511, 87512, 87660, 87661)

Proprietary Name and Clinical Laboratory or Manufacturer	Alpha-Numeric Code	Code Descriptor
▶Xpert® Xpress MVP, Cepheid®◀	●81515	▶Infectious disease, bacterial vaginosis and vaginitis, real-time PCR amplification of DNA markers for Atopobium vaginae, Atopobium species, Megasphaera type 1, and Bacterial Vaginosis Associated Bacteria-2 (BVAB-2), utilizing vaginal-fluid specimens, algorithm reported as positive or negative for high likelihood of bacterial vaginosis, includes separate detection of Trichomonas vaginalis and Candida species (C. albicans, C. tropicalis, C. parapsilosis, C. dubliniensis), Candida glabrata/Candida krusei, when reported◀
HCV FibroSURE™, FibroTest™, BioPredictive S.A.S.	#81596	Infectious disease, chronic hepatitis C virus (HCV) infection, six biochemical assays (ALT, A2-macroglobulin, apolipoprotein A-1, total bilirubin, GGT, and haptoglobin) utilizing serum, prognostic algorithm reported as scores for fibrosis and necroinflammatory activity in liver
Enhanced Liver Fibrosis™ (ELF™) Test, Siemens Healthcare Diagnostics Inc/Siemens Healthcare Laboratory LLC	81517	Liver disease, analysis of 3 biomarkers (hyaluronic acid [HA], procollagen III amino terminal peptide [PIIINP], tissue inhibitor of metalloproteinase 1 [TIMP-1]), using immunoassays, utilizing serum, prognostic algorithm reported as a risk score and risk of liver fibrosis and liver-related clinical events within 5 years (Do not report 81517 in conjunction with 83520 for identification of biomarkers included for liver disease analysis)
Breast Cancer Index, Biotheranostics, Inc	81518	Oncology (breast), mRNA, gene expression profiling by real-time RT-PCR of 11 genes (7 content and 4 housekeeping), utilizing formalin-fixed paraffin-embedded tissue, algorithms reported as percentage risk for metastatic recurrence and likelihood of benefit from extended endocrine therapy
EndoPredict®, Myriad Genetic Laboratories, Inc	#81522	Oncology (breast), mRNA, gene expression profiling by RT-PCR of 12 genes (8 content and 4 housekeeping), utilizing formalin-fixed paraffin-embedded tissue, algorithm reported as recurrence risk score
Oncotype DX®, Genomic Health	81519	Oncology (breast), mRNA, gene expression profiling by real-time RT-PCR of 21 genes, utilizing formalin-fixed paraffin-embedded tissue, algorithm reported as recurrence score
Prosigna® Breast Cancer Assay, NanoString Technologies, Inc	81520	Oncology (breast), mRNA gene expression profiling by hybrid capture of 58 genes (50 content and 8 housekeeping), utilizing formalin-fixed paraffin-embedded tissue, algorithm reported as a recurrence risk score

(Continued on page 208)

Proprietary Name and Clinical Laboratory or Manufacturer	Alpha-Numeric Code	Code Descriptor
MammaPrint®, Agendia, Inc	81521	Oncology (breast), mRNA, microarray gene expression profiling of 70 content genes and 465 housekeeping genes, utilizing fresh frozen or formalin-fixed paraffin-embedded tissue, algorithm reported as index related to risk of distant metastasis (Do not report 81521 in conjunction with 81523 for the same specimen)
MammaPrint®, Agendia, Inc	81523	Oncology (breast), mRNA, next-generation sequencing gene expression profiling of 70 content genes and 31 housekeeping genes, utilizing formalin-fixed paraffin-embedded tissue, algorithm reported as index related to risk to distant metastasis (Do not report 81523 in conjunction with 81521 for the same specimen)
Oncotype DX® Colon Cancer Assay, Genomic Health	81525	Oncology (colon), mRNA, gene expression profiling by real-time RT-PCR of 12 genes (7 content and 5 housekeeping), utilizing formalin-fixed paraffin-embedded tissue, algorithm reported as a recurrence score
Cologuard™, Exact Sciences, Inc	81528	Oncology (colorectal) screening, quantitative real-time target and signal amplification of 10 DNA markers (*KRAS* mutations, promoter methylation of *NDRG4* and *BMP3*) and fecal hemoglobin, utilizing stool, algorithm reported as a positive or negative result (Do not report 81528 in conjunction with 81275, 82274)
DecisionDx® Melanoma, Castle Biosciences, Inc	81529	Oncology (cutaneous melanoma), mRNA, gene expression profiling by real-time RT-PCR of 31 genes (28 content and 3 housekeeping), utilizing formalin-fixed paraffin-embedded tissue, algorithm reported as recurrence risk, including likelihood of sentinel lymph node metastasis
ChemoFX®, Helomics, Corp	81535 +81536	Oncology (gynecologic), live tumor cell culture and chemotherapeutic response by DAPI stain and morphology, predictive algorithm reported as a drug response score; first single drug or drug combination each additional single drug or drug combination (List separately in addition to code for primary procedure) (Use 81536 in conjunction with 81535)
VeriStrat, Biodesix, Inc	81538	Oncology (lung), mass spectrometric 8-protein signature, including amyloid A, utilizing serum, prognostic and predictive algorithm reported as good versus poor overall survival
Risk of Ovarian Malignancy Algorithm (ROMA)™, Fujirebio Diagnostics	#81500	Oncology (ovarian), biochemical assays of two proteins (CA-125 and HE4), utilizing serum, with menopausal status, algorithm reported as a risk score (Do not report 81500 in conjunction with 86304, 86305)

★=Telemedicine   ◀=Audio-only   +=Add-on code   ✒=FDA approval pending   #=Resequenced code   ⦸=Modifier 51 exempt

Proprietary Name and Clinical Laboratory or Manufacturer	Alpha-Numeric Code	Code Descriptor
OVA1™, Vermillion, Inc	#81503	Oncology (ovarian), biochemical assays of five proteins (CA-125, apolipoprotein A1, beta-2 microglobulin, transferrin, and pre-albumin), utilizing serum, algorithm reported as a risk score (Do not report 81503 in conjunction with 82172, 82232, 84134, 84466, 86304)
4Kscore test, OPKO Health, Inc	81539	Oncology (high-grade prostate cancer), biochemical assay of four proteins (Total PSA, Free PSA, Intact PSA, and human kallikrein-2 [hK2]), utilizing plasma or serum, prognostic algorithm reported as a probability score
Prolaris®, Myriad Genetic Laboratories, Inc	81541	Oncology (prostate), mRNA gene expression profiling by real-time RT-PCR of 46 genes (31 content and 15 housekeeping), utilizing formalin-fixed paraffin-embedded tissue, algorithm reported as a disease-specific mortality risk score
Decipher® Prostate, Decipher® Biosciences	81542	Oncology (prostate), mRNA, microarray gene expression profiling of 22 content genes, utilizing formalin-fixed paraffin-embedded tissue, algorithm reported as metastasis risk score
ConfirmMDx® for Prostate Cancer, MDxHealth, Inc	81551	Oncology (prostate), promoter methylation profiling by real-time PCR of 3 genes (GSTP1, APC, RASSF1), utilizing formalin-fixed paraffin-embedded tissue, algorithm reported as a likelihood of prostate cancer detection on repeat biopsy
Afirma® Genomic Sequencing Classifier, Veracyte, Inc	#81546	Oncology (thyroid), mRNA, gene expression analysis of 10,196 genes, utilizing fine needle aspirate, algorithm reported as a categorical result (eg, benign or suspicious)
Tissue of Origin Test Kit-FFPE, Cancer Genetics, Inc	#81504	Oncology (tissue of origin), microarray gene expression profiling of > 2000 genes, utilizing formalin-fixed paraffin-embedded tissue, algorithm reported as tissue similarity scores
CancerTYPE ID, bioTheranostics, Inc	#81540	Oncology (tumor of unknown origin), mRNA, gene expression profiling by real-time RT-PCR of 92 genes (87 content and 5 housekeeping) to classify tumor into main cancer type and subtype, utilizing formalin-fixed paraffin-embedded tissue, algorithm reported as a probability of a predicted main cancer type and subtype
DecisionDx®-UM test, Castle Biosciences, Inc	81552	Oncology (uveal melanoma), mRNA, gene expression profiling by real-time RT-PCR of 15 genes (12 content and 3 housekeeping), utilizing fine needle aspirate or formalin-fixed paraffin-embedded tissue, algorithm reported as risk of metastasis

(Continued on page 210)

Proprietary Name and Clinical Laboratory or Manufacturer	Alpha-Numeric Code	Code Descriptor
Envisia® Genomic Classifier, Veracyte, Inc	81554	Pulmonary disease (idiopathic pulmonary fibrosis [IPF]), mRNA, gene expression analysis of 190 genes, utilizing transbronchial biopsies, diagnostic algorithm reported as categorical result (eg, positive or negative for high probability of usual interstitial pneumonia [UIP])
▶TruGraf® Kidney, Eurofins Transplant Genomics, Inc◀	●81558	▶Transplantation medicine (allograft rejection, kidney), mRNA, gene expression profiling by quantitative polymerase chain reaction (qPCR) of 139 genes, utilizing whole blood, algorithm reported as a binary categorization as transplant excellence, which indicates immune quiescence, or not transplant excellence, indicating subclinical rejection◀
Pleximmune™, Plexision, Inc	81560	Transplantation medicine (allograft rejection, pediatric liver and small bowel), measurement of donor and third-party-induced CD154+T-cytotoxic memory cells, utilizing whole peripheral blood, algorithm reported as a rejection risk score (Do not report 81560 in conjunction with 85032, 86353, 86821, 88184, 88185, 88187, 88230, 88240, 88241, 0018M)
—	81599	Unlisted multianalyte assay with algorithmic analysis (Do not use 81599 for multianalyte assays with algorithmic analyses listed in Appendix O)
Proprietary Laboratory Analyses (PLA)		
PreciseType® HEA Test, Immucor, Inc	0001U	Red blood cell antigen typing, DNA, human erythrocyte antigen gene analysis of 35 antigens from 11 blood groups, utilizing whole blood, common RBC alleles reported
PolypDX™, Atlantic Diagnostic Laboratories, LLC, Metabolomic Technologies, Inc	0002U	Oncology (colorectal), quantitative assessment of three urine metabolites (ascorbic acid, succinic acid and carnitine) by liquid chromatography with tandem mass spectrometry (LC-MS/MS) using multiple reaction monitoring acquisition, algorithm reported as likelihood of adenomatous polyps
Overa (OVA1 Next Generation), Aspira Labs, Inc, Vermillion, Inc	0003U	Oncology (ovarian) biochemical assays of five proteins (apolipoprotein A-1, CA 125 II, follicle stimulating hormone, human epididymis protein 4, transferrin), utilizing serum, algorithm reported as a likelihood score
ExosomeDx® Prostate (IntelliScore), Exosome Diagnostics, Inc, Exosome Diagnostics, Inc	0005U	Oncology (prostate) gene expression profile by real-time RT-PCR of 3 genes (*ERG, PCA3,* and *SPDEF*), urine, algorithm reported as risk score
ToxProtect, Genotox Laboratories LTD	0007U	Drug test(s), presumptive, with definitive confirmation of positive results, any number of drug classes, urine, includes specimen verification including DNA authentication in comparison to buccal DNA, per date of service

★ = Telemedicine ◀ = Audio-only ✛ = Add-on code ⁄ = FDA approval pending # = Resequenced code ⊘ = Modifier 51 exempt

Proprietary Name and Clinical Laboratory or Manufacturer	Alpha-Numeric Code	Code Descriptor
AmHPR® H. pylori Antibiotic Resistance Panel, American Molecular Laboratories, Inc	0008U	Helicobacter pylori detection and antibiotic resistance, DNA, 16S and 23S rRNA, gyrA, pbp1, rdxA and rpoB, next generation sequencing, formalin-fixed paraffin-embedded or fresh tissue or fecal sample, predictive, reported as positive or negative for resistance to clarithromycin, fluoroquinolones, metronidazole, amoxicillin, tetracycline, and rifabutin
DEPArray™ HER2, PacificDx	0009U	Oncology (breast cancer), *ERBB2* (HER2) copy number by FISH, tumor cells from formalin-fixed paraffin-embedded tissue isolated using image-based dielectrophoresis (DEP) sorting, reported as *ERBB2* gene amplified or non-amplified
Bacterial Typing by Whole Genome Sequencing, Mayo Clinic	0010U	Infectious disease (bacterial), strain typing by whole genome sequencing, phylogenetic-based report of strain relatedness, per submitted isolate
Cordant CORE™, Cordant Health Solutions	0011U	Prescription drug monitoring, evaluation of drugs present by LC-MS/MS, using oral fluid, reported as a comparison to an estimated steady-state range, per date of service including all drug compounds and metabolites
—	(0012U has been deleted)	—
—	(0013U has been deleted)	—
—	(0014U has been deleted)	—
BCR-ABL1 major and minor breakpoint fusion transcripts, University of Iowa, Department of Pathology, Asuragen	0016U	Oncology (hematolymphoid neoplasia), RNA, *BCR/ABL1* major and minor breakpoint fusion transcripts, quantitative PCR amplification, blood or bone marrow, report of fusion not detected or detected with quantitation
JAK2 Mutation, University of Iowa, Department of Pathology	0017U	Oncology (hematolymphoid neoplasia), *JAK2* mutation, DNA, PCR amplification of exons 12-14 and sequence analysis, blood or bone marrow, report of *JAK2* mutation not detected or detected
ThyraMIR™, Interpace Diagnostics	0018U	Oncology (thyroid), microRNA profiling by RT-PCR of 10 microRNA sequences, utilizing fine needle aspirate, algorithm reported as a positive or negative result for moderate to high risk of malignancy
OncoTarget/OncoTreat, Columbia University Department of Pathology and Cell Biology, Darwin Health	0019U	Oncology, RNA, gene expression by whole transcriptome sequencing, formalin-fixed paraffin-embedded tissue or fresh frozen tissue, predictive algorithm reported as potential targets for therapeutic agents
Apifiny®, Armune BioScience, Inc	0021U	Oncology (prostate), detection of 8 autoantibodies (ARF 6, NKX3-1, 5'-UTR-BMI1, CEP 164, 3'-UTR-Ropporin, Desmocollin, AURKAIP-1, CSNK2A2), multiplexed immunoassay and flow cytometry serum, algorithm reported as risk score

(Continued on page 212)

▲ = Revised code   ● = New code   ▶ ◀ = Contains new or revised text   ✖ = Duplicate PLA test   ↕ = Category I PLA   American Medical Association   **211**

Proprietary Name and Clinical Laboratory or Manufacturer	Alpha-Numeric Code	Code Descriptor
Oncomine™ Dx Target Test, Thermo Fisher Scientific, Thermo Fisher Scientific	0022U	Targeted genomic sequence analysis panel, non-small cell lung neoplasia, DNA and RNA analysis, 23 genes, interrogation for sequence variants and rearrangements, reported as presence or absence of variants and associated therapy(ies) to consider
LeukoStrat® CDx *FLT3* Mutation Assay, LabPMM LLC, an Invivoscribe Technologies, Inc Company, Invivoscribe Technologies, Inc	0023U	Oncology (acute myelogenous leukemia), DNA, genotyping of internal tandem duplication, p.D835, p.I836, using mononuclear cells, reported as detection or non-detection of *FLT3* mutation and indication for or against the use of midostaurin
GlycA, Laboratory Corporation of America, Laboratory Corporation of America	0024U	Glycosylated acute phase proteins (GlycA), nuclear magnetic resonance spectroscopy, quantitative
UrSure Tenofovir Quantification Test, Synergy Medical Laboratories, UrSure Inc	0025U	Tenofovir, by liquid chromatography with tandem mass spectrometry (LC-MS/MS), urine, quantitative
Thyroseq Genomic Classifier, CBLPath, Inc, University of Pittsburgh Medical Center	0026U	Oncology (thyroid), DNA and mRNA of 112 genes, next-generation sequencing, fine needle aspirate of thyroid nodule, algorithmic analysis reported as a categorical result ("Positive, high probability of malignancy" or "Negative, low probability of malignancy")
JAK2 Exons 12 to 15 Sequencing, Mayo Clinic, Mayo Clinic	0027U	*JAK2 (Janus kinase 2)* (eg, myeloproliferative disorder) gene analysis, targeted sequence analysis exons 12-15
Focused Pharmacogenomics Panel, Mayo Clinic, Mayo Clinic	0029U	Drug metabolism (adverse drug reactions and drug response), targeted sequence analysis (ie, *CYP1A2, CYP2C19, CYP2C9, CYP2D6, CYP3A4, CYP3A5, CYP4F2, SLCO1B1, VKORC1* and rs12777823)
Warfarin Response Genotype, Mayo Clinic, Mayo Clinic	0030U	Drug metabolism (warfarin drug response), targeted sequence analysis (ie, *CYP2C9, CYP4F2, VKORC1,* rs12777823)
Cytochrome P450 1A2 Genotype, Mayo Clinic, Mayo Clinic	0031U	*CYP1A2 (cytochrome P450 family 1, subfamily A, member 2)* (eg, drug metabolism) gene analysis, common variants (ie, *1F, *1K, *6, *7)
Catechol-O-Methyltransferase (*COMT*) Genotype, Mayo Clinic, Mayo Clinic	0032U	*COMT (catechol-O-methyltransferase)* (eg, drug metabolism) gene analysis, c.472G>A (rs4680) variant
Serotonin Receptor Genotype (*HTR2A* and *HTR2C*), Mayo Clinic, Mayo Clinic	0033U	*HTR2A (5-hydroxytryptamine receptor 2A), HTR2C (5-hydroxytryptamine receptor 2C)* (eg, citalopram metabolism) gene analysis, common variants (ie, *HTR2A* rs7997012 [c.614-2211T>C], *HTR2C* rs3813929 [c.-759C>T] and rs1414334 [c.551-3008C>G])
Thiopurine Methyltransferase (*TPMT*) and Nudix Hydrolase (*NUDT15*) Genotyping, Mayo Clinic, Mayo Clinic	0034U	*TPMT (thiopurine S-methyltransferase), NUDT15 (nudix hydroxylase 15)* (eg, thiopurine metabolism) gene analysis, common variants (ie, *TPMT* *2, *3A, *3B, *3C, *4, *5, *6, *8, *12; *NUDT15* *3, *4, *5)

★ = Telemedicine   ◀ = Audio-only   ✛ = Add-on code   ✗ = FDA approval pending   # = Resequenced code   ⊘ = Modifier 51 exempt

Proprietary Name and Clinical Laboratory or Manufacturer	Alpha-Numeric Code	Code Descriptor
Real-time quaking-induced conversion for prion detection (RT-QuIC), National Prion Disease Pathology Surveillance Center	0035U	Neurology (prion disease), cerebrospinal fluid, detection of prion protein by quaking-induced conformational conversion, qualitative
EXaCT-1 Whole Exome Testing, Lab of Oncology-Molecular Detection, Weill Cornell Medicine-Clinical Genomics Laboratory	0036U	Exome (ie, somatic mutations), paired formalin-fixed paraffin-embedded tumor tissue and normal specimen, sequence analyses
FoundationOne CDx™ (F1CDx), Foundation Medicine, Inc, Foundation Medicine, Inc	0037U	Targeted genomic sequence analysis, solid organ neoplasm, DNA analysis of 324 genes, interrogation for sequence variants, gene copy number amplifications, gene rearrangements, microsatellite instability and tumor mutational burden
Sensieva™ Droplet 25OH Vitamin D2/D3 Microvolume LC/MS Assay, InSource Diagnostics, InSource Diagnostics	0038U	Vitamin D, 25 hydroxy D2 and D3, by LC-MS/MS, serum microsample, quantitative
Anti-dsDNA, High Salt/Avidity, University of Washington, Department of Laboratory Medicine, Bio-Rad	0039U	Deoxyribonucleic acid (DNA) antibody, double stranded, high avidity
MRDx BCR-ABL Test, MolecularMD, MolecularMD	0040U	*BCR/ABL1 (t(9;22))* (eg, chronic myelogenous leukemia) translocation analysis, major breakpoint, quantitative
Lyme ImmunoBlot IgM, IGeneX Inc, ID-FISH Technology Inc (ASR) (Lyme ImmunoBlot IgM Strips Only)	0041U	Borrelia burgdorferi, antibody detection of 5 recombinant protein groups, by immunoblot, IgM
Lyme ImmunoBlot IgG, IGeneX Inc, ID-FISH Technology Inc (ASR) (Lyme ImmunoBlot IgG Strips Only)	0042U	Borrelia burgdorferi, antibody detection of 12 recombinant protein groups, by immunoblot, IgG
Tick-Borne Relapsing Fever (TBRF) Borrelia ImmunoBlots IgM Test, IGeneX Inc, ID-FISH Technology (Provides TBRF ImmunoBlot IgM Strips)	0043U	Tick-borne relapsing fever Borrelia group, antibody detection to 4 recombinant protein groups, by immunoblot, IgM
Tick-Borne Relapsing Fever (TBRF) Borrelia ImmunoBlots IgG Test, IGeneX Inc, ID-FISH Technology Inc (Provides TBRF ImmunoBlot IgG Strips)	0044U	Tick-borne relapsing fever Borrelia group, antibody detection to 4 recombinant protein groups, by immunoblot, IgG
The Oncotype DX® Breast DCIS Score™ Test, Genomic Health, Inc, Genomic Health, Inc	0045U	Oncology (breast ductal carcinoma in situ), mRNA, gene expression profiling by real-time RT-PCR of 12 genes (7 content and 5 housekeeping), utilizing formalin-fixed paraffin-embedded tissue, algorithm reported as recurrence score
FLT3 ITD MRD by NGS, LabPMM LLC, an Invivoscribe Technologies, Inc Company	0046U	*FLT3 (fms-related tyrosine kinase 3)* (eg, acute myeloid leukemia) internal tandem duplication (ITD) variants, quantitative

(Continued on page 214)

Proprietary Name and Clinical Laboratory or Manufacturer	Alpha-Numeric Code	Code Descriptor
▶Genomic Prostate Score® (GPS) Test, MDxHealth, Inc, MDxHealth, Inc◀	0047U	Oncology (prostate), mRNA, gene expression profiling by real-time RT-PCR of 17 genes (12 content and 5 housekeeping), utilizing formalin-fixed paraffin-embedded tissue, algorithm reported as a risk score
MSK-IMPACT (Integrated Mutation Profiling of Actionable Cancer Targets), Memorial Sloan Kettering Cancer Center	0048U	Oncology (solid organ neoplasia), DNA, targeted sequencing of protein-coding exons of 468 cancer-associated genes, including interrogation for somatic mutations and microsatellite instability, matched with normal specimens, utilizing formalin-fixed paraffin-embedded tumor tissue, report of clinically significant mutation(s)
NPM1 MRD by NGS, LabPMM LLC, an Invivoscribe Technologies, Inc Company	0049U	*NPM1 (nucleophosmin)* (eg, acute myeloid leukemia) gene analysis, quantitative
MyAML NGS Panel, LabPMM LLC, an Invivoscribe Technologies, Inc Company	0050U	Targeted genomic sequence analysis panel, acute myelogenous leukemia, DNA analysis, 194 genes, interrogation for sequence variants, copy number variants or rearrangements
UCompliDx, Elite Medical Laboratory Solutions, LLC, Elite Medical Laboratory Solutions, LLC (LDT)	0051U	Prescription drug monitoring, evaluation of drugs present by liquid chromatography tandem mass spectrometry (LC-MS/MS), urine or blood, 31 drug panel, reported as quantitative results, detected or not detected, per date of service
VAP Cholesterol Test, VAP Diagnostics Laboratory, Inc, VAP Diagnostics Laboratory, Inc	0052U	Lipoprotein, blood, high resolution fractionation and quantitation of lipoproteins, including all five major lipoprotein classes and subclasses of HDL, LDL, and VLDL by vertical auto profile ultracentrifugation
—	(0053U has been deleted)	—
AssuranceRx Micro Serum, Firstox Laboratories, LLC, Firstox Laboratories, LLC	0054U	Prescription drug monitoring, 14 or more classes of drugs and substances, definitive tandem mass spectrometry with chromatography, capillary blood, quantitative report with therapeutic and toxic ranges, including steady-state range for the prescribed dose when detected, per date of service
myTAIHEART, TAI Diagnostics, Inc, TAI Diagnostics, Inc	0055U	Cardiology (heart transplant), cell-free DNA, PCR assay of 96 DNA target sequences (94 single nucleotide polymorphism targets and two control targets), plasma
—	(0056U has been deleted)	—
Merkel SmT Oncoprotein Antibody Titer, University of Washington, Department of Laboratory Medicine	0058U	Oncology (Merkel cell carcinoma), detection of antibodies to the Merkel cell polyoma virus oncoprotein (small T antigen), serum, quantitative
Merkel Virus VP1 Capsid Antibody, University of Washington, Department of Laboratory Medicine	0059U	Oncology (Merkel cell carcinoma), detection of antibodies to the Merkel cell polyoma virus capsid protein (VP1), serum, reported as positive or negative
Twins Zygosity PLA, Natera, Inc, Natera, Inc	0060U	Twin zygosity, genomic-targeted sequence analysis of chromosome 2, using circulating cell-free fetal DNA in maternal blood

★ = Telemedicine ◀ = Audio-only ✚ = Add-on code ✗ = FDA approval pending # = Resequenced code ⦸ = Modifier 51 exempt

Proprietary Name and Clinical Laboratory or Manufacturer	Alpha-Numeric Code	Code Descriptor
Transcutaneous multispectral measurement of tissue oxygenation and hemoglobin using spatial frequency domain imaging (SFDI), Modulated Imaging, Inc, Modulated Imaging, Inc	0061U	Transcutaneous measurement of five biomarkers (tissue oxygenation [StO_2], oxyhemoglobin [$ctHbO_2$], deoxyhemoglobin [ctHbR], papillary and reticular dermal hemoglobin concentrations [ctHb1 and ctHb2]), using spatial frequency domain imaging (SFDI) and multi-spectral analysis
SLE-key® Rule Out, Veracis Inc, Veracis Inc	0062U	Autoimmune (systemic lupus erythematosus), IgG and IgM analysis of 80 biomarkers, utilizing serum, algorithm reported with a risk score
NPDX ASD ADM Panel I, Stemina Biomarker Discovery, Inc, Stemina Biomarker Discovery, Inc d/b/a NeuroPointDX	0063U	Neurology (autism), 32 amines by LC-MS/MS, using plasma, algorithm reported as metabolic signature associated with autism spectrum disorder
BioPlex 2200 Syphilis Total & RPR Assay, Bio-Rad Laboratories, Bio-Rad Laboratories	0064U	Antibody, Treponema pallidum, total and rapid plasma reagin (RPR), immunoassay, qualitative
BioPlex 2200 RPR Assay, Bio-Rad Laboratories, Bio-Rad Laboratories	0065U	Syphilis test, non-treponemal antibody, immunoassay, qualitative (RPR)
—	(0066U has been deleted)	—
BBDRisk Dx™, Silbiotech, Inc, Silbiotech, Inc	0067U	Oncology (breast), immunohistochemistry, protein expression profiling of 4 biomarkers (matrix metalloproteinase-1 [MMP-1], carcinoembryonic antigen-related cell adhesion molecule 6 [CEACAM6], hyaluronoglucosaminidase [HYAL1], highly expressed in cancer protein [HEC1]), formalin-fixed paraffin-embedded precancerous breast tissue, algorithm reported as carcinoma risk score
MYCODART-PCR™ Dual Amplification Real Time PCR Panel for 6 Candida species, RealTime Laboratories, Inc/MycoDART, Inc, RealTime Laboratories, Inc	0068U	Candida species panel (C. albicans, C. glabrata, C. parapsilosis, C. kruseii, C. tropicalis, and C. auris), amplified probe technique with qualitative report of the presence or absence of each species
miR-31now™, GoPath Laboratories, GoPath Laboratories	0069U	Oncology (colorectal), microRNA, RT-PCR expression profiling of miR-31-3p, formalin-fixed paraffin-embedded tissue, algorithm reported as an expression score
CYP2D6 Common Variants and Copy Number, Mayo Clinic, Laboratory Developed Test	0070U	CYP2D6 (cytochrome P450, family 2, subfamily D, polypeptide 6) (eg, drug metabolism) gene analysis, common and select rare variants (ie, *2, *3, *4, *4N, *5, *6, *7, *8, *9, *10, *11, *12, *13, *14A, *14B, *15, *17, *29, *35, *36, *41, *57, *61, *63, *68, *83, *xN)
CYP2D6 Full Gene Sequencing, Mayo Clinic, Laboratory Developed Test	+0071U	CYP2D6 (cytochrome P450, family 2, subfamily D, polypeptide 6) (eg, drug metabolism) gene analysis, full gene sequence (List separately in addition to code for primary procedure) (Use 0071U in conjunction with 0070U)

(Continued on page 216)

Proprietary Name and Clinical Laboratory or Manufacturer	Alpha-Numeric Code	Code Descriptor
CYP2D6-2D7 Hybrid Gene Targeted Sequence Analysis, Mayo Clinic, Laboratory Developed Test	+0072U	*CYP2D6 (cytochrome P450, family 2, subfamily D, polypeptide 6)* (eg, drug metabolism) gene analysis, targeted sequence analysis (ie, *CYP2D6-2D7* hybrid gene) (List separately in addition to code for primary procedure) (Use 0072U in conjunction with 0070U)
CYP2D7-2D6 Hybrid Gene Targeted Sequence Analysis, Mayo Clinic, Laboratory Developed Test	+0073U	*CYP2D6 (cytochrome P450, family 2, subfamily D, polypeptide 6)* (eg, drug metabolism) gene analysis, targeted sequence analysis (ie, *CYP2D7-2D6* hybrid gene) (List separately in addition to code for primary procedure) (Use 0073U in conjunction with 0070U)
CYP2D6 trans-duplication/multiplication non-duplicated gene targeted sequence analysis, Mayo Clinic, Laboratory Developed Test	+0074U	*CYP2D6 (cytochrome P450, family 2, subfamily D, polypeptide 6)* (eg, drug metabolism) gene analysis, targeted sequence analysis (ie, non-duplicated gene when duplication/multiplication is trans) (List separately in addition to code for primary procedure) (Use 0074U in conjunction with 0070U)
CYP2D6 5' gene duplication/multiplication targeted sequence analysis, Mayo Clinic, Laboratory Developed Test	+0075U	*CYP2D6 (cytochrome P450, family 2, subfamily D, polypeptide 6)* (eg, drug metabolism) gene analysis, targeted sequence analysis (ie, 5' gene duplication/multiplication) (List separately in addition to code for primary procedure) (Use 0075U in conjunction with 0070U)
CYP2D6 3' gene duplication/multiplication targeted sequence analysis, Mayo Clinic, Laboratory Developed Test	+0076U	*CYP2D6 (cytochrome P450, family 2, subfamily D, polypeptide 6)* (eg, drug metabolism) gene analysis, targeted sequence analysis (ie, 3' gene duplication/multiplication) (List separately in addition to code for primary procedure) (Use 0076U in conjunction with 0070U)
M-Protein Detection and Isotyping by MALDI-TOF Mass Spectrometry, Mayo Clinic, Laboratory Developed Test	0077U	Immunoglobulin paraprotein (M-protein), qualitative, immunoprecipitation and mass spectrometry, blood or urine, including isotype
—	▶(0078U has been deleted)◀	—
ToxLok™, InSource Diagnostics, InSource Diagnostics	0079U	Comparative DNA analysis using multiple selected single-nucleotide polymorphisms (SNPs), urine and buccal DNA, for specimen identity verification
BDX-XL2, Biodesix®, Inc, Biodesix®, Inc	0080U	Oncology (lung), mass spectrometric analysis of galectin-3-binding protein and scavenger receptor cysteine-rich type 1 protein M130, with five clinical risk factors (age, smoking status, nodule diameter, nodule-spiculation status and nodule location), utilizing plasma, algorithm reported as a categorical probability of malignancy

★=Telemedicine ◀=Audio-only +=Add-on code ✗=FDA approval pending #=Resequenced code ⊘=Modifier 51 exempt

Proprietary Name and Clinical Laboratory or Manufacturer	Alpha-Numeric Code	Code Descriptor
NextGen Precision™ Testing, Precision Diagnostics, Precision Diagnostics LBN Precision Toxicology, LLC	0082U	Drug test(s), definitive, 90 or more drugs or substances, definitive chromatography with mass spectrometry, and presumptive, any number of drug classes, by instrument chemistry analyzer (utilizing immunoassay), urine, report of presence or absence of each drug, drug metabolite or substance with description and severity of significant interactions per date of service
Onco4D™, Animated Dynamics, Inc, Animated Dynamics, Inc	0083U	Oncology, response to chemotherapy drugs using motility contrast tomography, fresh or frozen tissue, reported as likelihood of sensitivity or resistance to drugs or drug combinations
BLOODchip® ID CORE XT™, Grifols Diagnostic Solutions Inc	0084U	Red blood cell antigen typing, DNA, genotyping of 10 blood groups with phenotype prediction of 37 red blood cell antigens
Accelerate PhenoTest™ BC kit, Accelerate Diagnostics, Inc	0086U	Infectious disease (bacterial and fungal), organism identification, blood culture, using rRNA FISH, 6 or more organism targets, reported as positive or negative with phenotypic minimum inhibitory concentration (MIC)-based antimicrobial susceptibility
Molecular Microscope® MMDx— Heart, Kashi Clinical Laboratories	0087U	Cardiology (heart transplant), mRNA gene expression profiling by microarray of 1283 genes, transplant biopsy tissue, allograft rejection and injury algorithm reported as a probability score
Molecular Microscope® MMDx— Kidney, Kashi Clinical Laboratories	0088U	Transplantation medicine (kidney allograft rejection), microarray gene expression profiling of 1494 genes, utilizing transplant biopsy tissue, algorithm reported as a probability score for rejection
Pigmented Lesion Assay (PLA), DermTech	0089U	Oncology (melanoma), gene expression profiling by RTqPCR, *PRAME* and *LINC00518*, superficial collection using adhesive patch(es)
myPath® Melanoma, Castle Biosciences, Inc	0090U	Oncology (cutaneous melanoma), mRNA gene expression profiling by RT-PCR of 23 genes (14 content and 9 housekeeping), utilizing formalin-fixed paraffin-embedded (FFPE) tissue, algorithm reported as a categorical result (ie, benign, intermediate, malignant)
FirstSight^CRC, CellMax Life	0091U	Oncology (colorectal) screening, cell enumeration of circulating tumor cells, utilizing whole blood, algorithm, for the presence of adenoma or cancer, reported as a positive or negative result
REVEAL Lung Nodule Characterization, MagArray, Inc	0092U	Oncology (lung), three protein biomarkers, immunoassay using magnetic nanosensor technology, plasma, algorithm reported as risk score for likelihood of malignancy
ComplyRX, Claro Labs	0093U	Prescription drug monitoring, evaluation of 65 common drugs by LC-MS/MS, urine, each drug reported detected or not detected

(Continued on page 218)

▲ = Revised code   ● = New code   ▶ ◀ = Contains new or revised text   ✕ = Duplicate PLA test   ⇅ = Category I PLA

Proprietary Name and Clinical Laboratory or Manufacturer	Alpha-Numeric Code	Code Descriptor
RCIGM Rapid Whole Genome Sequencing, Rady Children's Institute for Genomic Medicine (RCIGM)	0094U	Genome (eg, unexplained constitutional or heritable disorder or syndrome), rapid sequence analysis
Esophageal String Test™ (EST), Children's Hospital Colorado Department of Pathology and Laboratory Medicine	0095U	Eosinophilic esophagitis (Eotaxin-3 *[CCL26 {C-C motif chemokine ligand 26}]* and major basic protein *[PRG2 {proteoglycan 2, pro eosinophil major basic protein}]*), enzyme-linked immunosorbent assays (ELISA), specimen obtained by esophageal string test device, algorithm reported as probability of active or inactive eosinophilic esophagitis
HPV, High-Risk, Male Urine, Molecular Testing Labs	0096U	Human papillomavirus (HPV), high-risk types (ie, 16, 18, 31, 33, 35, 39, 45, 51, 52, 56, 58, 59, 66, 68), male urine
—	(0097U has been deleted)	—
ColoNext®, Ambry Genetics®, Ambry Genetics®	0101U	Hereditary colon cancer disorders (eg, Lynch syndrome, *PTEN* hamartoma syndrome, Cowden syndrome, familial adenomatosis polyposis), genomic sequence analysis panel utilizing a combination of NGS, Sanger, MLPA, and array CGH, with mRNA analytics to resolve variants of unknown significance when indicated (15 genes [sequencing and deletion/duplication], *EPCAM* and *GREM1* [deletion/duplication only])
BreastNext®, Ambry Genetics®, Ambry Genetics®	0102U	Hereditary breast cancer-related disorders (eg, hereditary breast cancer, hereditary ovarian cancer, hereditary endometrial cancer), genomic sequence analysis panel utilizing a combination of NGS, Sanger, MLPA, and array CGH, with mRNA analytics to resolve variants of unknown significance when indicated (17 genes [sequencing and deletion/duplication])
OvaNext®, Ambry Genetics®, Ambry Genetics®	0103U	Hereditary ovarian cancer (eg, hereditary ovarian cancer, hereditary endometrial cancer), genomic sequence analysis panel utilizing a combination of NGS, Sanger, MLPA, and array CGH, with mRNA analytics to resolve variants of unknown significance when indicated (24 genes [sequencing and deletion/duplication], *EPCAM* [deletion/duplication only])
KidneyIntelX™, RenalytixAI, RenalytixAI	0105U	Nephrology (chronic kidney disease), multiplex electrochemiluminescent immunoassay (ECLIA) of tumor necrosis factor receptor 1A, receptor superfamily 2 *(TNFR1, TNFR2),* and kidney injury molecule-1 (KIM-1) combined with longitudinal clinical data, including *APOL1* genotype if available, and plasma (isolated fresh or frozen), algorithm reported as probability score for rapid kidney function decline (RKFD)

★ = Telemedicine   ◀ = Audio-only   ✚ = Add-on code   ✗ = FDA approval pending   # = Resequenced code   ⊘ = Modifier 51 exempt

Proprietary Name and Clinical Laboratory or Manufacturer	Alpha-Numeric Code	Code Descriptor
13C-Spirulina Gastric Emptying Breath Test (GEBT), Cairn Diagnostics d/b/a Advanced Breath Diagnostics, LLC, Cairn Diagnostics d/b/a Advanced Breath Diagnostics, LLC	0106U	Gastric emptying, serial collection of 7 timed breath specimens, non-radioisotope carbon-13 (^{13}C) spirulina substrate, analysis of each specimen by gas isotope ratio mass spectrometry, reported as rate of $^{13}CO_2$ excretion
Singulex Clarity C. diff toxins A/B Assay, Singulex	0107U	Clostridium difficile toxin(s) antigen detection by immunoassay technique, stool, qualitative, multiple-step method
TissueCypher® Barrett's Esophagus Assay, Cernostics, Cernostics	0108U	Gastroenterology (Barrett's esophagus), whole slide–digital imaging, including morphometric analysis, computer-assisted quantitative immunolabeling of 9 protein biomarkers (p16, AMACR, p53, CD68, COX-2, CD45RO, HIF1a, HER-2, K20) and morphology, formalin-fixed paraffin-embedded tissue, algorithm reported as risk of progression to high-grade dysplasia or cancer
MYCODART Dual Amplification Real Time PCR Panel for 4 Aspergillus species, RealTime Laboratories, Inc/MycoDART, Inc	0109U	Infectious disease (Aspergillus species), real-time PCR for detection of DNA from 4 species *(A. fumigatus, A. terreus, A. niger, and A. flavus)*, blood, lavage fluid, or tissue, qualitative reporting of presence or absence of each species
Oral OncolyticAssuranceRX, Firstox Laboratories, LLC, Firstox Laboratories, LLC	0110U	Prescription drug monitoring, one or more oral oncology drug(s) and substances, definitive tandem mass spectrometry with chromatography, serum or plasma from capillary blood or venous blood, quantitative report with steady-state range for the prescribed drug(s) when detected
Praxis™ Extended RAS Panel, Illumina, Illumina	0111U	Oncology (colon cancer), targeted *KRAS* (codons 12, 13, and 61) and *NRAS* (codons 12, 13, and 61) gene analysis, utilizing formalin-fixed paraffin-embedded tissue
MicroGenDX qPCR & NGS For Infection, MicroGenDX, MicroGenDX	0112U	Infectious agent detection and identification, targeted sequence analysis (16S and 18S rRNA genes) with drug-resistance gene
MyProstateScore, Lynx DX, Lynx DX	0113U	Oncology (prostate), measurement of *PCA3* and *TMPRSS2-ERG* in urine and PSA in serum following prostatic massage, by RNA amplification and fluorescence-based detection, algorithm reported as risk score
EsoGuard™, Lucid Diagnostics, Lucid Diagnostics	0114U	Gastroenterology (Barrett's esophagus), *VIM* and *CCNA1* methylation analysis, esophageal cells, algorithm reported as likelihood for Barrett's esophagus
ePlex Respiratory Pathogen (RP) Panel, GenMark Diagnostics, Inc, GenMark Diagnostics, Inc	0115U	Respiratory infectious agent detection by nucleic acid (DNA and RNA), 18 viral types and subtypes and 2 bacterial targets, amplified probe technique, including multiplex reverse transcription for RNA targets, each analyte reported as detected or not detected

(Continued on page 220)

Appendix O

Proprietary Name and Clinical Laboratory or Manufacturer	Alpha-Numeric Code	Code Descriptor
Snapshot Oral Fluid Compliance, Ethos Laboratories	0116U	Prescription drug monitoring, enzyme immunoassay of 35 or more drugs confirmed with LC-MS/MS, oral fluid, algorithm results reported as a patient-compliance measurement with risk of drug to drug interactions for prescribed medications
Foundation PI^{SM}, Ethos Laboratories	0117U	Pain management, analysis of 11 endogenous analytes (methylmalonic acid, xanthurenic acid, homocysteine, pyroglutamic acid, vanilmandelate, 5-hydroxyindoleacetic acid, hydroxymethylglutarate, ethylmalonate, 3-hydroxypropyl mercapturic acid (3-HPMA), quinolinic acid, kynurenic acid), LC-MS/MS, urine, algorithm reported as a pain-index score with likelihood of atypical biochemical function associated with pain
►Eurofins TRAC™ dd-cfDNA, Transplant Genomics Inc, Transplant Genomics Inc◄	0118U	Transplantation medicine, quantification of donor-derived cell-free DNA using whole genome next-generation sequencing, plasma, reported as percentage of donor-derived cell-free DNA in the total cell-free DNA
MI-HEART Ceramides, Plasma, Mayo Clinic, Laboratory Developed Test	0119U	Cardiology, ceramides by liquid chromatography–tandem mass spectrometry, plasma, quantitative report with risk score for major cardiovascular events
Lymph3Cx Lymphoma Molecular Subtyping Assay, Mayo Clinic, Laboratory Developed Test	0120U	Oncology (B-cell lymphoma classification), mRNA, gene expression profiling by fluorescent probe hybridization of 58 genes (45 content and 13 housekeeping genes), formalin-fixed paraffin-embedded tissue, algorithm reported as likelihood for primary mediastinal B-cell lymphoma (PMBCL) and diffuse large B-cell lymphoma (DLBCL) with cell of origin subtyping in the latter (Do not report 0120U in conjunction with 0017M)
Flow Adhesion of Whole Blood on VCAM-1 (FAB-V), Functional Fluidics, Functional Fluidics	0121U	Sickle cell disease, microfluidic flow adhesion (VCAM-1), whole blood
Flow Adhesion of Whole Blood to P-SELECTIN (WB-PSEL), Functional Fluidics, Functional Fluidics	0122U	Sickle cell disease, microfluidic flow adhesion (P-Selectin), whole blood
Mechanical Fragility, RBC by shear stress profiling and spectral analysis, Functional Fluidics, Functional Fluidics	0123U	Mechanical fragility, RBC, shear stress and spectral analysis profiling
BRCAplus, Ambry Genetics	0129U	Hereditary breast cancer–related disorders (eg, hereditary breast cancer, hereditary ovarian cancer, hereditary endometrial cancer), genomic sequence analysis and deletion/duplication analysis panel (ATM, BRCA1, BRCA2, CDH1, CHEK2, PALB2, PTEN, and TP53)

★ =Telemedicine   ◀ =Audio-only   ✚ =Add-on code   ✖ =FDA approval pending   # =Resequenced code   ⊘ =Modifier 51 exempt

Appendix O

Proprietary Name and Clinical Laboratory or Manufacturer	Alpha-Numeric Code	Code Descriptor
+RNAinsight™ for ColoNext®, Ambry Genetics	✚0130U	Hereditary colon cancer disorders (eg, Lynch syndrome, PTEN hamartoma syndrome, Cowden syndrome, familial adenomatosis polyposis), targeted mRNA sequence analysis panel *(APC, CDH1, CHEK2, MLH1, MSH2, MSH6, MUTYH, PMS2, PTEN,* and *TP53)* (List separately in addition to code for primary procedure) (Use 0130U in conjunction with 81435, 0101U)
+RNAinsight™ for BreastNext®, Ambry Genetics	✚0131U	Hereditary breast cancer–related disorders (eg, hereditary breast cancer, hereditary ovarian cancer, hereditary endometrial cancer), targeted mRNA sequence analysis panel (13 genes) (List separately in addition to code for primary procedure) (Use 0131U in conjunction with 81162, 81432, 0102U)
+RNAinsight™ for OvaNext®, Ambry Genetics	✚0132U	Hereditary ovarian cancer–related disorders (eg, hereditary breast cancer, hereditary ovarian cancer, hereditary endometrial cancer), targeted mRNA sequence analysis panel (17 genes) (List separately in addition to code for primary procedure) (Use 0132U in conjunction with 81162, 81432, 0103U)
+RNAinsight™ for ProstateNext®, Ambry Genetics	✚0133U	Hereditary prostate cancer–related disorders, targeted mRNA sequence analysis panel (11 genes) (List separately in addition to code for primary procedure) (Use 0133U in conjunction with 81162)
+RNAinsight™ for CancerNext®, Ambry Genetics	✚0134U	Hereditary pan cancer (eg, hereditary breast and ovarian cancer, hereditary endometrial cancer, hereditary colorectal cancer), targeted mRNA sequence analysis panel (18 genes) (List separately in addition to code for primary procedure) (Use 0134U in conjunction with 81162, 81432, 81435)
+RNAinsight™ for GYNPlus®, Ambry Genetics	✚0135U	Hereditary gynecological cancer (eg, hereditary breast and ovarian cancer, hereditary endometrial cancer, hereditary colorectal cancer), targeted mRNA sequence analysis panel (12 genes) (List separately in addition to code for primary procedure) (Use 0135U in conjunction with 81162)
+RNAinsight™ for *ATM*, Ambry Genetics	✚0136U	*ATM (ataxia telangiectasia mutated)* (eg, ataxia telangiectasia) mRNA sequence analysis (List separately in addition to code for primary procedure) (Use 0136U in conjunction with 81408)
+RNAinsight™ for *PALB2*, Ambry Genetics	✚0137U	*PALB2 (partner and localizer of BRCA2)* (eg, breast and pancreatic cancer) mRNA sequence analysis (List separately in addition to code for primary procedure) (Use 0137U in conjunction with 81307)

(Continued on page 222)

Appendix O

Proprietary Name and Clinical Laboratory or Manufacturer	Alpha-Numeric Code	Code Descriptor
+RNAinsight™ for *BRCA1/2*, Ambry Genetics	+0138U	*BRCA1 (BRCA1, DNA repair associated), BRCA2 (BRCA2, DNA repair associated)* (eg, hereditary breast and ovarian cancer) mRNA sequence analysis (List separately in addition to code for primary procedure) (Use 0138U in conjunction with 81162)
ePlex® BCID Fungal Pathogens Panel, GenMark Diagnostics, Inc, GenMark Diagnostics, Inc	0140U	Infectious disease (fungi), fungal pathogen identification, DNA (15 fungal targets), blood culture, amplified probe technique, each target reported as detected or not detected
ePlex® BCID Gram-Positive Panel, GenMark Diagnostics, Inc, GenMark Diagnostics, Inc	0141U	Infectious disease (bacteria and fungi), gram-positive organism identification and drug resistance element detection, DNA (20 gram-positive bacterial targets, 4 resistance genes, 1 pan gram-negative bacterial target, 1 pan Candida target), blood culture, amplified probe technique, each target reported as detected or not detected
ePlex® BCID Gram-Negative Panel, GenMark Diagnostics, Inc, GenMark Diagnostics, Inc	0142U	Infectious disease (bacteria and fungi), gram-negative bacterial identification and drug resistance element detection, DNA (21 gram-negative bacterial targets, 6 resistance genes, 1 pan gram-positive bacterial target, 1 pan Candida target), amplified probe technique, each target reported as detected or not detected
—	(0143U has been deleted)	—
—	(0144U has been deleted)	—
—	(0145U has been deleted)	—
—	(0146U has been deleted)	—
—	(0147U has been deleted)	—
—	(0148U has been deleted)	—
—	(0149U has been deleted)	—
—	(0150U has been deleted)	—
—	(0151U has been deleted)	—
Karius® Test, Karius Inc, Karius Inc	0152U	Infectious disease (bacteria, fungi, parasites, and DNA viruses), microbial cell-free DNA, plasma, untargeted next-generation sequencing, report for significant positive pathogens
Insight TNBCtype™, Insight Molecular Labs	0153U	Oncology (breast), mRNA, gene expression profiling by next-generation sequencing of 101 genes, utilizing formalin-fixed paraffin-embedded tissue, algorithm reported as a triple negative breast cancer clinical subtype(s) with information on immune cell involvement
therascreen® *FGFR* RGQ RT-PCR Kit, QIAGEN, QIAGEN GmbH	0154U	Oncology (urothelial cancer), RNA, analysis by real-time RT-PCR of the *FGFR3 (fibroblast growth factor receptor 3)* gene analysis (ie, p.R248C [c.742C>T], p. S249C [c.746C>G], p.G370C [c.1108G>T], p. Y373C [c.1118A>G], FGFR3-TACC3v1, and FGFR3-TACC3v3), utilizing formalin-fixed paraffin-embedded urothelial cancer tumor tissue, reported as *FGFR* gene alteration status

Proprietary Name and Clinical Laboratory or Manufacturer	Alpha-Numeric Code	Code Descriptor
therascreen *PIK3CA* RGQ PCR Kit, QIAGEN, QIAGEN GmbH	0155U	Oncology (breast cancer), DNA, *PIK3CA (phosphatidylinositol-4,5-bisphosphate 3-kinase, catalytic subunit alpha)* (eg, breast cancer) gene analysis (ie, p.C420R, p.E542K, p.E545A, p.E545D [g.1635G>T only], p.E545G, p.E545K, p.Q546E, p.Q546R, p.H1047L, p.H1047R, p.H1047Y), utilizing formalin-fixed paraffin-embedded breast tumor tissue, reported as *PIK3CA* gene mutation status
SMASH™, New York Genome Center, Marvel Genomics™	0156U	Copy number (eg, intellectual disability, dysmorphology), sequence analysis
CustomNext + RNA: *APC*, Ambry Genetics®, Ambry Genetics®	+0157U	*APC (APC regulator of WNT signaling pathway)* (eg, familial adenomatosis polyposis [FAP]) mRNA sequence analysis (List separately in addition to code for primary procedure) (Use 0157U in conjunction with 81201)
CustomNext + RNA: *MLH1*, Ambry Genetics®, Ambry Genetics®	+0158U	*MLH1 (mutL homolog 1)* (eg, hereditary non-polyposis colorectal cancer, Lynch syndrome) mRNA sequence analysis (List separately in addition to code for primary procedure) (Use 0158U in conjunction with 81292)
CustomNext + RNA: *MSH2*, Ambry Genetics®, Ambry Genetics®	+0159U	*MSH2 (mutS homolog 2)* (eg, hereditary colon cancer, Lynch syndrome) mRNA sequence analysis (List separately in addition to code for primary procedure) (Use 0159U in conjunction with 81295)
CustomNext + RNA: *MSH6*, Ambry Genetics®, Ambry Genetics®	+0160U	*MSH6 (mutS homolog 6)* (eg, hereditary colon cancer, Lynch syndrome) mRNA sequence analysis (List separately in addition to code for primary procedure) (Use 0160U in conjunction with 81298)
CustomNext + RNA: *PMS2*, Ambry Genetics®, Ambry Genetics®	+0161U	*PMS2 (PMS1 homolog 2, mismatch repair system component)* (eg, hereditary non-polyposis colorectal cancer, Lynch syndrome) mRNA sequence analysis (List separately in addition to code for primary procedure) (Use 0161U in conjunction with 81317)
CustomNext + RNA: Lynch *(MLH1, MSH2, MSH6, PMS2)*, Ambry Genetics®, Ambry Genetics®	+0162U	Hereditary colon cancer (Lynch syndrome), targeted mRNA sequence analysis panel *(MLH1, MSH2, MSH6, PMS2)* (List separately in addition to code for primary procedure) (Use 0162U in conjunction with 81292, 81295, 81298, 81317, 81435)
BeScreened™-CRC, Beacon Biomedical Inc, Beacon Biomedical Inc	0163U	Oncology (colorectal) screening, biochemical enzyme-linked immunosorbent assay (ELISA) of 3 plasma or serum proteins (teratocarcinoma derived growth factor-1 [TDGF-1, Cripto-1], carcinoembryonic antigen [CEA], extracellular matrix protein [ECM]), with demographic data (age, gender, CRC-screening compliance) using a proprietary algorithm and reported as likelihood of CRC or advanced adenomas

(Continued on page 224)

Proprietary Name and Clinical Laboratory or Manufacturer	Alpha-Numeric Code	Code Descriptor
ibs-smart™, Gemelli Biotech, Gemelli Biotech	0164U	Gastroenterology (irritable bowel syndrome [IBS]), immunoassay for anti-CdtB and anti-vinculin antibodies, utilizing plasma, algorithm for elevated or not elevated qualitative results
VeriMAP™ Peanut Dx – Bead-based Epitope Assay, AllerGenis™ Clinical Laboratory, AllerGenis™ LLC	0165U	Peanut allergen-specific quantitative assessment of multiple epitopes using enzyme-linked immunosorbent assay (ELISA), blood, individual epitope results and probability of peanut allergy
LiverFASt™, Fibronostics	0166U	Liver disease, 10 biochemical assays (α2-macroglobulin, haptoglobin, apolipoprotein A1, bilirubin, GGT, ALT, AST, triglycerides, cholesterol, fasting glucose) and biometric and demographic data, utilizing serum, algorithm reported as scores for fibrosis, necroinflammatory activity, and steatosis with a summary interpretation
—	▶(0167U has been deleted)◀	—
NT (*NUDT15* and *TPMT*) genotyping panel, RPRD Diagnostics	0169U	*NUDT15 (nudix hydrolase 15)* and *TPMT (thiopurine S-methyltransferase)* (eg, drug metabolism) gene analysis, common variants
Clarifi™, Quadrant Biosciences, Inc, Quadrant Biosciences, Inc	0170U	Neurology (autism spectrum disorder [ASD]), RNA, next-generation sequencing, saliva, algorithmic analysis, and results reported as predictive probability of ASD diagnosis
MyMRD® NGS Panel, Laboratory for Personalized Molecular Medicine, Laboratory for Personalized Molecular Medicine	0171U	Targeted genomic sequence analysis panel, acute myeloid leukemia, myelodysplastic syndrome, and myeloproliferative neoplasms, DNA analysis, 23 genes, interrogation for sequence variants, rearrangements and minimal residual disease, reported as presence/absence
myChoice® CDx, Myriad Genetics Laboratories, Inc, Myriad Genetics Laboratories, Inc	0172U	Oncology (solid tumor as indicated by the label), somatic mutation analysis of *BRCA1 (BRCA1, DNA repair associated), BRCA2 (BRCA2, DNA repair associated)* and analysis of homologous recombination deficiency pathways, DNA, formalin-fixed paraffin-embedded tissue, algorithm quantifying tumor genomic instability score
Psych HealthPGx Panel, RPRD Diagnostics, RPRD Diagnostics	0173U	Psychiatry (ie, depression, anxiety), genomic analysis panel, includes variant analysis of 14 genes
LC-MS/MS Targeted Proteomic Assay, OncoOmicDx Laboratory, LDT	0174U	Oncology (solid tumor), mass spectrometric 30 protein targets, formalin-fixed paraffin-embedded tissue, prognostic and predictive algorithm reported as likely, unlikely, or uncertain benefit of 39 chemotherapy and targeted therapeutic oncology agents
Genomind® Professional PGx Express™ CORE, Genomind, Inc, Genomind, Inc	0175U	Psychiatry (eg, depression, anxiety), genomic analysis panel, variant analysis of 15 genes

★=Telemedicine ◀=Audio-only ✛=Add-on code ✗=FDA approval pending #=Resequenced code ⦸=Modifier 51 exempt

Proprietary Name and Clinical Laboratory or Manufacturer	Alpha-Numeric Code	Code Descriptor
IB*Schek*®, Commonwealth Diagnostics International, Inc, Commonwealth Diagnostics International, Inc	0176U	Cytolethal distending toxin B (CdtB) and vinculin IgG antibodies by immunoassay (ie, ELISA)
therascreen® *PIK3CA* RGQ PCR Kit, QIAGEN, QIAGEN GmbH	0177U	Oncology (breast cancer), DNA, *PIK3CA (phosphatidylinositol-4,5-bisphosphate 3-kinase catalytic subunit alpha)* gene analysis of 11 gene variants utilizing plasma, reported as *PIK3CA* gene mutation status
VeriMAP™ Peanut Reactivity Threshold–Bead Based Epitope Assay, AllerGenis™ Clinical Laboratory, AllerGenis™ LLC	0178U	Peanut allergen-specific quantitative assessment of multiple epitopes using enzyme-linked immunosorbent assay (ELISA), blood, report of minimum eliciting exposure for a clinical reaction
Resolution ctDx Lung™, Resolution Bioscience, Resolution Bioscience, Inc	0179U	Oncology (non-small cell lung cancer), cell-free DNA, targeted sequence analysis of 23 genes (single nucleotide variations, insertions and deletions, fusions without prior knowledge of partner/breakpoint, copy number variations), with report of significant mutation(s)
Navigator ABO Sequencing, Grifols Immunohematology Center, Grifols Immunohematology Center	0180U	Red cell antigen (ABO blood group) genotyping (ABO), gene analysis Sanger/chain termination/conventional sequencing, *ABO (ABO, alpha 1-3-N-acetylgalactosaminyltransferase and alpha 1-3-galactosyltransferase)* gene, including subtyping, 7 exons
Navigator CO Sequencing, Grifols Immunohematology Center, Grifols Immunohematology Center	0181U	Red cell antigen (Colton blood group) genotyping (CO), gene analysis, *AQP1 (aquaporin 1 [Colton blood group])* exon 1
Navigator CROM Sequencing, Grifols Immunohematology Center, Grifols Immunohematology Center	0182U	Red cell antigen (Cromer blood group) genotyping (CROM), gene analysis, *CD55 (CD55 molecule [Cromer blood group])* exons 1-10
Navigator DI Sequencing, Grifols Immunohematology Center, Grifols Immunohematology Center	0183U	Red cell antigen (Diego blood group) genotyping (DI), gene analysis, *SLC4A1 (solute carrier family 4 member 1 [Diego blood group])* exon 19
Navigator DO Sequencing, Grifols Immunohematology Center, Grifols Immunohematology Center	0184U	Red cell antigen (Dombrock blood group) genotyping (DO), gene analysis, *ART4 (ADP-ribosyltransferase 4 [Dombrock blood group])* exon 2
Navigator FUT1 Sequencing, Grifols Immunohematology Center, Grifols Immunohematology Center	0185U	Red cell antigen (H blood group) genotyping (FUT1), gene analysis, *FUT1 (fucosyltransferase 1 [H blood group])* exon 4
Navigator FUT2 Sequencing, Grifols Immunohematology Center, Grifols Immunohematology Center	0186U	Red cell antigen (H blood group) genotyping (FUT2), gene analysis, *FUT2 (fucosyltransferase 2)* exon 2
Navigator FY Sequencing, Grifols Immunohematology Center, Grifols Immunohematology Center	0187U	Red cell antigen (Duffy blood group) genotyping (FY), gene analysis, *ACKR1 (atypical chemokine receptor 1 [Duffy blood group])* exons 1-2
Navigator GE Sequencing, Grifols Immunohematology Center, Grifols Immunohematology Center	0188U	Red cell antigen (Gerbich blood group) genotyping (GE), gene analysis, *GYPC (glycophorin C [Gerbich blood group])* exons 1-4

(Continued on page 226)

▲ = Revised code ● = New code ▶ ◀ = Contains new or revised text ✕ = Duplicate PLA test ↑↓ = Category I PLA   American Medical Association **225**

Proprietary Name and Clinical Laboratory or Manufacturer	Alpha-Numeric Code	Code Descriptor
Navigator GYPA Sequencing, Grifols Immunohematology Center, Grifols Immunohematology Center	0189U	Red cell antigen (MNS blood group) genotyping (GYPA), gene analysis, *GYPA (glycophorin A [MNS blood group])* introns 1, 5, exon 2
Navigator GYPB Sequencing, Grifols Immunohematology Center, Grifols Immunohematology Center	0190U	Red cell antigen (MNS blood group) genotyping (GYPB), gene analysis, *GYPB (glycophorin B [MNS blood group])* introns 1, 5, pseudoexon 3
Navigator IN Sequencing, Grifols Immunohematology Center, Grifols Immunohematology Center	0191U	Red cell antigen (Indian blood group) genotyping (IN), gene analysis, *CD44 (CD44 molecule [Indian blood group])* exons 2, 3, 6
Navigator JK Sequencing, Grifols Immunohematology Center, Grifols Immunohematology Center	0192U	Red cell antigen (Kidd blood group) genotyping (JK), gene analysis, *SLC14A1 (solute carrier family 14 member 1 [Kidd blood group])* gene promoter, exon 9
Navigator JR Sequencing, Grifols Immunohematology Center, Grifols Immunohematology Center	0193U	Red cell antigen (JR blood group) genotyping (JR), gene analysis, *ABCG2 (ATP binding cassette subfamily G member 2 [Junior blood group])* exons 2-26
Navigator KEL Sequencing, Grifols Immunohematology Center, Grifols Immunohematology Center	0194U	Red cell antigen (Kell blood group) genotyping (KEL), gene analysis, *KEL (Kell metallo-endopeptidase [Kell blood group])* exon 8
Navigator *KLF1* Sequencing, Grifols Immunohematology Center, Grifols Immunohematology Center	0195U	*KLF1 (Kruppel-like factor 1)*, targeted sequencing (ie, exon 13)
Navigator LU Sequencing, Grifols Immunohematology Center, Grifols Immunohematology Center	0196U	Red cell antigen (Lutheran blood group) genotyping (LU), gene analysis, *BCAM (basal cell adhesion molecule [Lutheran blood group])* exon 3
Navigator LW Sequencing, Grifols Immunohematology Center, Grifols Immunohematology Center	0197U	Red cell antigen (Landsteiner-Wiener blood group) genotyping (LW), gene analysis, *ICAM4 (intercellular adhesion molecule 4 [Landsteiner-Wiener blood group])* exon 1
Navigator RHD/CE Sequencing, Grifols Immunohematology Center, Grifols Immunohematology Center	0198U	Red cell antigen (RH blood group) genotyping (RHD and RHCE), gene analysis Sanger/chain termination/conventional sequencing, *RHD (Rh blood group D antigen) exons 1-10 and RHCE (Rh blood group CcEe antigens)* exon 5
Navigator SC Sequencing, Grifols Immunohematology Center, Grifols Immunohematology Center	0199U	Red cell antigen (Scianna blood group) genotyping (SC), gene analysis, *ERMAP (erythroblast membrane associated protein [Scianna blood group])* exons 4, 12
Navigator XK Sequencing, Grifols Immunohematology Center, Grifols Immunohematology Center	0200U	Red cell antigen (Kx blood group) genotyping (XK), gene analysis, *XK (X-linked Kx blood group)* exons 1-3
Navigator YT Sequencing, Grifols Immunohematology Center, Grifols Immunohematology Center	0201U	Red cell antigen (Yt blood group) genotyping (YT), gene analysis, *ACHE (acetylcholinesterase [Cartwright blood group])* exon 2

★=Telemedicine   ◄=Audio-only   ✚=Add-on code   ✖=FDA approval pending   #=Resequenced code   ⊘=Modifier 51 exempt

Proprietary Name and Clinical Laboratory or Manufacturer	Alpha-Numeric Code	Code Descriptor
BioFire® Respiratory Panel 2.1 (RP2.1), BioFire® Diagnostics, BioFire® Diagnostics, LLC	✖0202U	Infectious disease (bacterial or viral respiratory tract infection), pathogen-specific nucleic acid (DNA or RNA), 22 targets including severe acute respiratory syndrome coronavirus 2 (SARS-CoV-2), qualitative RT-PCR, nasopharyngeal swab, each pathogen reported as detected or not detected

(For additional PLA code with identical clinical descriptor, see 0223U. See Appendix O or the most current listing on the AMA CPT website to determine appropriate code assignment) |
PredictSURE IBD™ Test, KSL Diagnostics, PredictImmune Ltd	0203U	Autoimmune (inflammatory bowel disease), mRNA, gene expression profiling by quantitative RT-PCR, 17 genes (15 target and 2 reference genes), whole blood, reported as a continuous risk score and classification of inflammatory bowel disease aggressiveness
—	▶(0204U has been deleted)◀	—
Vita Risk®, Arctic Medical Laboratories, Arctic Medical Laboratories	0205U	Ophthalmology (age-related macular degeneration), analysis of 3 gene variants (2 *CFH* gene, 1 *ARMS2* gene), using PCR and MALDI-TOF, buccal swab, reported as positive or negative for neovascular age-related macular-degeneration risk associated with zinc supplements
DISCERN™, NeuroDiagnostics, NeuroDiagnostics	0206U	Neurology (Alzheimer disease); cell aggregation using morphometric imaging and protein kinase C-epsilon (PKCe) concentration in response to amylospheroid treatment by ELISA, cultured skin fibroblasts, each reported as positive or negative for Alzheimer disease
	+0207U	quantitative imaging of phosphorylated *ERK1* and *ERK2* in response to bradykinin treatment by in situ immunofluorescence, using cultured skin fibroblasts, reported as a probability index for Alzheimer disease (List separately in addition to code for primary procedure)

(Use 0207U in conjunction with 0206U) |
—	(0208U has been deleted)	—
CNGnome™, PerkinElmer Genomics, PerkinElmer Genomics	0209U	Cytogenomic constitutional (genome-wide) analysis, interrogation of genomic regions for copy number, structural changes and areas of homozygosity for chromosomal abnormalities
BioPlex 2200 RPR Assay – Quantitative, Bio-Rad Laboratories, Bio-Rad Laboratories	0210U	Syphilis test, non-treponemal antibody, immunoassay, quantitative (RPR)
MI Cancer Seek™ - NGS Analysis, Caris MPI d/b/a Caris Life Sciences, Caris MPI d/b/a Caris Life Sciences	0211U	Oncology (pan-tumor), DNA and RNA by next-generation sequencing, utilizing formalin-fixed paraffin-embedded tissue, interpretative report for single nucleotide variants, copy number alterations, tumor mutational burden, and microsatellite instability, with therapy association

(Continued on page 228)

▲ = Revised code   ● = New code   ▶ ◀ = Contains new or revised text   ✖ = Duplicate PLA test   ↕ = Category I PLA

Proprietary Name and Clinical Laboratory or Manufacturer	Alpha-Numeric Code	Code Descriptor
Genomic Unity® Whole Genome Analysis – Proband, Variantyx Inc, Variantyx Inc	0212U	Rare diseases (constitutional/heritable disorders), whole genome and mitochondrial DNA sequence analysis, including small sequence changes, deletions, duplications, short tandem repeat gene expansions, and variants in non-uniquely mappable regions, blood or saliva, identification and categorization of genetic variants, proband (Do not report 0212U in conjunction with 81425)
Genomic Unity® Whole Genome Analysis – Comparator, Variantyx Inc, Variantyx Inc	0213U	Rare diseases (constitutional/heritable disorders), whole genome and mitochondrial DNA sequence analysis, including small sequence changes, deletions, duplications, short tandem repeat gene expansions, and variants in non-uniquely mappable regions, blood or saliva, identification and categorization of genetic variants, each comparator genome (eg, parent, sibling) (Do not report 0213U in conjunction with 81426)
Genomic Unity® Exome Plus Analysis – Proband, Variantyx Inc, Variantyx Inc	0214U	Rare diseases (constitutional/heritable disorders), whole exome and mitochondrial DNA sequence analysis, including small sequence changes, deletions, duplications, short tandem repeat gene expansions, and variants in non-uniquely mappable regions, blood or saliva, identification and categorization of genetic variants, proband (Do not report 0214U in conjunction with 81415)
Genomic Unity® Exome Plus Analysis – Comparator, Variantyx Inc, Variantyx Inc	0215U	Rare diseases (constitutional/heritable disorders), whole exome and mitochondrial DNA sequence analysis, including small sequence changes, deletions, duplications, short tandem repeat gene expansions, and variants in non-uniquely mappable regions, blood or saliva, identification and categorization of genetic variants, each comparator exome (eg, parent, sibling) (Do not report 0215U in conjunction with 81416)
Genomic Unity® Ataxia Repeat Expansion and Sequence Analysis, Variantyx Inc, Variantyx Inc	0216U	Neurology (inherited ataxias), genomic DNA sequence analysis of 12 common genes including small sequence changes, deletions, duplications, short tandem repeat gene expansions, and variants in non-uniquely mappable regions, blood or saliva, identification and categorization of genetic variants
Genomic Unity® Comprehensive Ataxia Repeat Expansion and Sequence Analysis, Variantyx Inc, Variantyx Inc	0217U	Neurology (inherited ataxias), genomic DNA sequence analysis of 51 genes including small sequence changes, deletions, duplications, short tandem repeat gene expansions, and variants in non-uniquely mappable regions, blood or saliva, identification and categorization of genetic variants
Genomic Unity® DMD Analysis, Variantyx Inc, Variantyx Inc	0218U	Neurology (muscular dystrophy), DMD gene sequence analysis, including small sequence changes, deletions, duplications, and variants in non-uniquely mappable regions, blood or saliva, identification and characterization of genetic variants

★=Telemedicine   ◀=Audio-only   ✚=Add-on code   ✗=FDA approval pending   #=Resequenced code   ⊘=Modifier 51 exempt

Proprietary Name and Clinical Laboratory or Manufacturer	Alpha-Numeric Code	Code Descriptor
Sentosa® SQ HIV-1 Genotyping Assay, Vela Diagnostics USA, Inc, Vela Operations Singapore Pte Ltd	0219U	Infectious agent (human immunodeficiency virus), targeted viral next-generation sequence analysis (ie, protease [PR], reverse transcriptase [RT], integrase [INT]), algorithm reported as prediction of antiviral drug susceptibility
PreciseDx™ Breast Cancer Test, PreciseDx, PreciseDx	0220U	Oncology (breast cancer), image analysis with artificial intelligence assessment of 12 histologic and immunohistochemical features, reported as a recurrence score
Navigator ABO Blood Group NGS, Grifols Immunohematology Center, Grifols Immunohematology Center	0221U	Red cell antigen (ABO blood group) genotyping (ABO), gene analysis, next-generation sequencing, *ABO (ABO, alpha 1-3-N-acetylgalactosaminyltransferase and alpha 1-3-galactosyltransferase) gene*
Navigator Rh Blood Group NGS, Grifols Immunohematology Center, Grifols Immunohematology Center	0222U	Red cell antigen (RH blood group) genotyping (RHD and RHCE), gene analysis, next-generation sequencing, RH proximal promoter, exons 1-10, portions of introns 2-3
QIAstat-Dx Respiratory SARS CoV-2 Panel, QIAGEN Sciences, QIAGEN GmbH	✂0223U	Infectious disease (bacterial or viral respiratory tract infection), pathogen-specific nucleic acid (DNA or RNA), 22 targets including severe acute respiratory syndrome coronavirus 2 (SARS-CoV-2), qualitative RT-PCR, nasopharyngeal swab, each pathogen reported as detected or not detected (For additional PLA code with identical clinical descriptor, see 0202U. See Appendix O or the most current listing on the AMA CPT website to determine appropriate code assignment)
COVID-19 Antibody Test, Mt Sinai, Mount Sinai Laboratory	0224U	Antibody, severe acute respiratory syndrome coronavirus 2 (SARS-CoV-2) (coronavirus disease [COVID-19]), includes titer(s), when performed (Do not report 0224U in conjunction with 86769)
ePlex® Respiratory Pathogen Panel 2, GenMark Dx, GenMark Diagnostics, Inc	0225U	Infectious disease (bacterial or viral respiratory tract infection) pathogen-specific DNA and RNA, 21 targets, including severe acute respiratory syndrome coronavirus 2 (SARS-CoV-2), amplified probe technique, including multiplex reverse transcription for RNA targets, each analyte reported as detected or not detected
Tru-Immune™, Ethos Laboratories, GenScript® USA Inc	0226U	Surrogate viral neutralization test (sVNT), severe acute respiratory syndrome coronavirus 2 (SARS-CoV-2) (coronavirus disease [COVID-19]), ELISA, plasma, serum
Comprehensive Screen, Aspenti Health	0227U	Drug assay, presumptive, 30 or more drugs or metabolites, urine, liquid chromatography with tandem mass spectrometry (LC-MS/MS) using multiple reaction monitoring (MRM), with drug or metabolite description, includes sample validation

(Continued on page 230)

Proprietary Name and Clinical Laboratory or Manufacturer	Alpha-Numeric Code	Code Descriptor
PanGIA Prostate, Genetics Institute of America, Entopsis, LLC	0228U	Oncology (prostate), multianalyte molecular profile by photometric detection of macromolecules adsorbed on nanosponge array slides with machine learning, utilizing first morning voided urine, algorithm reported as likelihood of prostate cancer
Colvera®, Clinical Genomics Pathology Inc	0229U	*BCAT1 (Branched chain amino acid transaminase 1)* and *IKZF1 (IKAROS family zinc finger 1)* (eg, colorectal cancer) promoter methylation analysis
Genomic Unity® AR Analysis, Variantyx Inc, Variantyx Inc	0230U	*AR (androgen receptor)* (eg, spinal and bulbar muscular atrophy, Kennedy disease, X chromosome inactivation), full sequence analysis, including small sequence changes in exonic and intronic regions, deletions, duplications, short tandem repeat (STR) expansions, mobile element insertions, and variants in non-uniquely mappable regions
Genomic Unity® CACNA1A Analysis, Variantyx Inc, Variantyx Inc	0231U	*CACNA1A (calcium voltage-gated channel subunit alpha 1A)* (eg, spinocerebellar ataxia), full gene analysis, including small sequence changes in exonic and intronic regions, deletions, duplications, short tandem repeat (STR) gene expansions, mobile element insertions, and variants in non-uniquely mappable regions
Genomic Unity® CSTB Analysis, Variantyx Inc, Variantyx Inc	0232U	*CSTB (cystatin B)* (eg, progressive myoclonic epilepsy type 1A, Unverricht-Lundborg disease), full gene analysis, including small sequence changes in exonic and intronic regions, deletions, duplications, short tandem repeat (STR) expansions, mobile element insertions, and variants in non-uniquely mappable regions
Genomic Unity® FXN Analysis, Variantyx Inc, Variantyx Inc	0233U	*FXN (frataxin)* (eg, Friedreich ataxia), gene analysis, including small sequence changes in exonic and intronic regions, deletions, duplications, short tandem repeat (STR) expansions, mobile element insertions, and variants in non-uniquely mappable regions
Genomic Unity® MECP2 Analysis, Variantyx Inc, Variantyx Inc	0234U	*MECP2 (methyl CpG binding protein 2)* (eg, Rett syndrome), full gene analysis, including small sequence changes in exonic and intronic regions, deletions, duplications, mobile element insertions, and variants in non-uniquely mappable regions
Genomic Unity® PTEN Analysis, Variantyx Inc, Variantyx Inc	0235U	*PTEN (phosphatase and tensin homolog)* (eg, Cowden syndrome, PTEN hamartoma tumor syndrome), full gene analysis, including small sequence changes in exonic and intronic regions, deletions, duplications, mobile element insertions, and variants in non-uniquely mappable regions
Genomic Unity® SMN1/2 Analysis, Variantyx Inc, Variantyx Inc	0236U	*SMN1 (survival of motor neuron 1, telomeric)* and *SMN2 (survival of motor neuron 2, centromeric)* (eg, spinal muscular atrophy) full gene analysis, including small sequence changes in exonic and intronic regions, duplications, deletions, and mobile element insertions

Proprietary Name and Clinical Laboratory or Manufacturer	Alpha-Numeric Code	Code Descriptor
Genomic Unity® Cardiac Ion Channelopathies Analysis, Variantyx Inc, Variantyx Inc	0237U	Cardiac ion channelopathies (eg, Brugada syndrome, long QT syndrome, short QT syndrome, catecholaminergic polymorphic ventricular tachycardia), genomic sequence analysis panel including *ANK2, CASQ2, CAV3, KCNE1, KCNE2, KCNH2, KCNJ2, KCNQ1, RYR2,* and *SCN5A,* including small sequence changes in exonic and intronic regions, deletions, duplications, mobile element insertions, and variants in non-uniquely mappable regions
Genomic Unity® Lynch Syndrome Analysis, Variantyx Inc, Variantyx Inc	0238U	Oncology (Lynch syndrome), genomic DNA sequence analysis of *MLH1, MSH2, MSH6, PMS2,* and *EPCAM,* including small sequence changes in exonic and intronic regions, deletions, duplications, mobile element insertions, and variants in non-uniquely mappable regions
FoundationOne® Liquid CDx, Foundation Medicine, Inc, Foundation Medicine, Inc	0239U	Targeted genomic sequence analysis panel, solid organ neoplasm, cell-free DNA, analysis of 311 or more genes, interrogation for sequence variants, including substitutions, insertions, deletions, select rearrangements, and copy number variations
Xpert® Xpress CoV-2/Flu/RSV plus (SARS-CoV-2 and Flu targets), Cepheid®	0240U	Infectious disease (viral respiratory tract infection), pathogen-specific RNA, 3 targets (severe acute respiratory syndrome coronavirus 2 [SARS-CoV-2], influenza A, influenza B), upper respiratory specimen, each pathogen reported as detected or not detected
Xpert® Xpress CoV-2/Flu/RSV plus (all targets), Cepheid®	0241U	Infectious disease (viral respiratory tract infection), pathogen-specific RNA, 4 targets (severe acute respiratory syndrome coronavirus 2 [SARS-CoV-2], influenza A, influenza B, respiratory syncytial virus [RSV]), upper respiratory specimen, each pathogen reported as detected or not detected
Guardant360® CDx, Guardant Health Inc, Guardant Health Inc	0242U	Targeted genomic sequence analysis panel, solid organ neoplasm, cell-free circulating DNA analysis of 55-74 genes, interrogation for sequence variants, gene copy number amplifications, and gene rearrangements
PlGF Preeclampsia Screen, PerkinElmer Genetics, PerkinElmer Genetics, Inc	0243U	Obstetrics (preeclampsia), biochemical assay of placental-growth factor, time-resolved fluorescence immunoassay, maternal serum, predictive algorithm reported as a risk score for preeclampsia
Oncotype MAP™ Pan-Cancer Tissue Test, Paradigm Diagnostics, Inc, Paradigm Diagnostics, Inc	0244U	Oncology (solid organ), DNA, comprehensive genomic profiling, 257 genes, interrogation for single-nucleotide variants, insertions/deletions, copy number alterations, gene rearrangements, tumor-mutational burden and microsatellite instability, utilizing formalin-fixed paraffin-embedded tumor tissue
ThyGeNEXT® Thyroid Oncogene Panel, Interpace Diagnostics, Interpace Diagnostics	0245U	Oncology (thyroid), mutation analysis of 10 genes and 37 RNA fusions and expression of 4 mRNA markers using next-generation sequencing, fine needle aspirate, report includes associated risk of malignancy expressed as a percentage

(Continued on page 232)

Proprietary Name and Clinical Laboratory or Manufacturer	Alpha-Numeric Code	Code Descriptor
PrecisionBlood™, San Diego Blood Bank, San Diego Blood Bank	0246U	Red blood cell antigen typing, DNA, genotyping of at least 16 blood groups with phenotype prediction of at least 51 red blood cell antigens
PreTRM®, Sera Prognostics, Sera Prognostics, Inc®	0247U	Obstetrics (preterm birth), insulin-like growth factor–binding protein 4 (IBP4), sex hormone–binding globulin (SHBG), quantitative measurement by LC-MS/MS, utilizing maternal serum, combined with clinical data, reported as predictive-risk stratification for spontaneous preterm birth
3D Predict Glioma, KIYATEC®, Inc	▲0248U	▶Oncology, spheroid cell culture in 3D microenvironment, 12-drug panel, brain- or brain metastasis–response prediction for each drug◀
Theralink® Reverse Phase Protein Array (RPPA), Theralink® Technologies, Inc, Theralink® Technologies, Inc	0249U	Oncology (breast), semiquantitative analysis of 32 phosphoproteins and protein analytes, includes laser capture microdissection, with algorithmic analysis and interpretative report
PGDx elio™ tissue complete, Personal Genome Diagnostics, Inc, Personal Genome Diagnostics, Inc	0250U	Oncology (solid organ neoplasm), targeted genomic sequence DNA analysis of 505 genes, interrogation for somatic alterations (SNVs [single nucleotide variant], small insertions and deletions, one amplification, and four translocations), microsatellite instability and tumor-mutation burden
Intrinsic Hepcidin IDx™ Test, IntrinsicDx, Intrinsic LifeSciences™ LLC	0251U	Hepcidin-25, enzyme-linked immunosorbent assay (ELISA), serum or plasma
POC (Products of Conception), Igenomix®, Igenomix® USA	0252U	Fetal aneuploidy short tandem–repeat comparative analysis, fetal DNA from products of conception, reported as normal (euploidy), monosomy, trisomy, or partial deletion/duplication, mosaicism, and segmental aneuploidy
ERA® (Endometrial Receptivity Analysis), Igenomix®, Igenomix® USA	0253U	Reproductive medicine (endometrial receptivity analysis), RNA gene expression profile, 238 genes by next-generation sequencing, endometrial tissue, predictive algorithm reported as endometrial window of implantation (eg, pre-receptive, receptive, post-receptive)
SMART PGT-A (Pre-implantation Genetic Testing - Aneuploidy), Igenomix®, Igenomix® USA	0254U	Reproductive medicine (preimplantation genetic assessment), analysis of 24 chromosomes using embryonic DNA genomic sequence analysis for aneuploidy, and a mitochondrial DNA score in euploid embryos, results reported as normal (euploidy), monosomy, trisomy, or partial deletion/duplication, mosaicism, and segmental aneuploidy, per embryo tested
Cap-Score™ Test, Androvia LifeSciences, Avantor Clinical Services (previously known as Therapak)	0255U	Andrology (infertility), sperm-capacitation assessment of ganglioside GM1 distribution patterns, fluorescence microscopy, fresh or frozen specimen, reported as percentage of capacitated sperm and probability of generating a pregnancy score

★ = Telemedicine   ◀ = Audio-only   ✚ = Add-on code   𝗡 = FDA approval pending   # = Resequenced code   ⊘ = Modifier 51 exempt

Proprietary Name and Clinical Laboratory or Manufacturer	Alpha-Numeric Code	Code Descriptor
Trimethylamine (TMA) and TMA N-Oxide, Children's Hospital Colorado Laboratory	0256U	Trimethylamine/trimethylamine N-oxide (TMA/TMAO) profile, tandem mass spectrometry (MS/MS), urine, with algorithmic analysis and interpretive report
Very-Long Chain Acyl-CoA Dehydrogenase (VLCAD) Enzyme Activity, Children's Hospital Colorado Laboratory	0257U	Very long chain acyl-coenzyme A (CoA) dehydrogenase (VLCAD), leukocyte enzyme activity, whole blood
Mind.Px, Mindera, Mindera Corporation	0258U	Autoimmune (psoriasis), mRNA, next-generation sequencing, gene expression profiling of 50-100 genes, skin-surface collection using adhesive patch, algorithm reported as likelihood of response to psoriasis biologics
GFR by NMR, Labtech™ Diagnostics	0259U	Nephrology (chronic kidney disease), nuclear magnetic resonance spectroscopy measurement of myo-inositol, valine, and creatinine, algorithmically combined with cystatin C (by immunoassay) and demographic data to determine estimated glomerular filtration rate (GFR), serum, quantitative
Augusta Optical Genome Mapping, Georgia Esoteric and Molecular (GEM) Laboratory, LLC, Bionano Genomics Inc	✄0260U	Rare diseases (constitutional/heritable disorders), identification of copy number variations, inversions, insertions, translocations, and other structural variants by optical genome mapping (For additional PLA codes with identical clinical descriptor, see 0264U, 0454U. See Appendix O or the most current listing on the AMA CPT website to determine appropriate code assignment)
Immunoscore®, HalioDx, HalioDx	0261U	Oncology (colorectal cancer), image analysis with artificial intelligence assessment of 4 histologic and immunohistochemical features (CD3 and CD8 within tumor-stroma border and tumor core), tissue, reported as immune response and recurrence-risk score
OncoSignal 7 Pathway Signal, Protean BioDiagnostics, Philips Electronics Nederland BV	0262U	Oncology (solid tumor), gene expression profiling by real-time RT-PCR of 7 gene pathways (ER, AR, PI3K, MAPK, HH, TGFB, Notch), formalin-fixed paraffin-embedded (FFPE), algorithm reported as gene pathway activity score
NPDX ASD and Central Carbon Energy Metabolism, Stemina Biomarker Discovery, Inc, Stemina Biomarker Discovery, Inc	0263U	Neurology (autism spectrum disorder [ASD]), quantitative measurements of 16 central carbon metabolites (ie, α-ketoglutarate, alanine, lactate, phenylalanine, pyruvate, succinate, carnitine, citrate, fumarate, hypoxanthine, inosine, malate, S-sulfocysteine, taurine, urate, and xanthine), liquid chromatography tandem mass spectrometry (LC-MS/MS), plasma, algorithmic analysis with result reported as negative or positive (with metabolic subtypes of ASD)

(Continued on page 234)

▲ = Revised code   ● = New code   ▶◀ = Contains new or revised text   ✄ = Duplicate PLA test   ↑↓ = Category I PLA   American Medical Association   **233**

Proprietary Name and Clinical Laboratory or Manufacturer	Alpha-Numeric Code	Code Descriptor
Praxis Optical Genome Mapping, Praxis Genomics LLC	✳0264U	Rare diseases (constitutional/heritable disorders), identification of copy number variations, inversions, insertions, translocations, and other structural variants by optical genome mapping (For additional PLA codes with identical clinical descriptor, see 0260U, 0454U. See Appendix O or the most current listing on the AMA CPT website to determine appropriate code assignment)
Praxis Whole Genome Sequencing, Praxis Genomics LLC	0265U	Rare constitutional and other heritable disorders, whole genome and mitochondrial DNA sequence analysis, blood, frozen and formalin-fixed paraffin-embedded (FFPE) tissue, saliva, buccal swabs or cell lines, identification of single nucleotide and copy number variants
Praxis Transcriptome, Praxis Genomics LLC	0266U	Unexplained constitutional or other heritable disorders or syndromes, tissue-specific gene expression by whole-transcriptome and next-generation sequencing, blood, formalin-fixed paraffin-embedded (FFPE) tissue or fresh frozen tissue, reported as presence or absence of splicing or expression changes
Praxis Combined Whole Genome Sequencing and Optical Genome Mapping, Praxis Genomics LLC	0267U	Rare constitutional and other heritable disorders, identification of copy number variations, inversions, insertions, translocations, and other structural variants by optical genome mapping and whole genome sequencing
Versiti™ aHUS Genetic Evaluation, Versiti™ Diagnostic Laboratories, Versiti™	0268U	Hematology (atypical hemolytic uremic syndrome [aHUS]), genomic sequence analysis of 15 genes, blood, buccal swab, or amniotic fluid
Versiti™ Autosomal Dominant Thrombocytopenia Panel, Versiti™ Diagnostic Laboratories, Versiti™	0269U	Hematology (autosomal dominant congenital thrombocytopenia), genomic sequence analysis of 22 genes, blood, buccal swab, or amniotic fluid
Versiti™ Coagulation Disorder Panel, Versiti™ Diagnostic Laboratories, Versiti™	0270U	Hematology (congenital coagulation disorders), genomic sequence analysis of 20 genes, blood, buccal swab, or amniotic fluid
Versiti™ Congenital Neutropenia Panel, Versiti™ Diagnostic Laboratories, Versiti™	0271U	Hematology (congenital neutropenia), genomic sequence analysis of 24 genes, blood, buccal swab, or amniotic fluid
Versiti™ Comprehensive Bleeding Disorder Panel, Versiti™ Diagnostic Laboratories, Versiti™	0272U	Hematology (genetic bleeding disorders), genomic sequence analysis of 60 genes and duplication/deletion of PLAU, blood, buccal swab, or amniotic fluid, comprehensive
Versiti™ Fibrinolytic Disorder Panel, Versiti™ Diagnostic Laboratories, Versiti™	0273U	Hematology (genetic hyperfibrinolysis, delayed bleeding), analysis of 9 genes (F13A1, F13B, FGA, FGB, FGG, SERPINA1, SERPINE1, SERPINF2 by next-generation sequencing, and PLAU by array comparative genomic hybridization), blood, buccal swab, or amniotic fluid

Proprietary Name and Clinical Laboratory or Manufacturer	Alpha-Numeric Code	Code Descriptor
Versiti™ Comprehensive Platelet Disorder Panel, Versiti™ Diagnostic Laboratories, Versiti™	0274U	Hematology (genetic platelet disorders), genomic sequence analysis of 62 genes and duplication/deletion of *PLAU*, blood, buccal swab, or amniotic fluid
Versiti™ Heparin-Induced Thrombocytopenia Evaluation – PEA, Versiti™ Diagnostic Laboratories, Versiti™	0275U	Hematology (heparin-induced thrombocytopenia), platelet antibody reactivity by flow cytometry, serum
Versiti™ Inherited Thrombocytopenia Panel, Versiti™ Diagnostic Laboratories, Versiti™	0276U	Hematology (inherited thrombocytopenia), genomic sequence analysis of 42 genes, blood, buccal swab, or amniotic fluid
Versiti™ Platelet Function Disorder Panel, Versiti™ Diagnostic Laboratories, Versiti™	0277U	Hematology (genetic platelet function disorder), genomic sequence analysis of 40 genes and duplication/deletion of *PLAU*, blood, buccal swab, or amniotic fluid
Versiti™ Thrombosis Panel, Versiti™ Diagnostic Laboratories, Versiti™	0278U	Hematology (genetic thrombosis), genomic sequence analysis of 14 genes, blood, buccal swab, or amniotic fluid
Versiti™ VWF Collagen III Binding, Versiti™ Diagnostic Laboratories, Versiti™	0279U	Hematology (von Willebrand disease [VWD]), von Willebrand factor (VWF) and collagen III binding by enzyme-linked immunosorbent assays (ELISA), plasma, report of collagen III binding
Versiti™ VWF Collagen IV Binding, Versiti™ Diagnostic Laboratories, Versiti™	0280U	Hematology (von Willebrand disease [VWD]), von Willebrand factor (VWF) and collagen IV binding by enzyme-linked immunosorbent assays (ELISA), plasma, report of collagen IV binding
Versiti™ VWF Propeptide Antigen, Versiti™ Diagnostic Laboratories, Versiti™	0281U	Hematology (von Willebrand disease [VWD]), von Willebrand propeptide, enzyme-linked immunosorbent assays (ELISA), plasma, diagnostic report of von Willebrand factor (VWF) propeptide antigen level
Versiti™ Red Cell Genotyping Panel, Versiti™ Diagnostic Laboratories, Versiti™	0282U	Red blood cell antigen typing, DNA, genotyping of 12 blood group system genes to predict 44 red blood cell antigen phenotypes
Versiti™ VWD Type 2B Evaluation, Versiti™ Diagnostic Laboratories, Versiti™	0283U	von Willebrand factor (VWF), type 2B, platelet-binding evaluation, radioimmunoassay, plasma
Versiti™ VWD Type 2N Binding, Versiti™ Diagnostic Laboratories, Versiti™	0284U	von Willebrand factor (VWF), type 2N, factor VIII and VWF binding evaluation, enzyme-linked immunosorbent assays (ELISA), plasma
RadTox™ cfDNA test, DiaCarta Clinical Lab, DiaCarta Inc	0285U	Oncology, response to radiation, cell-free DNA, quantitative branched chain DNA amplification, plasma, reported as a radiation toxicity score
CNT (*CEP72, TPMT* and *NUDT15*) genotyping panel, RPRD Diagnostics	0286U	*CEP72 (centrosomal protein, 72-KDa), NUDT15 (nudix hydrolase 15)* and *TPMT (thiopurine S-methyltransferase)* (eg, drug metabolism) gene analysis, common variants

(Continued on page 236)

Appendix O

Proprietary Name and Clinical Laboratory or Manufacturer	Alpha-Numeric Code	Code Descriptor
ThyroSeq® CRC, CBLPath, Inc, University of Pittsburgh Medical Center	0287U	Oncology (thyroid), DNA and mRNA, next-generation sequencing analysis of 112 genes, fine needle aspirate or formalin-fixed paraffin-embedded (FFPE) tissue, algorithmic prediction of cancer recurrence, reported as a categorical risk result (low, intermediate, high)
DetermaRx™, Oncocyte Corporation	0288U	Oncology (lung), mRNA, quantitative PCR analysis of 11 genes (BAG1, BRCA1, CDC6, CDK2AP1, ERBB3, FUT3, IL11, LCK, RND3, SH3BGR, WNT3A) and 3 reference genes (ESD, TBP, YAP1), formalin-fixed paraffin-embedded (FFPE) tumor tissue, algorithmic interpretation reported as a recurrence risk score
MindX Blood Test™ - Memory/Alzheimer's, MindX Sciences™ Laboratory, MindX Sciences™ Inc	0289U	Neurology (Alzheimer disease), mRNA, gene expression profiling by RNA sequencing of 24 genes, whole blood, algorithm reported as predictive risk score
MindX Blood Test™ - Pain, MindX Sciences™ Laboratory, MindX Sciences™ Inc	0290U	Pain management, mRNA, gene expression profiling by RNA sequencing of 36 genes, whole blood, algorithm reported as predictive risk score
MindX Blood Test™ - Mood, MindX Sciences™ Laboratory, MindX Sciences™ Inc	0291U	Psychiatry (mood disorders), mRNA, gene expression profiling by RNA sequencing of 144 genes, whole blood, algorithm reported as predictive risk score
MindX Blood Test™ - Stress, MindX Sciences™ Laboratory, MindX Sciences™ Inc	0292U	Psychiatry (stress disorders), mRNA, gene expression profiling by RNA sequencing of 72 genes, whole blood, algorithm reported as predictive risk score
MindX Blood Test™ - Suicidality, MindX Sciences™ Laboratory, MindX Sciences™ Inc	0293U	Psychiatry (suicidal ideation), mRNA, gene expression profiling by RNA sequencing of 54 genes, whole blood, algorithm reported as predictive risk score
MindX Blood Test™ - Longevity, MindX Sciences™ Laboratory, MindX Sciences™ Inc	0294U	Longevity and mortality risk, mRNA, gene expression profiling by RNA sequencing of 18 genes, whole blood, algorithm reported as predictive risk score
DCISionRT®, PreludeDx™, Prelude Corporation	0295U	Oncology (breast ductal carcinoma in situ), protein expression profiling by immunohistochemistry of 7 proteins (COX2, FOXA1, HER2, Ki-67, p16, PR, SIAH2), with 4 clinicopathologic factors (size, age, margin status, palpability), utilizing formalin-fixed paraffin-embedded (FFPE) tissue, algorithm reported as a recurrence risk score
mRNA CancerDetect™, Viome Life Sciences, Inc, Viome Life Sciences, Inc	0296U	Oncology (oral and/or oropharyngeal cancer), gene expression profiling by RNA sequencing of at least 20 molecular features (eg, human and/or microbial mRNA), saliva, algorithm reported as positive or negative for signature associated with malignancy
Praxis Somatic Whole Genome Sequencing, Praxis Genomics LLC	0297U	Oncology (pan tumor), whole genome sequencing of paired malignant and normal DNA specimens, fresh or formalin-fixed paraffin-embedded (FFPE) tissue, blood or bone marrow, comparative sequence analyses and variant identification

★ = Telemedicine   ◀ = Audio-only   ✛ = Add-on code   ✗ = FDA approval pending   # = Resequenced code   ⊘ = Modifier 51 exempt

Proprietary Name and Clinical Laboratory or Manufacturer	Alpha-Numeric Code	Code Descriptor
Praxis Somatic Transcriptome, Praxis Genomics LLC	0298U	Oncology (pan tumor), whole transcriptome sequencing of paired malignant and normal RNA specimens, fresh or formalin-fixed paraffin-embedded (FFPE) tissue, blood or bone marrow, comparative sequence analyses and expression level and chimeric transcript identification
Praxis Somatic Optical Genome Mapping, Praxis Genomics LLC	0299U	Oncology (pan tumor), whole genome optical genome mapping of paired malignant and normal DNA specimens, fresh frozen tissue, blood, or bone marrow, comparative structural variant identification
Praxis Somatic Combined Whole Genome Sequencing and Optical Genome Mapping, Praxis Genomics LLC	0300U	Oncology (pan tumor), whole genome sequencing and optical genome mapping of paired malignant and normal DNA specimens, fresh tissue, blood, or bone marrow, comparative sequence analyses and variant identification
Bartonella ddPCR, Galaxy Diagnostics, Inc	0301U	Infectious agent detection by nucleic acid (DNA or RNA), Bartonella henselae and Bartonella quintana, droplet digital PCR (ddPCR);
	0302U	following liquid enrichment
Hypoxic BioChip Adhesion, BioChip Labs™, BioChip Labs™	0303U	Hematology, red blood cell (RBC) adhesion to endothelial/subendothelial adhesion molecules, functional assessment, whole blood, with algorithmic analysis and result reported as an RBC adhesion index; hypoxic
	0304U	normoxic
Ektacytometry, BioChip Labs™, BioChip Labs™	0305U	Hematology, red blood cell (RBC) functionality and deformity as a function of shear stress, whole blood, reported as a maximum elongation index
Invitae PCM Tissue Profiling and MRD Baseline Assay, Invitae Corporation, Invitae Corporation	0306U	Oncology (minimal residual disease [MRD]), next-generation targeted sequencing analysis, cell-free DNA, initial (baseline) assessment to determine a patient-specific panel for future comparisons to evaluate for MRD (Do not report 0306U in conjunction with 0307U)
Invitae PCM MRD Monitoring, Invitae Corporation, Invitae Corporation	0307U	Oncology (minimal residual disease [MRD]), next-generation targeted sequencing analysis of a patient-specific panel, cell-free DNA, subsequent assessment with comparison to previously analyzed patient specimens to evaluate for MRD (Do not report 0307U in conjunction with 0306U)
HART CADhs®, Atlas Genomics, Prevencio, Inc	0308U	Cardiology (coronary artery disease [CAD]), analysis of 3 proteins (high sensitivity [hs] troponin, adiponectin, and kidney injury molecule-1 [KIM-1]) with 3 clinical parameters (age, sex, history of cardiac intervention), plasma, algorithm reported as a risk score for obstructive CAD

(Continued on page 238)

▲ = Revised code   ● = New code   ▶ ◀ = Contains new or revised text   ✕ = Duplicate PLA test   ⇅ = Category I PLA   American Medical Association   **237**

Appendix O

Appendix O

Proprietary Name and Clinical Laboratory or Manufacturer	Alpha-Numeric Code	Code Descriptor
HART CVE®, Atlas Genomics, Prevencio, Inc	0309U	Cardiology (cardiovascular disease), analysis of 4 proteins (NT-proBNP, osteopontin, tissue inhibitor of metalloproteinase-1 [TIMP-1], and kidney injury molecule-1 [KIM-1]), plasma, algorithm reported as a risk score for major adverse cardiac event
HART KD®, Atlas Genomics, Prevencio, Inc	0310U	Pediatrics (vasculitis, Kawasaki disease [KD]), analysis of 3 biomarkers (NT-proBNP, C-reactive protein, and T-uptake), plasma, algorithm reported as a risk score for KD
Accelerate PhenoTest® BC kit, AST configuration, Accelerate Diagnostics, Inc, Accelerate Diagnostics, Inc	0311U	Infectious disease (bacterial), quantitative antimicrobial susceptibility reported as phenotypic minimum inhibitory concentration (MIC)–based antimicrobial susceptibility for each organism identified (Do not report 0311U in conjunction with 87076, 87077, 0086U)
Avise® Lupus, Exagen Inc, Exagen Inc	0312U	Autoimmune diseases (eg, systemic lupus erythematosus [SLE]), analysis of 8 IgG autoantibodies and 2 cell-bound complement activation products using enzyme-linked immunosorbent immunoassay (ELISA), flow cytometry and indirect immunofluorescence, serum, or plasma and whole blood, individual components reported along with an algorithmic SLE-likelihood assessment
PancreaSeq® Genomic Classifier, Molecular and Genomic Pathology Laboratory, University of Pittsburgh Medical Center	0313U	Oncology (pancreas), DNA and mRNA next-generation sequencing analysis of 74 genes and analysis of CEA (CEACAM5) gene expression, pancreatic cyst fluid, algorithm reported as a categorical result (ie, negative, low probability of neoplasia or positive, high probability of neoplasia)
DecisionDx® DiffDx™-Melanoma, Castle Biosciences, Inc, Castle Biosciences, Inc	0314U	Oncology (cutaneous melanoma), mRNA gene expression profiling by RT-PCR of 35 genes (32 content and 3 housekeeping), utilizing formalin-fixed paraffin-embedded (FFPE) tissue, algorithm reported as a categorical result (ie, benign, intermediate, malignant)
DecisionDx®-SCC, Castle Biosciences, Inc, Castle Biosciences, Inc	0315U	Oncology (cutaneous squamous cell carcinoma), mRNA gene expression profiling by RT-PCR of 40 genes (34 content and 6 housekeeping), utilizing formalin-fixed paraffin-embedded (FFPE) tissue, algorithm reported as a categorical risk result (ie, Class 1, Class 2A, Class 2B)
Lyme Borrelia Nanotrap® Urine Antigen Test, Galaxy Diagnostics Inc	0316U	Borrelia burgdorferi (Lyme disease), OspA protein evaluation, urine
LungLB®, LungLife AI®, LungLife AI®	0317U	Oncology (lung cancer), four-probe FISH (3q29, 3p22.1, 10q22.3, 10cen) assay, whole blood, predictive algorithm-generated evaluation reported as decreased or increased risk for lung cancer

★ =Telemedicine   ◀ =Audio-only   ✛ =Add-on code   ⁄ =FDA approval pending   # =Resequenced code   ⦶ =Modifier 51 exempt

Proprietary Name and Clinical Laboratory or Manufacturer	Alpha-Numeric Code	Code Descriptor
EpiSign Complete, Greenwood Genetic Center	0318U	Pediatrics (congenital epigenetic disorders), whole genome methylation analysis by microarray for 50 or more genes, blood
Clarava™, Verici Dx, Verici Dx, Inc	0319U	Nephrology (renal transplant), RNA expression by select transcriptome sequencing, using pretransplant peripheral blood, algorithm reported as a risk score for early acute rejection
Tuteva™, Verici Dx, Verici Dx, Inc	0320U	Nephrology (renal transplant), RNA expression by select transcriptome sequencing, using posttransplant peripheral blood, algorithm reported as a risk score for acute cellular rejection
Bridge Urinary Tract Infection Detection and Resistance Test, Bridge Diagnostics	0321U	Infectious agent detection by nucleic acid (DNA or RNA), genitourinary pathogens, identification of 20 bacterial and fungal organisms and identification of 16 associated antibiotic-resistance genes, multiplex amplified probe technique
NPDX ASD Test Panel III, Stemina Biomarker Discovery d/b/a NeuroPointDX, Stemina Biomarker Discovery d/b/a NeuroPointDX	0322U	Neurology (autism spectrum disorder [ASD]), quantitative measurements of 14 acyl carnitines and microbiome-derived metabolites, liquid chromatography with tandem mass spectrometry (LC-MS/MS), plasma, results reported as negative or positive for risk of metabolic subtypes associated with ASD
Johns Hopkins Metagenomic Next-Generation Sequencing Assay for Infectious Disease Diagnostics, Johns Hopkins Medical Microbiology Laboratory	0323U	Infectious agent detection by nucleic acid (DNA and RNA), central nervous system pathogen, metagenomic next-generation sequencing, cerebrospinal fluid (CSF), identification of pathogenic bacteria, viruses, parasites, or fungi
—	(0324U has been deleted)	—
—	(0325U has been deleted)	—
Guardant360®, Guardant Health, Inc, Guardant Health, Inc	0326U	Targeted genomic sequence analysis panel, solid organ neoplasm, cell-free circulating DNA analysis of 83 or more genes, interrogation for sequence variants, gene copy number amplifications, gene rearrangements, microsatellite instability and tumor mutational burden
Vasistera™, Natera, Inc, Natera, Inc	0327U	Fetal aneuploidy (trisomy 13, 18, and 21), DNA sequence analysis of selected regions using maternal plasma, algorithm reported as a risk score for each trisomy, includes sex reporting, if performed
CareView360, Newstar Medical Laboratories, LLC, Newstar Medical Laboratories, LLC	0328U	Drug assay, definitive, 120 or more drugs and metabolites, urine, quantitative liquid chromatography with tandem mass spectrometry (LC-MS/MS), includes specimen validity and algorithmic analysis describing drug or metabolite and presence or absence of risks for a significant patient-adverse event, per date of service

(Continued on page 240)

Proprietary Name and Clinical Laboratory or Manufacturer	Alpha-Numeric Code	Code Descriptor
Oncomap™ ExTra, Exact Sciences, Inc, Genomic Health Inc	0329U	Oncology (neoplasia), exome and transcriptome sequence analysis for sequence variants, gene copy number amplifications and deletions, gene rearrangements, microsatellite instability and tumor mutational burden utilizing DNA and RNA from tumor with DNA from normal blood or saliva for subtraction, report of clinically significant mutation(s) with therapy associations
Bridge Women's Health Infectious Disease Detection Test, Bridge Diagnostics, Thermo Fisher and Hologic Test Kit on Panther Instrument	0330U	Infectious agent detection by nucleic acid (DNA or RNA), vaginal pathogen panel, identification of 27 organisms, amplified probe technique, vaginal swab
Augusta Hematology Optical Genome Mapping, Georgia Esoteric and Molecular Labs, Augusta University, Bionano	0331U	Oncology (hematolymphoid neoplasia), optical genome mapping for copy number alterations and gene rearrangements utilizing DNA from blood or bone marrow, report of clinically significant alterations
EpiSwitch® CiRT (Checkpoint-inhibitor Response Test), Next Bio-Research Services, LLC, Oxford BioDynamics, PLC	0332U	Oncology (pan-tumor), genetic profiling of 8 DNA-regulatory (epigenetic) markers by quantitative polymerase chain reaction (qPCR), whole blood, reported as a high or low probability of responding to immune checkpoint–inhibitor therapy
HelioLiver™ Test, Fulgent Genetics, LLC, Helio Health, Inc	0333U	Oncology (liver), surveillance for hepatocellular carcinoma (HCC) in high-risk patients, analysis of methylation patterns on circulating cell-free DNA (cfDNA) plus measurement of serum of AFP/AFP-L3 and oncoprotein des-gamma-carboxy-prothrombin (DCP), algorithm reported as normal or abnormal result
Guardant360 TissueNext™, Guardant Health, Inc, Guardant Health, Inc	0334U	Oncology (solid organ), targeted genomic sequence analysis, formalin-fixed paraffin-embedded (FFPE) tumor tissue, DNA analysis, 84 or more genes, interrogation for sequence variants, gene copy number amplifications, gene rearrangements, microsatellite instability and tumor mutational burden
IriSight™ Prenatal Analysis – Proband, Variantyx, Inc, Variantyx, Inc	0335U	Rare diseases (constitutional/heritable disorders), whole genome sequence analysis, including small sequence changes, copy number variants, deletions, duplications, mobile element insertions, uniparental disomy (UPD), inversions, aneuploidy, mitochondrial genome sequence analysis with heteroplasmy and large deletions, short tandem repeat (STR) gene expansions, fetal sample, identification and categorization of genetic variants

(Do not report 0335U in conjunction with 81425, 0212U) |

★ = Telemedicine   ◀ = Audio-only   ✚ = Add-on code   ✗ = FDA approval pending   # = Resequenced code   ⊘ = Modifier 51 exempt

Appendix O

Proprietary Name and Clinical Laboratory or Manufacturer	Alpha-Numeric Code	Code Descriptor
IriSight™ Prenatal Analysis – Comparator, Variantyx, Inc, Variantyx, Inc	0336U	Rare diseases (constitutional/heritable disorders), whole genome sequence analysis, including small sequence changes, copy number variants, deletions, duplications, mobile element insertions, uniparental disomy (UPD), inversions, aneuploidy, mitochondrial genome sequence analysis with heteroplasmy and large deletions, short tandem repeat (STR) gene expansions, blood or saliva, identification and categorization of genetic variants, each comparator genome (eg, parent) (Do not report 0336U in conjunction with 81426, 0213U)
CELLSEARCH® Circulating Multiple Myeloma Cell (CMMC) Test, Menarini Silicon Biosystems, Inc, Menarini Silicon Biosystems, Inc	0337U	Oncology (plasma cell disorders and myeloma), circulating plasma cell immunologic selection, identification, morphological characterization, and enumeration of plasma cells based on differential CD138, CD38, CD19, and CD45 protein biomarker expression, peripheral blood
CELLSEARCH® HER2 Circulating Tumor Cell (CTC-HER2) Test, Menarini Silicon Biosystems, Inc, Menarini Silicon Biosystems, Inc	0338U	Oncology (solid tumor), circulating tumor cell selection, identification, morphological characterization, detection and enumeration based on differential EpCAM, cytokeratins 8, 18, and 19, and CD45 protein biomarkers, and quantification of HER2 protein biomarker–expressing cells, peripheral blood
SelectMDx® for Prostate Cancer, MDxHealth®, Inc, MDxHealth®, Inc	0339U	Oncology (prostate), mRNA expression profiling of HOXC6 and DLX1, reverse transcription polymerase chain reaction (RT-PCR), first-void urine following digital rectal examination, algorithm reported as probability of high-grade cancer
Signatera™, Natera, Inc, Natera, Inc	0340U	Oncology (pan-cancer), analysis of minimal residual disease (MRD) from plasma, with assays personalized to each patient based on prior next-generation sequencing of the patient's tumor and germline DNA, reported as absence or presence of MRD, with disease-burden correlation, if appropriate
Single Cell Prenatal Diagnosis (SCPD) Test, Luna Genetics, Inc, Luna Genetics, Inc	0341U	Fetal aneuploidy DNA sequencing comparative analysis, fetal DNA from products of conception, reported as normal (euploidy), monosomy, trisomy, or partial deletion/duplication, mosaicism, and segmental aneuploid
IMMray® PanCan-d, Immunovia, Inc, Immunovia, Inc	0342U	Oncology (pancreatic cancer), multiplex immunoassay of C5, C4, cystatin C, factor B, osteoprotegerin (OPG), gelsolin, IGFBP3, CA125 and multiplex electrochemiluminescent immunoassay (ECLIA) for CA19-9, serum, diagnostic algorithm reported qualitatively as positive, negative, or borderline

(Continued on page 242)

Proprietary Name and Clinical Laboratory or Manufacturer	Alpha-Numeric Code	Code Descriptor
miR Sentinel™ Prostate Cancer Test, miR Scientific, LLC, miR Scientific, LLC	0343U	Oncology (prostate), exosome-based analysis of 442 small noncoding RNAs (sncRNAs) by quantitative reverse transcription polymerase chain reaction (RT-qPCR), urine, reported as molecular evidence of no-, low-, intermediate- or high-risk of prostate cancer
OWLiver®, CIMA Sciences, LLC	0344U	Hepatology (nonalcoholic fatty liver disease [NAFLD]), semiquantitative evaluation of 28 lipid markers by liquid chromatography with tandem mass spectrometry (LC-MS/MS), serum, reported as at-risk for nonalcoholic steatohepatitis (NASH) or not NASH
GeneSight® Psychotropic, Assurex Health, Inc, Myriad Genetics, Inc	⋕0345U	Psychiatry (eg, depression, anxiety, attention deficit hyperactivity disorder [ADHD]), genomic analysis panel, variant analysis of 15 genes, including deletion/duplication analysis of *CYP2D6* (For additional PLA code with identical clinical descriptor, see 0411U. See Appendix O to determine appropriate code assignment)
QUEST AD-Detect™, Beta-Amyloid 42/40 Ratio, Plasma, Quest Diagnostics	0346U	Beta amyloid, Aβ40 and Aβ42 by liquid chromatography with tandem mass spectrometry (LC-MS/MS), ratio, plasma
RightMed® PGx16 Test, OneOme®, OneOme®, LLC	0347U	Drug metabolism or processing (multiple conditions), whole blood or buccal specimen, DNA analysis, 16 gene report, with variant analysis and reported phenotypes
RightMed® Comprehensive Test Exclude F2 and F5, OneOme®, OneOme®, LLC	0348U	Drug metabolism or processing (multiple conditions), whole blood or buccal specimen, DNA analysis, 25 gene report, with variant analysis and reported phenotypes
RightMed® Comprehensive Test, OneOme®, OneOme®, LLC	0349U	Drug metabolism or processing (multiple conditions), whole blood or buccal specimen, DNA analysis, 27 gene report, with variant analysis, including reported phenotypes and impacted gene-drug interactions
RightMed® Gene Report, OneOme®, OneOme®, LLC	0350U	Drug metabolism or processing (multiple conditions), whole blood or buccal specimen, DNA analysis, 27 gene report, with variant analysis and reported phenotypes
MeMed BV®, MeMed Diagnostics, Ltd, MeMed Diagnostics, Ltd	▲0351U	▶Infectious disease (bacterial or viral), biochemical assays, tumor necrosis factor-related apoptosis-inducing ligand (TRAIL), interferon gamma-induced protein-10 (IP-10), and C-reactive protein, serum, or venous whole blood, algorithm reported as likelihood of bacterial infection◀

★ = Telemedicine   ◀ = Audio-only   ✚ = Add-on code   ✗ = FDA approval pending   # = Resequenced code   ⊘ = Modifier 51 exempt

Proprietary Name and Clinical Laboratory or Manufacturer	Alpha-Numeric Code	Code Descriptor
—	▶(0352U has been deleted. To report infectious disease, bacterial vaginosis and vaginitis, real-time PCR amplification of DNA markers for algorithm reported as high likelihood of bacterial vaginosis, use 81515)◀	—
—	▶(0353U has been deleted)◀	—
—	▶(0354U has been deleted)◀	—
Apolipoprotein L1 *(APOL1)* Renal Risk Variant Genotyping, Quest Diagnostics®, Quest Diagnostics®	0355U	*APOL1 (apolipoprotein L1)* (eg, chronic kidney disease), risk variants (G1, G2)
NavDx®, Naveris, Inc, Naveris, Inc	▲0356U	▶Oncology (oropharyngeal or anal), evaluation of 17 DNA biomarkers using droplet digital PCR (ddPCR), cell-free DNA, algorithm reported as a prognostic risk score for cancer recurrence◀
—	(0357U has been deleted)	—
Lumipulse® G β-Amyloid Ratio (1-42/1-40) Test, Fujirebio Diagnostics, Inc, Fujirebio Diagnostics, Inc	0358U	Neurology (mild cognitive impairment), analysis of β-amyloid 1-42 and 1-40, chemiluminescence enzyme immunoassay, cerebral spinal fluid, reported as positive, likely positive, or negative
IsoPSA®, Cleveland Diagnostics, Inc, Cleveland Diagnostics, Inc	0359U	Oncology (prostate cancer), analysis of all prostate-specific antigen (PSA) structural isoforms by phase separation and immunoassay, plasma, algorithm reports risk of cancer
Nodify CDT®, Biodesix, Inc, Biodesix, Inc	0360U	Oncology (lung), enzyme-linked immunosorbent assay (ELISA) of 7 autoantibodies (p53, NY-ESO-1, CAGE, GBU4-5, SOX2, MAGE A4, and HuD), plasma, algorithm reported as a categorical result for risk of malignancy
Neurofilament Light Chain (NfL), Mayo Clinic, Mayo Clinic	0361U	Neurofilament light chain, digital immunoassay, plasma, quantitative
Thyroid GuidePx®, Protean BioDiagnostics, Qualisure Diagnostics	0362U	Oncology (papillary thyroid cancer), gene-expression profiling via targeted hybrid capture–enrichment RNA sequencing of 82 content genes and 10 housekeeping genes, fine needle aspirate or formalin-fixed paraffin-embedded (FFPE) tissue, algorithm reported as one of three molecular subtypes

(*Continued on page 244*)

Proprietary Name and Clinical Laboratory or Manufacturer	Alpha-Numeric Code	Code Descriptor
Cxbladder™ Triage, Pacific Edge Diagnostics USA, Ltd, Pacific Edge Diagnostics USA, Ltd	0363U	Oncology (urothelial), mRNA, gene-expression profiling by real-time quantitative PCR of 5 genes (*MDK, HOXA13, CDC2 [CDK1], IGFBP5,* and *CXCR2*), utilizing urine, algorithm incorporates age, sex, smoking history, and macrohematuria frequency, reported as a risk score for having urothelial carcinoma
clonoSEQ® Assay, Adaptive Biotechnologies	0364U	Oncology (hematolymphoid neoplasm), genomic sequence analysis using multiplex (PCR) and next-generation sequencing with algorithm, quantification of dominant clonal sequence(s), reported as presence or absence of minimal residual disease (MRD) with quantitation of disease burden, when appropriate
Oncuria® Detect, DiaCarta Clinical Lab, DiaCarta, Inc	0365U	Oncology (bladder), analysis of 10 protein biomarkers (A1AT, ANG, APOE, CA9, IL8, MMP9, MMP10, PAI1, SDC1, and VEGFA) by immunoassays, urine, algorithm reported as a probability of bladder cancer
Oncuria® Monitor, DiaCarta Clinical Lab, DiaCarta, Inc	0366U	Oncology (bladder), analysis of 10 protein biomarkers (A1AT, ANG, APOE, CA9, IL8, MMP9, MMP10, PAI1, SDC1, and VEGFA) by immunoassays, urine, algorithm reported as a probability of recurrent bladder cancer
Oncuria® Predict, DiaCarta Clinical Lab, DiaCarta, Inc	0367U	Oncology (bladder), analysis of 10 protein biomarkers (A1AT, ANG, APOE, CA9, IL8, MMP9, MMP10, PAI1, SDC1, and VEGFA) by immunoassays, urine, diagnostic algorithm reported as a risk score for probability of rapid recurrence of recurrent or persistent cancer following transurethral resection
ColoScape™ Colorectal Cancer Detection, DiaCarta Clinical Lab, DiaCarta, Inc	0368U	Oncology (colorectal cancer), evaluation for mutations of *APC, BRAF, CTNNB1, KRAS, NRAS, PIK3CA, SMAD4,* and *TP53,* and methylation markers (MYO1G, KCNQ5, C9ORF50, FLI1, CLIP4, ZNF132, and TWIST1), multiplex quantitative polymerase chain reaction (qPCR), circulating cell-free DNA (cfDNA), plasma, report of risk score for advanced adenoma or colorectal cancer
GI assay (Gastrointestinal Pathogen with ABR), Lab Genomics LLC, Thermo Fisher Scientific	0369U	Infectious agent detection by nucleic acid (DNA and RNA), gastrointestinal pathogens, 31 bacterial, viral, and parasitic organisms and identification of 21 associated antibiotic-resistance genes, multiplex amplified probe technique
Lesion Infection (Wound), Lab Genomics LLC, Thermo Fisher Scientific	0370U	Infectious agent detection by nucleic acid (DNA and RNA), surgical wound pathogens, 34 microorganisms and identification of 21 associated antibiotic-resistance genes, multiplex amplified probe technique, wound swab

★ = Telemedicine   ◀ = Audio-only   + = Add-on code   ⊬ = FDA approval pending   # = Resequenced code   ⊘ = Modifier 51 exempt

Proprietary Name and Clinical Laboratory or Manufacturer	Alpha-Numeric Code	Code Descriptor
Qlear UTI, Lifescan Labs of Illinois, Thermo Fisher Scientific	0371U	Infectious agent detection by nucleic acid (DNA or RNA), genitourinary pathogen, semiquantitative identification, DNA from 16 bacterial organisms and 1 fungal organism, multiplex amplified probe technique via quantitative polymerase chain reaction (qPCR), urine
Qlear UTI - Reflex ABR, Lifescan Labs of Illinois, Thermo Fisher Scientific	0372U	Infectious disease (genitourinary pathogens), antibiotic-resistance gene detection, multiplex amplified probe technique, urine, reported as an antimicrobial stewardship risk score
Respiratory Pathogen with ABR (RPX), Lab Genomics LLC, Thermo Fisher Scientific	0373U	Infectious agent detection by nucleic acid (DNA and RNA), respiratory tract infection, 17 bacteria, 8 fungus, 13 virus, and 16 antibiotic-resistance genes, multiplex amplified probe technique, upper or lower respiratory specimen
Urogenital Pathogen with Rx Panel (UPX), Lab Genomics LLC, Thermo Fisher Scientific	0374U	Infectious agent detection by nucleic acid (DNA or RNA), genitourinary pathogens, identification of 21 bacterial and fungal organisms and identification of 21 associated antibiotic-resistance genes, multiplex amplified probe technique, urine
OvaWatch^{SM}, Aspira Women's Health^{SM}, Aspira Labs, Inc	0375U	Oncology (ovarian), biochemical assays of 7 proteins (follicle stimulating hormone, human epididymis protein 4, apolipoprotein A-1, transferrin, beta-2 macroglobulin, prealbumin [ie, transthyretin], and cancer antigen 125), algorithm reported as ovarian cancer risk score
ArteraAI Prostate Test, Artera Inc®, Artera Inc®	0376U	Oncology (prostate cancer), image analysis of at least 128 histologic features and clinical factors, prognostic algorithm determining the risk of distant metastases, and prostate cancer-specific mortality, includes predictive algorithm to androgen deprivation-therapy response, if appropriate
Liposcale®, CIMA Sciences, LLC	0377U	Cardiovascular disease, quantification of advanced serum or plasma lipoprotein profile, by nuclear magnetic resonance (NMR) spectrometry with report of a lipoprotein profile (including 23 variables)
UCGSL *RFC1* Repeat Expansion Test, University of Chicago Genetic Services Laboratories	0378U	*RFC1 (replication factor C subunit 1),* repeat expansion variant analysis by traditional and repeat-primed PCR, blood, saliva, or buccal swab
Solid Tumor Expanded Panel, Quest Diagnostics®, Quest Diagnostics®	0379U	Targeted genomic sequence analysis panel, solid organ neoplasm, DNA (523 genes) and RNA (55 genes) by next-generation sequencing, interrogation for sequence variants, gene copy number amplifications, gene rearrangements, microsatellite instability, and tumor mutational burden
PersonalisedRX, Lab Genomics LLC, Agena Bioscience, Inc	0380U	Drug metabolism (adverse drug reactions and drug response), targeted sequence analysis, 20 gene variants and *CYP2D6* deletion or duplication analysis with reported genotype and phenotype

(Continued on page 246)

Appendix O

Proprietary Name and Clinical Laboratory or Manufacturer	Alpha-Numeric Code	Code Descriptor
Branched-Chain Amino Acids, Self-Collect, Blood Spot, Mayo Clinic, Laboratory Developed Test	0381U	Maple syrup urine disease monitoring by patient-collected blood card sample, quantitative measurement of allo-isoleucine, leucine, isoleucine, and valine, liquid chromatography with tandem mass spectrometry (LC-MS/MS)
Phenylalanine and Tyrosine, Self-Collect, Blood Spot, Mayo Clinic, Laboratory Developed Test	0382U	Hyperphenylalaninemia monitoring by patient-collected blood card sample, quantitative measurement of phenylalanine and tyrosine, liquid chromatography with tandem mass spectrometry (LC-MS/MS)
Tyrosinemia Follow-Up Panel, Self-Collect, Blood Spot, Mayo Clinic, Laboratory Developed Test	0383U	Tyrosinemia type I monitoring by patient-collected blood card sample, quantitative measurement of tyrosine, phenylalanine, methionine, succinylacetone, nitisinone, liquid chromatography with tandem mass spectrometry (LC-MS/MS)
NaviDKD™ Predictive Diagnostic Screening for Kidney Health, Journey Biosciences, Inc, Journey Biosciences, Inc	0384U	Nephrology (chronic kidney disease), carboxymethyllysine, methylglyoxal hydroimidazolone, and carboxyethyl lysine by liquid chromatography with tandem mass spectrometry (LC-MS/MS) and HbA1c and estimated glomerular filtration rate (GFR), with risk score reported for predictive progression to high-stage kidney disease
PromarkerD, Sonic Reference Laboratory, Proteomics International Pty Ltd	0385U	Nephrology (chronic kidney disease), apolipoprotein A4 (ApoA4), CD5 antigen-like (CD5L), and insulin-like growth factor binding protein 3 (IGFBP3) by enzyme-linked immunoassay (ELISA), plasma, algorithm combining results with HDL, estimated glomerular filtration rate (GFR) and clinical data reported as a risk score for developing diabetic kidney disease
—	(0386U has been deleted)	—
AMBLor® melanoma prognostic test, Avero® Diagnostics	0387U	Oncology (melanoma), autophagy and beclin 1 regulator 1 (AMBRA1) and loricrin (AMLo) by immunohistochemistry, formalin-fixed paraffin-embedded (FFPE) tissue, report for risk of progression (Do not report 0387U in conjunction with 88341, 88342)
InVisionFirst®-Lung Liquid Biopsy, Inivata, Inc, Inivata, Inc	0388U	Oncology (non-small cell lung cancer), next-generation sequencing with identification of single nucleotide variants, copy number variants, insertions and deletions, and structural variants in 37 cancer-related genes, plasma, with report for alteration detection
KawasakiDx, OncoOmicsDx Laboratory, mProbe	0389U	Pediatric febrile illness (Kawasaki disease [KD]), interferon alpha-inducible protein 27 (IFI27) and mast cell-expressed membrane protein 1 (MCEMP1), RNA, using quantitative reverse transcription polymerase chain reaction (RT-qPCR), blood, reported as a risk score for KD

★ = Telemedicine ◀ = Audio-only ✚ = Add-on code ✔ = FDA approval pending # = Resequenced code ⊘ = Modifier 51 exempt

Appendix O

Proprietary Name and Clinical Laboratory or Manufacturer	Alpha-Numeric Code	Code Descriptor
PEPredictDx, OncoOmicsDx Laboratory, mProbe	0390U	Obstetrics (preeclampsia), kinase insert domain receptor (KDR), Endoglin (ENG), and retinol-binding protein 4 (RBP4), by immunoassay, serum, algorithm reported as a risk score
Strata Select™, Strata Oncology, Inc, Strata Oncology, Inc	0391U	Oncology (solid tumor), DNA and RNA by next-generation sequencing, utilizing formalin-fixed paraffin-embedded (FFPE) tissue, 437 genes, interpretive report for single nucleotide variants, splice-site variants, insertions/deletions, copy number alterations, gene fusions, tumor mutational burden, and microsatellite instability, with algorithm quantifying immunotherapy response score
Medication Management Neuropsychiatric Panel, RCA Laboratory Services LLC d/b/a GENETWORx, GENETWORx	0392U	Drug metabolism (depression, anxiety, attention deficit hyperactivity disorder [ADHD]), gene-drug interactions, variant analysis of 16 genes, including deletion/duplication analysis of *CYP2D6*, reported as impact of gene-drug interaction for each drug
SYNTap® Biomarker Test, Amprion Clinical Laboratory, Amprion Clinical Laboratory	0393U	Neurology (eg, Parkinson disease, dementia with Lewy bodies), cerebrospinal fluid (CSF), detection of misfolded α-synuclein protein by seed amplification assay, qualitative
PFAS Testing & PFASure™, National Medical Services, NMS Labs, Inc	0394U	Perfluoroalkyl substances (PFAS) (eg, perfluorooctanoic acid, perfluorooctane sulfonic acid), 16 PFAS compounds by liquid chromatography with tandem mass spectrometry (LC-MS/MS), plasma or serum, quantitative
OncobiotaLUNG, Micronoma™, Micronoma™	0395U	Oncology (lung), multi-omics (microbial DNA by shotgun next-generation sequencing and carcinoembryonic antigen and osteopontin by immunoassay), plasma, algorithm reported as malignancy risk for lung nodules in early-stage disease
—	▶(0396U has been deleted)◀	—
—	(0397U has been deleted)	—
ESOPREDICT® Barrett's Esophagus Risk Classifier Assay, Capsulomics, Inc d/b/a Previse	0398U	Gastroenterology (Barrett's esophagus), *P16, RUNX3, HPP1,* and *FBN1* DNA methylation analysis using PCR, formalin-fixed paraffin-embedded (FFPE) tissue, algorithm reported as risk score for progression to high-grade dysplasia or cancer
FRAT® (Folate Receptor Antibody Test), Religen Inc, Religen Inc	0399U	Neurology (cerebral folate deficiency), serum, detection of anti-human folate receptor IgG-binding antibody and blocking autoantibodies by enzyme-linked immunoassay (ELISA), qualitative, and blocking autoantibodies, using a functional blocking assay for IgG or IgM, quantitative, reported as positive or not detected
Genesys Carrier Panel, Genesys Diagnostics, Inc	0400U	Obstetrics (expanded carrier screening), 145 genes by next-generation sequencing, fragment analysis and multiplex ligation-dependent probe amplification, DNA, reported as carrier positive or negative

(Continued on page 248)

▲ = Revised code   ● = New code   ▶ ◀ = Contains new or revised text   ✕ = Duplicate PLA test   ↑↓ = Category I PLA   American Medical Association   **247**

Appendix O

Proprietary Name and Clinical Laboratory or Manufacturer	Alpha-Numeric Code	Code Descriptor
CARDIO inCode-Score (CIC-SCORE), GENinCode U.S. Inc, GENinCode U.S. Inc	0401U	Cardiology (coronary heart disease [CHD]), 9 genes (12 variants), targeted variant genotyping, blood, saliva, or buccal swab, algorithm reported as a genetic risk score for a coronary event
Abbott Alinity™ m STI Assay, Abbott Molecular, Inc	0402U	Infectious agent (sexually transmitted infection), Chlamydia trachomatis, Neisseria gonorrhoeae, Trichomonas vaginalis, Mycoplasma genitalium, multiplex amplified probe technique, vaginal, endocervical, or male urine, each pathogen reported as detected or not detected
MyProstateScore 2.0, LynxDX, LynxDX	▲0403U	▶Oncology (prostate), mRNA, gene expression profiling of 18 genes, first-catch urine, algorithm reported as percentage of likelihood of detecting clinically significant prostate cancer◀
DiviTum®TKa, Biovica Inc, Biovica International AB	0404U	Oncology (breast), semiquantitative measurement of thymidine kinase activity by immunoassay, serum, results reported as risk of disease progression
BTG Early Detection of Pancreatic Cancer, Breakthrough Genomics, Breakthrough Genomics	0405U	Oncology (pancreatic), 59 methylation haplotype block markers, next-generation sequencing, plasma, reported as cancer signal detected or not detected
CyPath® Lung, Precision Pathology Services, bioAffinity Technologies, Inc	0406U	Oncology (lung), flow cytometry, sputum, 5 markers (meso-tetra [4-carboxyphenyl] porphyrin [TCPP], CD206, CD66b, CD3, CD19), algorithm reported as likelihood of lung cancer
▶kidneyintelX.dkd™◀, Renalytix Inc, Renalytix Inc, NYC, NY	0407U	Nephrology (diabetic chronic kidney disease [CKD]), multiplex electrochemiluminescent immunoassay (ECLIA) of soluble tumor necrosis factor receptor 1 (sTNFR1), soluble tumor necrosis receptor 2 (sTNFR2), and kidney injury molecule 1 (KIM-1) combined with clinical data, plasma, algorithm reported as risk for progressive decline in kidney function
Omnia™ SARS-CoV-2 Antigen Test, Qorvo Biotechnologies, Qorvo Biotechnologies	0408U	Infectious agent antigen detection by bulk acoustic wave biosensor immunoassay, severe acute respiratory syndrome coronavirus 2 (SARS-CoV-2) (coronavirus disease [COVID-19])
LiquidHALLMARK®, Lucence Health, Inc	0409U	Oncology (solid tumor), DNA (80 genes) and RNA (36 genes), by next-generation sequencing from plasma, including single nucleotide variants, insertions/deletions, copy number alterations, microsatellite instability, and fusions, report showing identified mutations with clinical actionability
Avantect™ Pancreatic Cancer Test, ClearNote™ Health, ClearNote™ Health	0410U	Oncology (pancreatic), DNA, whole genome sequencing with 5-hydroxymethylcytosine enrichment, whole blood or plasma, algorithm reported as cancer detected or not detected

★ = Telemedicine   ◀ = Audio-only   ✛ = Add-on code   ✗ = FDA approval pending   # = Resequenced code   ⊘ = Modifier 51 exempt

Proprietary Name and Clinical Laboratory or Manufacturer	Alpha-Numeric Code	Code Descriptor
IDgenetix®, Castle Biosciences, Inc, Castle Biosciences, Inc	✕0411U	Psychiatry (eg, depression, anxiety, attention deficit hyperactivity disorder [ADHD]), genomic analysis panel, variant analysis of 15 genes, including deletion/duplication analysis of *CYP2D6* (For additional PLA code with identical clinical descriptor, see 0345U. See Appendix O to determine appropriate code assignment)
PrecivityAD® blood test, C2N Diagnostics LLC, C2N Diagnostics LLC	0412U	Beta amyloid, Aβ42/40 ratio, immunoprecipitation with quantitation by liquid chromatography with tandem mass spectrometry (LC-MS/MS) and qualitative ApoE isoform-specific proteotyping, plasma combined with age, algorithm reported as presence or absence of brain amyloid pathology
DH Optical Genome Mapping/Digital Karyotyping Assay, The Clinical Genomics and Advanced Technology (CGAT) Laboratory at Dartmouth Health, Bionano Genomics	0413U	Oncology (hematolymphoid neoplasm), optical genome mapping for copy number alterations, aneuploidy, and balanced/complex structural rearrangements, DNA from blood or bone marrow, report of clinically significant alterations
LungOI, Imagene	0414U	Oncology (lung), augmentative algorithmic analysis of digitized whole slide imaging for 8 genes *(ALK, BRAF, EGFR, ERBB2, MET, NTRK1-3, RET, ROS1)*, and *KRAS* G12C and PD-L1, if performed, formalin-fixed paraffin-embedded (FFPE) tissue, reported as positive or negative for each biomarker
SmartHealth Vascular Dx™, Morningstar Laboratories, LLC, SmartHealth DX	0415U	Cardiovascular disease (acute coronary syndrome [ACS]), IL-16, FAS, FASLigand, HGF, CTACK, EOTAXIN, and MCP-3 by immunoassay combined with age, sex, family history, and personal history of diabetes, blood, algorithm reported as a 5-year (deleted risk) score for ACS
—	►(0416U has been deleted)◄	—
Genomic Unity® Comprehensive Mitochondrial Disorders Analysis, Variantyx Inc, Variantyx Inc	0417U	Rare diseases (constitutional/heritable disorders), whole mitochondrial genome sequence with heteroplasmy detection and deletion analysis, nuclear-encoded mitochondrial gene analysis of 335 nuclear genes, including sequence changes, deletions, insertions, and copy number variants analysis, blood or saliva, identification and categorization of mitochondrial disorder–associated genetic variants
PreciseDx Breast Biopsy Test, PreciseDx, PreciseDx, Inc NYC, NY	0418U	Oncology (breast), augmentative algorithmic analysis of digitized whole slide imaging of 8 histologic and immunohistochemical features, reported as a recurrence score
Tempus nP, Tempus Labs, Inc, Tempus Labs, Inc	0419U	Neuropsychiatry (eg, depression, anxiety), genomic sequence analysis panel, variant analysis of 13 genes, saliva or buccal swab, report of each gene phenotype

(*Continued on page 250*)

Proprietary Name and Clinical Laboratory or Manufacturer	Alpha-Numeric Code	Code Descriptor
▶Cxbladder Detect+, Pacific Edge Diagnostics USA LTD, Pacific Edge Diagnostics USA LTD◀	●0420U	▶Oncology (urothelial), mRNA expression profiling by real-time quantitative PCR of *MDK, HOXA13, CDC2, IGFBP5,* and *CXCR2* in combination with droplet digital PCR (ddPCR) analysis of 6 single-nucleotide polymorphisms (SNPs) of genes *TERT* and *FGFR3*, urine, algorithm reported as a risk score for urothelial carcinoma◀
▶Colosense™, Geneoscopy, Inc, Geneoscopy, Inc◀	●0421U	▶Oncology (colorectal) screening, quantitative real-time target and signal amplification of 8 RNA markers *(GAPDH, SMAD4, ACY1, AREG, CDH1, KRAS, TNFRSF10B, EGLN2)* and fecal hemoglobin, algorithm reported as a positive or negative for colorectal cancer risk◀
▶Guardant360 Response™, Guardant Health, Inc, Guardant Health, Inc◀	●0422U	▶Oncology (pan-solid tumor), analysis of DNA biomarker response to anti-cancer therapy using cell-free circulating DNA, biomarker comparison to a previous baseline pre-treatment cell-free circulating DNA analysis using next-generation sequencing, algorithm reported as a quantitative change from baseline, including specific alterations, if appropriate◀
▶Genomind® Pharmacogenetics Report – Full, Genomind®, Inc, Genomind®, Inc◀	●0423U	▶Psychiatry (eg, depression, anxiety), genomic analysis panel, including variant analysis of 26 genes, buccal swab, report including metabolizer status and risk of drug toxicity by condition◀
▶miR Sentinel™ Prostate Cancer Test, miR Scientific®, LLC, miR Scientific®, LLC◀	●0424U	▶Oncology (prostate), exosome-based analysis of 53 small noncoding RNAs (sncRNAs) by quantitative reverse transcription polymerase chain reaction (RT-qPCR), urine, reported as no molecular evidence, low-, moderate-, or elevated-risk of prostate cancer◀
▶RCIGM Rapid Whole Genome Sequencing, Comparator Genome, Rady Children's Institute for Genomic Medicine, Rady Children's Institute for Genomic Medicine◀	●0425U	▶Genome (eg, unexplained constitutional or heritable disorder or syndrome), rapid sequence analysis, each comparator genome (eg, parents, siblings)◀
▶RCIGM Ultra-Rapid Whole Genome Sequencing, Rady Children's Institute for Genomic Medicine, Rady Children's Institute for Genomic Medicine◀	●0426U	▶Genome (eg, unexplained constitutional or heritable disorder or syndrome), ultra-rapid sequence analysis◀
▶Early Sepsis Indicator, Beckman Coulter, Inc◀	✚●0427U	▶Monocyte distribution width, whole blood (List separately in addition to code for primary procedure)◀ ▶(Use 0427U in conjunction with 85004, 85025)◀

★ = Telemedicine   ◀ = Audio-only   ✚ = Add-on code   ✗ = FDA approval pending   # = Resequenced code   ⊘ = Modifier 51 exempt

Proprietary Name and Clinical Laboratory or Manufacturer	Alpha-Numeric Code	Code Descriptor
▶Epic Sciences ctDNA Metastatic Breast Cancer Panel, Epic Sciences, Inc, Epic Sciences, Inc◀	●0428U	▶Oncology (breast), targeted hybrid-capture genomic sequence analysis panel, circulating tumor DNA (ctDNA) analysis of 56 or more genes, interrogation for sequence variants, gene copy number amplifications, gene rearrangements, microsatellite instability, and tumor mutation burden◀
▶Omnipathology Oropharyngeal HPV PCR Test, OmniPathology Solutions, Medical Corporation, OmniPathology Solutions, Medical Corporation◀	●0429U	▶Human papillomavirus (HPV), oropharyngeal swab, 14 high-risk types (ie, 16, 18, 31, 33, 35, 39, 45, 51, 52, 56, 58, 59, 66, and 68)◀
▶Malabsorption Evaluation Panel, Mayo Clinic/Mayo Clinic Laboratories, Mayo Clinic/Mayo Clinic Laboratories◀	●0430U	▶Gastroenterology, malabsorption evaluation of alpha-1-antitrypsin, calprotectin, pancreatic elastase and reducing substances, feces, quantitative◀
▶Glycine Receptor Alpha1 IgG, Mayo Clinic/Mayo Clinic Laboratories, Mayo Clinic/Mayo Clinic Laboratories◀	●0431U	▶Glycine receptor alpha1 IgG, serum or cerebrospinal fluid (CSF), live cell-binding assay (LCBA), qualitative◀
▶Kelch-Like Protein 11 Antibody, Mayo Clinic/Mayo Clinic Laboratories, Mayo Clinic/Mayo Clinic Laboratories◀	●0432U	▶Kelch-like protein 11 (KLHL11) antibody, serum or cerebrospinal fluid (CSF), cell-binding assay, qualitative◀
▶EpiSwitch® Prostate Screening Test (PSE), Oxford BioDynamics Inc, Oxford BioDynamics PLC◀	●0433U	▶Oncology (prostate), 5 DNA regulatory markers by quantitative PCR, whole blood, algorithm, including prostate-specific antigen, reported as likelihood of cancer◀
▶RightMed® Gene Test Exclude F2 and F5, OneOme® LLC, OneOme® LLC◀	●0434U	▶Drug metabolism (adverse drug reactions and drug response), genomic analysis panel, variant analysis of 25 genes with reported phenotypes◀
▶ChemoID®, ChemoID® Lab, Cordgenics, LLC◀	●0435U	▶Oncology, chemotherapeutic drug cytotoxicity assay of cancer stem cells (CSCs), from cultured CSCs and primary tumor cells, categorical drug response reported based on cytotoxicity percentage observed, minimum of 14 drugs or drug combinations◀
▶PROphet® NSCLC Test, OncoHost, Inc, OncoHost, Inc◀	●0436U	▶Oncology (lung), plasma analysis of 388 proteins, using aptamer-based proteomics technology, predictive algorithm reported as clinical benefit from immune checkpoint inhibitor therapy◀
▶MindX One™ Blood Test – Anxiety, MindX Sciences, MindX Sciences◀	●0437U	▶Psychiatry (anxiety disorders), mRNA, gene expression profiling by RNA sequencing of 15 biomarkers, whole blood, algorithm reported as predictive risk score◀
▶EffectiveRX™ Comprehensive Panel, RCA Laboratory Services LLC d/b/a GENETWORx, GENETWORx◀	●0438U	▶Drug metabolism (adverse drug reactions and drug response), buccal specimen, gene-drug interactions, variant analysis of 33 genes, including deletion/duplication analysis of *CYP2D6,* including reported phenotypes and impacted gene-drug interactions◀

(*Continued on page 252*)

▲=Revised code   ●=New code   ▶ ◀=Contains new or revised text   ✕=Duplicate PLA test   ↕=Category I PLA   American Medical Association   **251**

Proprietary Name and Clinical Laboratory or Manufacturer	Alpha-Numeric Code	Code Descriptor
▶Epi+Gen CHD™, Cardio Diagnostics, Inc, Cardio Diagnostics, Inc◀	●0439U	▶Cardiology (coronary heart disease [CHD]), DNA, analysis of 5 single-nucleotide polymorphisms (SNPs) (rs11716050 [LOC105376934], rs6560711 [WDR37], rs3735222 [SCIN/LOC107986769], rs6820447 [intergenic], and rs9638144 [ESYT2]) and 3 DNA methylation markers (cg00300879 [transcription start site {TSS200} of CNKSR1], cg09552548 [intergenic], and cg14789911 [body of SPATC1L]), qPCR and digital PCR, whole blood, algorithm reported as a 4-tiered risk score for a 3-year risk of symptomatic CHD◀
▶PrecisionCHD™, Cardio Diagnostics, Inc, Cardio Diagnostics, Inc◀	●0440U	▶Cardiology (coronary heart disease [CHD]), DNA, analysis of 10 single-nucleotide polymorphisms (SNPs) (rs710987 [LINC010019], rs1333048 [CDKN2B-AS1], rs12129789 [KCND3], rs942317 [KTN1-AS1], rs1441433 [PPP3CA], rs2869675 [PREX1], rs4639796 [ZBTB41], rs4376434 [LINC00972], rs12714414 [TMEM18], and rs7585056 [TMEM18]) and 6 DNA methylation markers (cg03725309 [SARS1], cg12586707 [CXCL1], cg04988978 [MPO], cg17901584 [DHCR24-DT], cg21161138 [AHRR], and cg12655112 [EHD4]), qPCR and digital PCR, whole blood, algorithm reported as detected or not detected for CHD◀
▶IntelliSep® test, Cytovale®◀	●0441U	▶Infectious disease (bacterial, fungal, or viral infection), semiquantitative biomechanical assessment (via deformability cytometry), whole blood, with algorithmic analysis and result reported as an index◀
▶FebriDx® Bacterial/Non-Bacterial Point-of-Care Assay, Lumos Diagnostics, LLC, Lumos Diagnostics, LLC◀	●0442U	▶Infectious disease (respiratory infection), Myxovirus resistance protein A (MxA) and C-reactive protein (CRP), fingerstick whole blood specimen, each biomarker reported as present or absent◀
▶Neurofilament Light Chain (NfL), Neuromuscular Clinical Laboratory at Washington University in St. Louis School of Medicine, Neuromuscular Clinical Laboratory at Washington University in St. Louis School of Medicine◀	●0443U	▶Neurofilament light chain (NfL), ultra-sensitive immunoassay, serum or cerebrospinal fluid◀
▶Aventa FusionPlus™, Aventa Genomics, LLC◀	●0444U	▶Oncology (solid organ neoplasia), targeted genomic sequence analysis panel of 361 genes, interrogation for gene fusions, translocations, or other rearrangements, using DNA from formalin-fixed paraffin-embedded (FFPE) tumor tissue, report of clinically significant variant(s)◀

★=Telemedicine ◀=Audio-only ✛=Add-on code ✗=FDA approval pending #=Resequenced code ⊘=Modifier 51 exempt

Proprietary Name and Clinical Laboratory or Manufacturer	Alpha-Numeric Code	Code Descriptor
►Elecsys® Phospho-Tau (181P) CSF (pTau181) and β-Amyloid (1-42) CSF II (Abeta 42) Ratio, Roche Diagnostics Operations, Inc (US owner/operator)◄	●0445U	►β-amyloid (Abeta42) and phospho tau (181P) (pTau181), electrochemiluminescent immunoassay (ECLIA), cerebral spinal fluid, ratio reported as positive or negative for amyloid pathology◄
►aisle® DX Disease Activity Index, Progentec Diagnostics, Inc, Progentec Diagnostics, Inc◄	●0446U	►Autoimmune diseases (systemic lupus erythematosus [SLE]), analysis of 10 cytokine soluble mediator biomarkers by immunoassay, plasma, individual components reported with an algorithmic risk score for current disease activity◄
►aisle® DX Flare Risk Index, Progentec Diagnostics, Inc, Progentec Diagnostics, Inc◄	●0447U	►Autoimmune diseases (systemic lupus erythematosus [SLE]), analysis of 11 cytokine soluble mediator biomarkers by immunoassay, plasma, individual components reported with an algorithmic prognostic risk score for developing a clinical flare◄
►oncoReveal™ DX Lung and Colon Cancer Assay, Pillar® Biosciences, Pillar® Biosciences◄	●0448U	►Oncology (lung and colon cancer), DNA, qualitative, next-generation sequencing detection of single-nucleotide variants and deletions in *EGFR* and *KRAS* genes, formalin-fixed paraffin-embedded (FFPE) solid tumor samples, reported as presence or absence of targeted mutation(s), with recommended therapeutic options◄
►UNITY Carrier Screen™, BillionToOne Laboratory, BillionToOne, Inc◄	●0449U	►Carrier screening for severe inherited conditions (eg, cystic fibrosis, spinal muscular atrophy, beta hemoglobinopathies [including sickle cell disease], alpha thalassemia), regardless of race or self-identified ancestry, genomic sequence analysis panel, must include analysis of 5 genes *(CFTR, SMN1, HBB, HBA1, HBA2)*◄
►M-inSight® Patient Definition Assay, Corgenix Clinical Laboratory, Sebia◄	●0450U	►Oncology (multiple myeloma), liquid chromatography with tandem mass spectrometry (LC-MS/MS), monoclonal paraprotein sequencing analysis, serum, results reported as baseline presence or absence of detectable clonotypic peptides◄
►M-inSight® Patient Follow-Up Assessment, Corgenix Clinical Laboratory, Sebia◄	●0451U	►Oncology (multiple myeloma), LC-MS/MS, peptide ion quantification, serum, results compared with baseline to determine monoclonal paraprotein abundance◄
►EarlyTect® Bladder Cancer Detection (EarlyTect® BCD), Promis Diagnostics, Inc, Promis Diagnostics, Inc◄	●0452U	►Oncology (bladder), methylated *PENK* DNA detection by linear target enrichment-quantitative methylation-specific real-time PCR (LTE-qMSP), urine, reported as likelihood of bladder cancer◄
►ColonAiQ®, Breakthrough Genomics, Singlera Genomics, Inc◄	●0453U	►Oncology (colorectal cancer), cell-free DNA (cfDNA), methylation-based quantitative PCR assay *(SEPTIN9, IKZF1, BCAT1,* Septin9-2, *VAV3, BCAN),* plasma, reported as presence or absence of circulating tumor DNA (ctDNA)◄

(Continued on page 254)

▲ = Revised code   ● = New code   ► ◄ = Contains new or revised text   ✕ = Duplicate PLA test   ↕ = Category I PLA

Appendix O

Proprietary Name and Clinical Laboratory or Manufacturer	Alpha-Numeric Code	Code Descriptor
▶Chromosome Genome Mapping, UR Medicine Labs, Bionano Genomics, Inc◀	✕●0454U	▶Rare diseases (constitutional/heritable disorders), identification of copy number variations, inversions, insertions, translocations, and other structural variants by optical genome mapping◀ ▶(For additional PLA codes with identical clinical descriptor, see 0260U, 0264U. See Appendix O or the most current listing on the AMA CPT website to determine appropriate code assignment)◀
▶Abbott Alinity™ m STI Assay, Abbott Molecular, Inc◀	●0455U	▶Infectious agents (sexually transmitted infection), Chlamydia trachomatis, Neisseria gonorrhoeae, and Trichomonas vaginalis, multiplex amplified probe technique, vaginal, endocervical, gynecological specimens, oropharyngeal swabs, rectal swabs, female or male urine, each pathogen reported as detected or not detected◀
▶PrismRA®, Scipher Medicine®, Scipher Medicine®◀	●0456U	▶Autoimmune (rheumatoid arthritis), next-generation sequencing (NGS), gene expression testing of 19 genes, whole blood, with analysis of anti-cyclic citrullinated peptides (CCP) levels, combined with sex, patient global assessment, and body mass index (BMI), algorithm reported as a score that predicts nonresponse to tumor necrosis factor inhibitor (TNFi) therapy◀
▶PFAS (Forever Chemicals) 9 Panel, Quest Diagnostics®, Quest Diagnostics®◀	●0457U	▶Perfluoroalkyl substances (PFAS) (eg, perfluorooctanoic acid, perfluorooctane sulfonic acid), 9 PFAS compounds by LC-MS/MS, plasma or serum, quantitative◀
▶Auria®, Namida Lab, Inc, Namida Lab, Inc◀	●0458U	▶Oncology (breast cancer), S100A8 and S100A9, by enzyme-linked immunosorbent assay (ELISA), tear fluid with age, algorithm reported as a risk score◀
▶Elecsys® Total Tau CSF (tTau) and β-Amyloid (1-42) CSF II (Abeta 42) Ratio, Roche Diagnostics Operations, Inc (US owner/operator)◀	●0459U	▶β-amyloid (Abeta42) and total tau (tTau), electrochemiluminescent immunoassay (ECLIA), cerebral spinal fluid, ratio reported as positive or negative for amyloid pathology◀
▶RightMed® Oncology Gene Report, OneOme® LLC, OneOme® LLC◀	●0460U	▶Oncology, whole blood or buccal, DNA single-nucleotide polymorphism (SNP) genotyping by real-time PCR of 24 genes, with variant analysis and reported phenotypes◀
▶RightMed® Oncology Medication Report, OneOme® LLC, OneOme® LLC◀	●0461U	▶Oncology, pharmacogenomic analysis of single-nucleotide polymorphism (SNP) genotyping by real-time PCR of 24 genes, whole blood or buccal swab, with variant analysis, including impacted gene-drug interactions and reported phenotypes◀
▶Salimetrics® Salivary Melatonin Profile (Circadian Phase Assessment), Salimetrics® Clinical Laboratory, Salimetrics®, LLC◀	●0462U	▶Melatonin levels test, sleep study, 7 or 9 sample melatonin profile (cortisol optional), enzyme-linked immunosorbent assay (ELISA), saliva, screening/preliminary◀

★=Telemedicine　◀=Audio-only　✚=Add-on code　✗=FDA approval pending　#=Resequenced code　⊘=Modifier 51 exempt

Proprietary Name and Clinical Laboratory or Manufacturer	Alpha-Numeric Code	Code Descriptor
►Proofer '7 HPV mRNA E6 and E7 Biomarker Test, Global Diagnostics Labs, LLC, PreTect AS, a Mel-Mont Medical, Inc, wholly owned subsidiary◄	●0463U	►Oncology (cervix), mRNA gene expression profiling of 14 biomarkers (E6 and E7 of the highest-risk human papillomavirus [HPV] types 16, 18, 31, 33, 45, 52, 58), by real-time nucleic acid sequence-based amplification (NASBA), exo- or endocervical epithelial cells, algorithm reported as positive or negative for increased risk of cervical dysplasia or cancer for each biomarker◄
►Cologuard Plus™, Exact Sciences Laboratories, LLC, Exact Sciences Corporation◄	●0464U	►Oncology (colorectal) screening, quantitative real-time target and signal amplification, methylated DNA markers, including LASS4, LRRC4 and PPP2R5C, a reference marker ZDHHC1, and a protein marker (fecal hemoglobin), utilizing stool, algorithm reported as a positive or negative result◄
►UriFind® Urothelial Carcinoma Assay, DiaCarta, Inc, AnchorDx◄	●0465U	►Oncology (urothelial carcinoma), DNA, quantitative methylation-specific PCR of 2 genes (ONECUT2, VIM), algorithmic analysis reported as positive or negative◄
►CardioRisk+, Gene by Gene, Ltd, OpenDNA, Ltd◄	●0466U	►Cardiology (coronary artery disease [CAD]), DNA, genome-wide association studies (564856 single-nucleotide polymorphisms [SNPs], targeted variant genotyping), patient lifestyle and clinical data, buccal swab, algorithm reported as polygenic risk to acquired heart disease◄
►UroAmp MRD, Convergent Genomics, Inc, Convergent Genomics, Inc◄	●0467U	►Oncology (bladder), DNA, next-generation sequencing (NGS) of 60 genes and whole genome aneuploidy, urine, algorithms reported as minimal residual disease (MRD) status positive or negative and quantitative disease burden◄
►NASHnext™(NIS4™), Labcorp, Labcorp◄	●0468U	►Hepatology (nonalcoholic steatohepatitis [NASH]), miR-34a-5p, alpha 2-macroglobulin, YKL40, HbA1c, serum and whole blood, algorithm reported as a single score for NASH activity and fibrosis◄
►IriSight™ CNV Analysis, Variantyx Inc, Variantyx Inc◄	●0469U	►Rare diseases (constitutional/heritable disorders), whole genome sequence analysis for chromosomal abnormalities, copy number variants, duplications/deletions, inversions, unbalanced translocations, regions of homozygosity (ROH), inheritance pattern that indicate uniparental disomy (UPD), and aneuploidy, fetal sample (amniotic fluid, chorionic villus sample, or products of conception), identification and categorization of genetic variants, diagnostic report of fetal results based on phenotype with maternal sample and paternal sample, if performed, as comparators and/or maternal cell contamination◄
►HPV-SEQ Test, Sysmex Inostics, Inc, Sysmex Inostics, Inc◄	●0470U	►Oncology (oropharyngeal), detection of minimal residual disease by next-generation sequencing (NGS) based quantitative evaluation of 8 DNA targets, cell-free HPV 16 and 18 DNA from plasma◄

(Continued on page 256)

Proprietary Name and Clinical Laboratory or Manufacturer	Alpha-Numeric Code	Code Descriptor
▶CRCdx® RAS Mutation Detection Kit, EntroGen, Inc, EntroGen, Inc◀	●0471U	▶Oncology (colorectal cancer), qualitative real-time PCR of 35 variants of *KRAS* and *NRAS* genes (exons 2, 3, 4), formalin-fixed paraffin-embedded (FFPE), predictive, identification of detected mutations◀
▶Early Sjögren's Syndrome Profile, Immco Diagnostics, Inc, Immco Diagnostics, Inc◀	●0472U	▶Carbonic anhydrase VI (CA VI), parotid specific/secretory protein (PSP) and salivary protein (SP1) IgG, IgM, and IgA antibodies, enzyme-linked immunosorbent assay (ELISA), semiqualitative, blood, reported as predictive evidence of early Sjögren's syndrome◀
▶xT CDx, Tempus AI, Inc, Tempus AI, Inc◀	●0473U	▶Oncology (solid tumor), next-generation sequencing (NGS) of DNA from formalin-fixed paraffin-embedded (FFPE) tissue with comparative sequence analysis from a matched normal specimen (blood or saliva), 648 genes, interrogation for sequence variants, insertion and deletion alterations, copy number variants, rearrangements, microsatellite instability, and tumor-mutation burden◀
▶GeneticsNow® Comprehensive Germline Panel, GoPath Diagnostics, Inc, GoPath Diagnostics, Inc◀	●0474U	▶Hereditary pan-cancer (eg, hereditary sarcomas, hereditary endocrine tumors, hereditary neuroendocrine tumors, hereditary cutaneous melanoma), genomic sequence analysis panel of 88 genes with 20 duplications/deletions using next-generation sequencing (NGS), Sanger sequencing, blood or saliva, reported as positive or negative for germline variants, each gene◀
▶ProstateNow™ Prostate Germline Panel, GoPath Diagnostics, Inc, GoPath Diagnostics, Inc◀	●0475U	▶Hereditary prostate cancer-related disorders, genomic sequence analysis panel using next-generation sequencing (NGS), Sanger sequencing, multiplex ligation-dependent probe amplification (MLPA), and array comparative genomic hybridization (CGH), evaluation of 23 genes and duplications/deletions when indicated, pathologic mutations reported with a genetic risk score for prostate cancer◀
▶RightMed® Mental Health Gene Report, OneOme, LLC, OneOme, LLC◀	●0476U	▶Drug metabolism, psychiatry (eg, major depressive disorder, general anxiety disorder, attention deficit hyperactivity disorder [ADHD], schizophrenia), whole blood, buccal swab, and pharmacogenomic genotyping of 14 genes and *CYP2D6* copy number variant analysis and reported phenotypes◀
▶RightMed® Mental Health Medication Report, OneOme, LLC, OneOme, LLC◀	●0477U	▶Drug metabolism, psychiatry (eg, major depressive disorder, general anxiety disorder, attention deficit hyperactivity disorder [ADHD], schizophrenia), whole blood, buccal swab, and pharmacogenomic genotyping of 14 genes and *CYP2D6* copy number variant analysis, including impacted gene-drug interactions and reported phenotypes◀

★=Telemedicine ◀=Audio-only ✚=Add-on code ✗=FDA approval pending #=Resequenced code ⊘=Modifier 51 exempt

Proprietary Name and Clinical Laboratory or Manufacturer	Alpha-Numeric Code	Code Descriptor
▶Lung HDPCR™, Protean BioDiagnostics, Protean BioDiagnostics◀	●0478U	▶Oncology (non-small cell lung cancer), DNA and RNA, digital PCR analysis of 9 genes *(EGFR, KRAS, BRAF, ALK, ROS1, RET, NTRK 1/2/3, ERBB2,* and *MET)* in formalin-fixed paraffin-embedded (FFPE) tissue, interrogation for single-nucleotide variants, insertions/deletions, gene rearrangements, and reported as actionable detected variants for therapy selection◀
▶ALZpath pTau217, Neurocode USA, Inc, Quanterix/ALZpath◀	●0479U	▶Tau, phosphorylated, pTau217◀
▶Bacteria, Viruses, Fungus, and Parasite Metagenomic Sequencing, Spinal Fluid (MSCSF), Mayo Clinic, Laboratory Developed Test◀	●0480U	▶Infectious disease (bacteria, viruses, fungi, and parasites), cerebrospinal fluid (CSF), metagenomic next-generation sequencing (DNA and RNA), bioinformatic analysis, with positive pathogen identification◀
▶IDH1, IDH2, and TERT Mutation Analysis, Next-Generation Sequencing, Tumor (IDTRT), Mayo Clinic, Laboratory Developed Test◀	●0481U	▶*IDH1 (isocitrate dehydrogenase 1 [NADP+]), IDH2 (isocitrate dehydrogenase 2 [NADP+]),* and *TERT (telomerase reverse transcriptase)* promoter (eg, central nervous system [CNS] tumors), next-generation sequencing (single-nucleotide variants [SNV], deletions, and insertions)◀
▶Preeclampsia sFlt-1/PlGF Ratio (PERA), Mayo Clinic, Laboratory Developed Test◀	●0482U	▶Obstetrics (preeclampsia), biochemical assay of soluble fms-like tyrosine kinase 1 (sFlt-1) and placental growth factor (PlGF), serum, ratio reported for sFlt-1/PlGF, with risk of progression for preeclampsia with severe features within 2 weeks◀
▶Ciprofloxacin Susceptibility of Neisseria gonorrhoeae, MedArbor Diagnostics, SpeeDx, Inc◀	●0483U	▶Infectious disease (Neisseria gonorrhoeae), sensitivity, ciprofloxacin resistance (gyrA S91F point mutation), oral, rectal, or vaginal swab, algorithm reported as probability of fluoroquinolone resistance◀
▶Macrolide Resistance of Mycoplasma genitalium, MedArbor Diagnostics, SpeeDx, Inc◀	●0484U	▶Infectious disease (Mycoplasma genitalium), macrolide sensitivity (23S rRNA point mutation), oral, rectal, or vaginal swab, algorithm reported as probability of macrolide resistance◀
▶Caris Assure™, Caris MPI, Inc d/b/a Caris Life Sciences®, Caris MPI, Inc d/b/a Caris Life Sciences®◀	●0485U	▶Oncology (solid tumor), cell-free DNA and RNA by next-generation sequencing, interpretative report for germline mutations, clonal hematopoiesis of indeterminate potential, and tumor-derived single-nucleotide variants, small insertions/deletions, copy number alterations, fusions, microsatellite instability, and tumor mutational burden◀
▶Northstar Response™, BillionToOne Laboratory, BillionToOne, Inc◀	●0486U	▶Oncology (pan-solid tumor), next-generation sequencing analysis of tumor methylation markers present in cell-free circulating tumor DNA, algorithm reported as quantitative measurement of methylation as a correlate of tumor fraction◀

(Continued on page 258)

▲ = Revised code   ● = New code   ▶ ◀ = Contains new or revised text   ✕ = Duplicate PLA test   ↑↓ = Category I PLA   American Medical Association   **257**

Appendix O

Proprietary Name and Clinical Laboratory or Manufacturer	Alpha-Numeric Code	Code Descriptor
▶Northstar Select™, BillionToOne Laboratory, BillionToOne, Inc◀	●0487U	▶Oncology (solid tumor), cell-free circulating DNA, targeted genomic sequence analysis panel of 84 genes, interrogation for sequence variants, aneuploidy-corrected gene copy number amplifications and losses, gene rearrangements, and microsatellite instability◀
▶UNITY Fetal Antigen™ NIPT, BillionToOne Laboratory, BillionToOne, Inc◀	●0488U	▶Obstetrics (fetal antigen noninvasive prenatal test), cell-free DNA sequence analysis for detection of fetal presence or absence of 1 or more of the Rh, C, c, D, E, Duffy (Fya), or Kell (K) antigen in alloimmunized pregnancies, reported as selected antigen(s) detected or not detected◀
▶UNITY Fetal Risk Screen™, BillionToOne Laboratory, BillionToOne, Inc◀	●0489U	▶Obstetrics (single-gene noninvasive prenatal test), cell-free DNA sequence analysis of 1 or more targets (eg, *CFTR, SMN1, HBB, HBA1, HBA2*) to identify paternally inherited pathogenic variants, and relative mutation-dosage analysis based on molecular counts to determine fetal inheritance of maternal mutation, algorithm reported as a fetal risk score for the condition (eg, cystic fibrosis, spinal muscular atrophy, beta hemoglobinopathies [including sickle cell disease], alpha thalassemia)◀
▶CELLSEARCH® Circulating Melanoma Cell (CMC) Test, Menarini Silicon Biosystems Inc, Menarini Silicon Biosystems Inc◀	●0490U	▶Oncology (cutaneous or uveal melanoma), circulating tumor cell selection, morphological characterization and enumeration based on differential CD146, high molecular–weight melanoma-associated antigen, CD34 and CD45 protein biomarkers, peripheral blood◀
▶CELLSEARCH® ER Circulating Tumor Cell (CTC-ER) Test, Menarini Silicon Biosystems Inc, Menarini Silicon Biosystems Inc◀	●0491U	▶Oncology (solid tumor), circulating tumor cell selection, morphological characterization and enumeration based on differential epithelial cell adhesion molecule (EpCAM), cytokeratins 8, 18, and 19, CD45 protein biomarkers, and quantification of estrogen receptor (ER) protein biomarker–expressing cells, peripheral blood◀
▶CELLSEARCH® PD-L1 Circulating Tumor Cell (CTC-PD-L1) Test, Menarini Silicon Biosystems Inc, Menarini Silicon Biosystems Inc◀	●0492U	▶Oncology (solid tumor), circulating tumor cell selection, morphological characterization and enumeration based on differential epithelial cell adhesion molecule (EpCAM), cytokeratins 8, 18, and 19, CD45 protein biomarkers, and quantification of PD-L1 protein biomarker–expressing cells, peripheral blood◀
▶Prospera™, Natera™◀	●0493U	▶Transplantation medicine, quantification of donor-derived cell-free DNA (cfDNA) using next-generation sequencing, plasma, reported as percentage of donor-derived cell-free DNA◀
▶Rh Test, Natera™◀	●0494U	▶Red blood cell antigen (fetal RhD gene analysis), next-generation sequencing of circulating cell-free DNA (cfDNA) of blood in pregnant individuals known to be RhD negative, reported as positive or negative◀

★ = Telemedicine   ◀ = Audio-only   ✚ = Add-on code   ✖ = FDA approval pending   # = Resequenced code   ⊘ = Modifier 51 exempt

Proprietary Name and Clinical Laboratory or Manufacturer	Alpha-Numeric Code	Code Descriptor
▶Stockholm3, BioAgilytix Diagnostics◀	●0495U	▶Oncology (prostate), analysis of circulating plasma proteins (tPSA, fPSA, KLK2, PSP94, and GDF15), germline polygenic risk score (60 variants), clinical information (age, family history of prostate cancer, prior negative prostate biopsy), algorithm reported as risk of likelihood of detecting clinically significant prostate cancer◀
▶ColoScape™ PLUS, DiaCarta, Inc, DiaCarta, Inc◀	●0496U	▶Oncology (colorectal), cell-free DNA, 8 genes for mutations, 7 genes for methylation by real-time RT-PCR, and 4 proteins by enzyme-linked immunosorbent assay, blood, reported positive or negative for colorectal cancer or advanced adenoma risk◀
▶OncoAssure™ Prostate, DiaCarta, Inc, DiaCarta, Inc◀	●0497U	▶Oncology (prostate), mRNA gene-expression profiling by real-time RT-PCR of 6 genes (FOXM1, MCM3, MTUS1, TTC21B, ALAS1, and PPP2CA), utilizing formalin-fixed paraffin-embedded (FFPE) tissue, algorithm reported as a risk score for prostate cancer◀
▶OptiSeq™ Colorectal Cancer NGS Panel, DiaCarta, Inc, DiaCarta, Inc◀	●0498U	▶Oncology (colorectal), next-generation sequencing for mutation detection in 43 genes and methylation pattern in 45 genes, blood, and formalin-fixed paraffin-embedded (FFPE) tissue, report of variants and methylation pattern with interpretation◀
▶OptiSeq™ Dual Cancer Panel Kit, DiaCarta, Inc, DiaCarta, Inc◀	●0499U	▶Oncology (colorectal and lung), DNA from formalin-fixed paraffin-embedded (FFPE) tissue, next-generation sequencing of 8 genes (NRAS, EGFR, CTNNB1, PIK3CA, APC, BRAF, KRAS, and TP53), mutation detection◀
▶QClamp® Plex VEXAS UBA1 Mutation Test, DiaCarta, Inc, DiaCarta, Inc◀	●0500U	▶Autoinflammatory disease (VEXAS syndrome), DNA, UBA1 gene mutations, targeted variant analysis (M41T, M41V, M41L, c.118-2A>C, c.118-1G>C, c.118-9_118-2del, S56F, S621C)◀
▶QuantiDNA™ Colorectal Cancer Triage Test, DiaCarta, Inc, DiaCarta, Inc◀	●0501U	▶Oncology (colorectal), blood, quantitative measurement of cell-free DNA (cfDNA)◀
▶QuantiVirus™ HPV E6/E7 mRNA Test for Cervical Cancer, DiaCarta, Inc, DiaCarta, Inc◀	●0502U	▶Human papillomavirus (HPV), E6/E7 markers for high-risk types (16, 18, 31, 33, 35, 39, 45, 51, 52, 56, 58, 59, 66, and 68), cervical cells, branched-chain capture hybridization, reported as negative or positive for high risk for HPV◀
▶PrecivityAD2™, C2N Diagnostics, LLC, C2N Diagnostics, LLC◀	●0503U	▶Neurology (Alzheimer disease), beta amyloid (Aβ40, Aβ42, Aβ42/40 ratio) and tau-protein (ptau217, np-tau217, ptau217/np-tau217 ratio), blood, immunoprecipitation with quantitation by liquid chromatography with tandem mass spectrometry (LC-MS/MS), algorithm score reported as likelihood of positive or negative for amyloid plaques◀

(Continued on page 260)

▲ = Revised code   ● = New code   ▶ ◀ = Contains new or revised text   ✳ = Duplicate PLA test   ↕ = Category I PLA   American Medical Association   **259**

Proprietary Name and Clinical Laboratory or Manufacturer	Alpha-Numeric Code	Code Descriptor
▶Urinary Tract Infection Testing, NxGen MDx LLC, NxGen MDx LLC◀	●0504U	▶Infectious disease (urinary tract infection), identification of 17 pathologic organisms, urine, real-time PCR, reported as positive or negative for each organism◀
▶Vaginal Infection Testing, NxGen MDx LLC, NxGen MDx LLC◀	●0505U	▶Infectious disease (vaginal infection), identification of 32 pathogenic organisms, swab, real-time PCR, reported as positive or negative for each organism◀
▶EndoSign® Barrett's Esophagus Test, Cyted Health Inc, Cyted Health Inc◀	●0506U	▶Gastroenterology (Barrett's esophagus), esophageal cells, DNA methylation analysis by next-generation sequencing of at least 89 differentially methylated genomic regions, algorithm reported as likelihood for Barrett's esophagus◀
▶Avantect Ovarian Cancer Test, ClearNote® Health◀	●0507U	▶Oncology (ovarian), DNA, whole-genome sequencing with 5-hydroxymethylcytosine (5hmC) enrichment, using whole blood or plasma, algorithm reported as cancer detected or not detected◀
▶VitaGraft™ Kidney Baseline + 1st Plasma Test, Oncocyte Corporation, Oncocyte Corporation◀	●0508U	▶Transplantation medicine, quantification of donor-derived cell-free DNA using 40 single-nucleotide polymorphisms (SNPs), plasma, and urine, initial evaluation reported as percentage of donor-derived cell-free DNA with risk for active rejection◀
▶VitaGraft™ Kidney Subsequent, Oncocyte Corporation, Oncocyte Corporation◀	●0509U	▶Transplantation medicine, quantification of donor-derived cell-free DNA using up to 12 single-nucleotide polymorphisms (SNPs) previously identified, plasma, reported as percentage of donor-derived cell-free DNA with risk for active rejection◀
▶PurIST℠, Tempus AI, Inc, Tempus AI, Inc◀	●0510U	▶Oncology (pancreatic cancer), augmentative algorithmic analysis of 16 genes from previously sequenced RNA whole-transcriptome data, reported as probability of predicted molecular subtype◀
▶PARIS, Tempus AI, Inc, Tempus AI, Inc (by its wholly owned subsidiary SEngine Precision Medicine, LLC)◀	●0511U	▶Oncology (solid tumor), tumor cell culture in 3D microenvironment, 36 or more drug panel, reported as tumor-response prediction for each drug◀
▶Tempus p-MSI, Tempus AI, Inc, Tempus AI, Inc◀	●0512U	▶Oncology (prostate), augmentative algorithmic analysis of digitized whole-slide imaging of histologic features for microsatellite instability (MSI) status, formalin-fixed paraffin-embedded (FFPE) tissue, reported as increased or decreased probability of MSI-high (MSI-H)◀
▶Tempus p-Prostate, Tempus AI, Inc, Tempus AI, Inc◀	●0513U	▶Oncology (prostate), augmentative algorithmic analysis of digitized whole-slide imaging of histologic features for microsatellite instability (MSI) and homologous recombination deficiency (HRD) status, formalin-fixed paraffin-embedded (FFPE) tissue, reported as increased or decreased probability of each biomarker◀

★=Telemedicine   ◀=Audio-only   ✚=Add-on code   ✗=FDA approval pending   #=Resequenced code   ⦸=Modifier 51 exempt

Proprietary Name and Clinical Laboratory or Manufacturer	Alpha-Numeric Code	Code Descriptor
▶Procise ADL™, ProciseDx Inc◀	●0514U	▶Gastroenterology (irritable bowel disease [IBD]), immunoassay for quantitative determination of adalimumab (ADL) levels in venous serum in patients undergoing adalimumab therapy, results reported as a numerical value as micrograms per milliliter (µg/mL)◀
▶Procise IFX™, ProciseDx Inc◀	●0515U	▶Gastroenterology (irritable bowel disease [IBD]), immunoassay for quantitative determination of infliximab (IFX) levels in venous serum in patients undergoing infliximab therapy, results reported as a numerical value as micrograms per milliliter (µg/mL)◀
▶MyGenVar Pharmacogenomics Test, Geisinger Medical Laboratories, Geisinger Medical Laboratories◀	●0516U	▶Drug metabolism, whole blood, pharmacogenomic genotyping of 40 genes and *CYP2D6* copy number variant analysis, reported as metabolizer status◀
▶PrecisView® CNS, Phenomics Health™ Inc, Phenomics Health™ Inc◀	●0517U	▶Therapeutic drug monitoring, 80 or more psychoactive drugs or substances, LC-MS/MS, plasma, qualitative and quantitative therapeutic minimally and maximally effective dose of prescribed and non-prescribed medications◀
▶SyncView® Pain, Phenomics Health™ Inc, Phenomics Health™ Inc◀	●0518U	▶Therapeutic drug monitoring, 90 or more pain and mental health drugs or substances, LC-MS/MS, plasma, qualitative and quantitative therapeutic minimally effective range of prescribed and non-prescribed medications◀
▶SyncView® PainPlus, Phenomics Health™ Inc, Phenomics Health™ Inc◀	●0519U	▶Therapeutic drug monitoring, medications specific to pain, depression, and anxiety, LC-MS/MS, plasma, 110 or more drugs or substances, qualitative and quantitative therapeutic minimally effective range of prescribed, non-prescribed, and illicit medications in circulation◀
▶SyncView® Rx, Phenomics Health™ Inc, Phenomics Health™ Inc◀	●0520U	▶Therapeutic drug monitoring, 200 or more drugs or substances, LC-MS/MS, plasma, qualitative and quantitative therapeutic minimally effective range of prescribed and non-prescribed medications◀

Rationale

In accordance with the changes made in the Pathology and Laboratory section, including the code additions, revisions, and deletions, Appendix O has been revised. One new administrative multianalyte assay with algorithmic analysis (MAAA) code (0020M), two new Category I MAAA codes (81515, 81558), and 101 new Proprietary Laboratory Analyses (PLA) codes (0420U-0520U) have been added.

A new administrative MAAA code (0020M) has been established to report an oncology analysis for the central nervous system (CNS) of 30000 DNA methylation loci by methylation array using a diagnostic algorithm reported as the probability of matching a reference tumor subclass. This procedure combines a conventional DNA methylation measurement method with an algorithm to diagnose and subtype brain and other CNS tumors by comparing against a unique reference dataset. The algorithm generates a probability score or likelihood of the test sample matching a reference tumor subclass. The molecular diagnosis resulting from the algorithmic analysis is used to make treatment decisions because it identifies tumor subtypes with an increased risk of recurrence that may need more aggressive therapy, as well as subtypes with a lower risk of recurrence that may be appropriately managed by surgery and observation.

A total of 101 new PLA codes have been established for the CPT 2025 code set. PLA codes are released and published on a quarterly basis (fall, winter, spring, and summer) at https://www.ama-assn.org/practice-management/cpt/cpt-pla-codes. New codes are effective the quarter following their online publication. Other changes include the deletion of eight codes (0078U, 0167U, 0204U, 0352U-0354U, 0396U, 0416U); the revision of four codes (0248U, 0351U, 0356U, 0403U); the editorial revision of one test name (0407U); and the revision of the test, laboratory, and manufacturer names for codes 0047U and 0118U.

Refer to the codebook and the Rationale for codes 81515, 81558, and 0420U-0520U for a full discussion of these changes.

Clinical Example (0020M)

A 17-year-old female presents with a pleomorphic tumor with focal papillary architecture. The primary diagnosis is a grade 4 malignant neuroepithelial tumor. Because the diagnosis is inconclusive, pathology tissue slides are sent for assessment using the methylation classifier.

Description of Procedure (0020M)

Perform tumor methylation classifier analysis on bisulfite-converted DNA extracted from tumor tissue using the methylation profiling microarray kit and array scanner. Upload the DNA methylation signature into the tumor classifier, and generate a classification score that indicates the probability of a match to one of the central nervous system tumor classes. A pathologist or medical laboratory director reviews and reports the results.

★ = Telemedicine ◀ = Audio-only ✚ = Add-on code ✗ = FDA approval pending # = Resequenced code ⊘ = Modifier 51 exempt

Appendix Q

Severe Acute Respiratory Syndrome Coronavirus 2 (SARS-CoV-2) (coronavirus disease [COVID-19]) Vaccines

▶The crosswalk of COVID-19 vaccine and administration codes and their associated patient age, vaccine manufacturer, vaccine name(s), NDC Labeler Product ID, and interval between doses instructions (formerly Appendix Q) have been removed from the CPT code set. For information and guidance on reporting for COVID-19 immunization services, refer to the E/M and Medicine section guidelines.◀

Rationale

To accommodate the deletion of codes that were previously used to report coronavirus disease 2019 (COVID-19) products and their administrations, except for code 91304, Appendix Q has been deleted.

Refer to the codebook and the Rationale for codes 90480 and 91318-91322 for a full discussion of the changes.

Notes

Appendix R

Digital Medicine–Services Taxonomy

Appendix R is a listing of digital medicine services described in the CPT code set. The digital medicine–services taxonomy table in this appendix classifies CPT codes that are related to digital medicine services into discrete categories of clinician-to-patient services (eg, visit), clinician-to-clinician services (eg, consultation), patient-monitoring services, and digital diagnostic services. The clinician-to-patient services and clinician-to-clinician services categories are differentiated by the nature of their services, ie, synchronous and asynchronous communication. The patient-monitoring services represent ongoing, extended monitoring that produces data that require physician assessment and interpretation and are further categorized into device/software set-up and education, data transfer, and data-interpretation services. The digital diagnostic services differentiate automated/autonomous, algorithmically enabled diagnostic-support services into patient-directed and image/specimen-directed services. The term "clinician" in the table represents a physician or other qualified health care professional (QHP) who may use the specific code(s).

This taxonomy is intended to support increased awareness and understanding of approaches to patient care through the multifaceted digital medicine services available for reporting in the CPT code set. The taxonomy is not intended to be a complete representation of all applicable digital medicine service codes in the CPT code set and does not supersede specific coding guidance listed in specific sections of the CPT code set. Furthermore, the table does not denote services that are currently payable through coverage policies by either public or commercial payers.

For purposes of this appendix, the following terms should be understood as:

- Digital medicine services represent the use of technologies for measurement and intervention in the service of patient health.
- Synchronous services represent real-time interactions between a distant-site physician or other QHP and a patient and/or family located at a remote originating site.
- Asynchronous services represent store-and-forward transmissions of health information over periods of time using a secure Web server, encrypted email, specially designed store-and-forward software, or electronic health record. Asynchronous services enable a patient to share health information for later review by the physician or other QHP. These services also allow a physician or other QHP to share a patient's medical history, images, physiologic/non-physiologic clinical data and/or pathology and laboratory reports with a specialist physician for diagnostic and treatment expertise.

Digital Medicine–Services Taxonomy*
(*Note that the codes listed in this table are examples and not meant to be an exhaustive list)

	Clinician*-to-Patient Services (Eg, visit)		Clinician-to-Clinician Services (Eg, consultation)		Patient Monitoring and/or Therapeutic Services			Digital Diagnostic Services	
	Synchronous	Asynchronous	Synchronous	Asynchronous	Device/Software Set-Up and Education	Data Transfer	Data Interpretation	Patient Directed	Image/Specimen Directed
Encounter Activity	Real-time audiovisual interaction	Store-and-forward digital communication	Real-time consultative communication between requesting and consulting clinicians	Store-and-forward consultative digital exchange of clinical information between requesting and consulting clinicians	In-person, virtual face-to-face, telephone, or other modalities of communication with patient to support device set-up education/supply	Acquisition of patient data with transfer to managing or interpreting physician/other QHP/clinical staff	Data review, interpretation, and patient management by clinical staff/physician/other QHP with associated patient communication	Automated and autonomous algorithmically enabled diagnostic support	
CPT Service	▲Synchronous audio-video visit (98000-98007)▼; ▲Synchronous audio-only visit (98008-98015) Brief communication technology-based service (98016)▼	Online digital evaluation & management (99421-99423) (98970-98972)	Interprofessional telephone/Internet/EHR consultation (Typically via telephone) (99446-99449, 99451); If patient is present at originating site→ transition to virtual face-to-face E/M consultation (Use modifier 95)	Interprofessional telephone/Internet/EHR consultation (99446-99449, 99451, 99452)	Remote physiologic monitoring initial set-up/education (99453)	Remote physiologic monitoring device supply (99454)	Physiologic data collection/interpretation by physician/other QHP (99091); Remote physiologic monitoring treatment management by clinical staff/physician/other QHP (99457, 99458)	Autonomous retinopathy screening (92229)	Multianalyte assays with algorithmic analyses (MAAA)

★ = Telemedicine ◄ = Audio-only ✚ = Add-on code ✗ = FDA approval pending # = Resequenced code ⊘ = Modifier 51 exempt

Digital Medicine—Services Taxonomy* (cont'd)
(*Note that the codes listed in this table are examples and not meant to be an exhaustive list)

	Clinician*-to-Patient Services (Eg. visit)		Clinician-to-Clinician Services (Eg. consultation)		Patient Monitoring and/or Therapeutic Services			Digital Diagnostic Services	
	Synchronous	Asynchronous	Synchronous	Asynchronous	Device/Software Set-Up and Education	Data Transfer	Data Interpretation	Patient Directed	Image/Specimen Directed
CPT Service					Remote therapeutic monitoring initial set-up/education (98975)	Remote therapeutic monitoring device supply (98976 for respiratory system; 98977 for musculo-skeletal system)	Remote therapeutic monitoring treatment management by physician/other QHP (98980, 98981)		Computer-aided detection (CAD) imaging (77048, 77049, 77065-77067, 0042T, 0174T, 0175T)
					Remote pulmonary artery pressure sensor monitoring treatment management by physician/other QHP (93264)				
					Ambulatory continuous glucose monitoring hook-up, education, recording print-out (95250 for office-equipped; 95249 for patient-equipped)		Ambulatory continuous glucose monitoring analysis (95251)		
					External electrocardiographic recording (Recording) (93224, 93225, 93241, 93242, 93245, 93246)	External electrocardiographic recording (Recording, scanning analysis with report, review and interpretation) (93224, 93241, 93245)	External electrocardiographic recording (Review and interpretation) (93224, 93227, 93241, 93244, 93245, 93248)	External electrocardiographic recording (Autonomous algorithms used to analyze/create report) (93241-93243, 93245-93247)	
						External electrocardiographic recording (Scanning analysis with report only) (93226, 93241, 93243, 93247)			

(Continued on page 268)

Appendix R

Appendix R

Digital Medicine–Services Taxonomy* (cont'd)
(*Note that the codes listed in this table are examples and not meant to be an exhaustive list)

CPT Service	Clinician*-to-Patient Services (Eg. visit)		Clinician-to-Clinician Services (Eg. consultation)		Patient Monitoring and/or Therapeutic Services			Digital Diagnostic Services	
	Synchronous	Asynchronous	Synchronous	Asynchronous	Device/Software Set-Up and Education	Data Transfer	Data Interpretation	Patient Directed	Image/Specimen Directed
					External mobile cardiovascular telemetry technical support (93229)		External mobile cardiovascular telemetry review and interpretation (93228)		
					Digital amblyopia services (0704T for initial set-up/education; 0705T for surveillance center technical support, including data transmission)		Digital amblyopia services (Assessment of patient performance, program data) (0706T)		
							Automated analysis of CT study (Data preparation, interpretation and report) (0691T)		

*The term "clinician" in the table represents a physician or other qualified health care professional (QHP) by whom the specific code may be used.

★ = Telemedicine   ◀ = Audio-only   + = Add-on code   N = FDA approval pending   # = Resequenced code   ⊘ = Modifier 51 exempt

Rationale

In accordance with the deletion of codes 99441-99443 and the establishment of codes 98000-98016, the Digital Medicine–Services Taxonomy table in Appendix R has been revised to reflect these changes.

Refer to the codebook and the Rationale for codes 98000-98016 for a full discussion of these changes.

Appendix R

Notes

Indexes

Instructions for the Use of the Changes Indexes

The Changes Indexes are not a substitute for the main text of *CPT Changes 2025* or the main text of the CPT codebook. The changes indexes consist of two types of content—coding changes and modifiers—all of which are intended to assist users in searching and locating information quickly within *CPT Changes 2025*.

Index of Coding Changes

The Index of Coding Changes lists new, revised, and deleted codes, and/or some codes that may be affected by revised and/or new guidelines and parenthetical notes. This index enables users to quickly search and locate the codes within a page(s), in addition to discerning the status of a code (new, revised, deleted, or textually changed) because the status of each new, revised, or deleted code is noted in parentheses next to the code number:

Index of Modifiers

The Index of Modifiers does not list all modifiers unless they are new, revised, or deleted, and/or if the modifier may be affected by revised and/or new codes, guidelines, and parenthetical notes. A limited Index of Modifiers, ie, limited to only those modifiers that appear in the Rationales and new or revised guidelines and/or parenthetical notes, is provided to help users quickly locate these modifiers and to know where in the book these modifiers are listed or mentioned.

Indexes

★ = Telemedicine ◀ = Audio-only ✚ = Add-on code ✎ = FDA approval pending # = Resequenced code ⊘ = Modifier 51 exempt

Index of Coding Changes

Codes in this index are in numerical order, with the four-digit alphanumeric codes first:

Category III changes (a four-digit code followed by the letter "T"); changes to administrative codes for multianalyte assays with algorithmic analyses (MAAA) (a four-digit code followed by the letter "M"); and changes to proprietary laboratory analysis (PLA) codes (a four-digit code followed by the letter "U"). Five-digit CPT codes follow.

▲ = Revised code　　● = New code　　▶◀ = Contains new or revised text　　✕ = Duplicate PLA test　　⇅ = Category I PLA　　　American Medical Association　**273**

★ = Telemedicine   ◀ = Audio-only   ➕ = Add-on code   ✚ = FDA approval pending   # = Resequenced code   ⊘ = Modifier 51 exempt

★ = Telemedicine   ◀ = Audio-only   ✚ = Add-on code   ✎ = FDA approval pending   # = Resequenced code   ⊘ = Modifier 51 exempt

★ = Telemedicine   ◀ = Audio-only   ✛ = Add-on code   ✗ = FDA approval pending   # = Resequenced code   ⃠ = Modifier 51 exempt

★ = Telemedicine   ◀ = Audio-only   ✦ = Add-on code   ✎ = FDA approval pending   # = Resequenced code   ⊘ = Modifier 51 exempt

Indexes

★ = Telemedicine   ◀ = Audio-only   ✛ = Add-on code   ⁄ = FDA approval pending   # = Resequenced code   ⃠ = Modifier 51 exempt

Indexes

★ = Telemedicine ◀ = Audio-only ✚ = Add-on code ✚ = FDA approval pending # = Resequenced code ⦸ = Modifier 51 exempt

★ = Telemedicine   ◀ = Audio-only   ✚ = Add-on code   𝒩 = FDA approval pending   # = Resequenced code   ⊘ = Modifier 51 exempt

Indexes

★ = Telemedicine   ◀ = Audio-only   ✚ = Add-on code   ⊮ = FDA approval pending   # = Resequenced code   ⊘ = Modifier 51 exempt

Indexes

Index of Modifiers

The modifiers in this Index of Modifiers is limited to only the modifiers that appear in the Rationales and in the new or revised guidelines and/or parenthetical notes.

Modifier, Descriptor

Page Numbers

NOTES

NOTES

NOTES

NOTES

NOTES